Injury
Epidemiology

Research and Control Strategies

SECOND EDITION

LEON S. ROBERTSON

New York   Oxford
OXFORD UNIVERSITY PRESS
1998

Oxford University Press

Oxford   New York
Athens   Auckland   Bangkok   Bogota
Bombay   Buenos Aires   Calcutta   Cape Town
Dar es Salaam   Delhi   Florence   Hong Kong   Istanbul
Karachi   Kuala Lumpur   Madras   Madrid
Melbourne   Mexico City   Nairobi   Paris
Singapore   Taipei   Tokyo   Toronto   Warsaw

and associated companies in
Berlin   Ibadan

Copyright © 1992, 1998 by Oxford University Press, Inc.

Published by Oxford University Press, Inc.
198 Madison Avenue, New York, New York 10016

Oxford is a registered trademark of Oxford University Press

Library of Congress Cataloging-in-Publication Data
Robertson, Leon S.
Injury epidemiology : research and control strategies /
Leon S. Robertson. – 2nd ed.
p.   cm.   Includes bibliographical references and index.
ISBN 0-19-512202-X
1. Wounds and injuries—United States—Epidemiology.
2. Wounds and injuries—Epidemiology—Research—Methodology.
I. Title.
RD93.8.R64   1998   614.5'99—DC21   97-35804
                                              CIP

9 8 7 6 5 4 3 2 1

Printed in the United States of America
on acid-free paper

Robertson, Leon S. *Injury Epidemiology: Research and Control Strategies,* Second Edition. ERRATUM, p. 238–239

Because of an error in computer programming, the ratios of certain injuries, hospital days, and lost workdays in rollovers are incorrect. The following text and table replace the paragraph beginning at the bottom of p. 238 and Table 10.4, p. 240. Nonfatal spine and brain injuries are combined here because the sample size on spinal injury was too small for confidence in a stable ratio.

During 1989–91, a death count from the FARS data indicates a total of 28,347 people died in rollovers of passenger cars, vans, utility vehicles, and light trucks. The analysis of the national sample of all rollovers in such vehicles during 1989–91, with ratio to deaths in parentheses, indicated 29,874 nonfatal, hospitalized spinal cord or brain injuries (1.054), 487,256 hospital days (17.19), and 1.16 million lost workdays (40.91) among those employed. Using the ratios times the deaths preventable by increased stability (columns 2–4 in Table 10.4), it is expected that failure to adopt a standard applicable in 1990 models will result in approximately 5300 nonfatal, hospitalized spinal cord or brain injuries, 86,473 hospital days, and 205,672 lost workdays in the vehicles in Table 10.4 manufactured through 1994.

TABLE 10.4. Projected Rollover Outcomes Preventable by a *T/2H* of 1.2 in 20 Years' Use, 1990–94 Models

MAKE/MODEL	DEATHS	NONFATAL SPINAL/ BRAIN	HOSPITAL DAYS	LOST WORKDAYS
Amigo	23	24	394	938
4Runner	135	142	2322	5522
Rodeo/Passport	66	69	1130	2687
Tracker	49	51	838	1993
Wrangler	64	67	1094	2603
Ranger Pickup	736	776	12,668	30,130
Blazer/Jimmy(S/T)	696	734	11,969	28,468
Nissan Pickup	144	152	2485	5911
Pathfinder	131	138	2252	5357
S10/S15 Pickup	340	359	5855	13,926
GM Light Pickups	592	624	10,175	24,201
F250 Pickup	178	188	3065	7290
Astro/Safari Van	327	345	5623	13,373
Bronco	108	114	1864	4433
Aerostar Van	312	329	5367	12,765
Explorer/Navajo	590	622	10,145	24,129
F150 Pickup	315	332	5411	12,871
Mazda MPV	26	27	445	1058
Lumina Van	78	82	1334	3173
Caravan/Voyager	118	125	2037	4844
Total	5028	5300	86,473	205,672

PREFACE

Injury Epidemiology, the first edition of this book, considered implications for injury control. The subtitle of the second edition, *Research and Control Strategies,* reflects this emphasis. Many new sections and references on those subjects have been added.

While the reception of the first edition by students and reviewers was mostly favorable, some readers were apparently confused or misled by the cryptic treatment given certain topics. Where this was made known to me, the sections have been rewritten or augmented in a quest for clarity. Some reviewers considered my criticism of certain studies or organizations harsh, and one accused me of favoring the U.S. auto industry, despite numerous criticisms of some of the actions and products of U.S.-based manufacturers. The sad facts are that some researchers produce invalid or misleading research reports, the products of many corporations are unnecessarily hazardous, and government agencies fail to act or enforce laws and standards. Reluctance to criticize invites continuation of these practices and failures. If injury control is to reach its full potential, we need not less, but more, harsh criticism of researchers and organizations that do not do their jobs.

Epidemiologic studies of injuries have increased more rapidly in quantity than in quality in the 1990s. The collection of data with no clear research question or potentially useful results remains all too common. The revised first chapter of this book delineates specific objectives of epidemiologic studies and the data and study designs needed to attain those objectives. Each subsequent chapter has been revised and expanded with these objectives in mind to provide a more progressive step-by-step development of topics.

New analyses and updates include details on potential years of life lost from injuries, cardiovascular diseases, and cancers (Chapter 2); effective uses of surveillance systems (Chapter 3); clarification of the relevance of causal thinking for prevention (Chapter 4); the misuse of behavioral inference in cases such as the C/K pickup truck fire issue (Chapter 5); recent studies of legal interventions (Chapter 6); the effects of motor vehicle crashworthiness relative to other factors (Chapter 7); questions for research in prevention and rehabilitation (Chapter 8); illustrations of cost–benefit, risk–benefit, and cost–savings analyses and evidence of confounding of estimates of effects of alcohol and seat belt use (Chapter 9); and the effect of regulatory failure on rollovers of top-heavy vehicles and fuel economy as well as alternatives to regulation (Chapter 10).

A number of new books that are worthwhile additions to class reading lists have appeared since the first edition was published. They are listed in the references for relevant chapters. To my knowledge, this remains the only textbook setting out general principles for research in injury epidemiology and evaluation of injury control. Good links to internet sites are found at http://www.injurycontrol.com.

Branford, Conn.   L.S.R.
May 1997

INJURY EPIDEMIOLOGY

PREFACE TO THE FIRST EDITION

Writing a book entails a certain amount of arrogance. The writer must believe that the content will be different, or will be presented in a different and more useful format, from that which other books provide. In this case, no textbook of injury epidemiology has appeared before, and general epidemiology texts seldom mention injury.

Several books devoted to injury data, injury control, and public policy were published in the 1980s. "The Injury Fact Book" by Susan Baker and colleagues is an excellent source of information on the distribution of injuries providing a variety of available data and cogent commentary. *Injury Control* by Julian Waller describes various ways to conceptualize the problem and suggests an enormous variety of programs for potential use in injury control. *Injury Prevention: Meeting the Challenge* by the National Committee for Injury Prevention and Control gives guidance to health agencies on the practical aspects of starting injury control programs. My *Injuries: Causes, Control Strategies and Public Policy* is an analysis of causal concepts and an evaluation of the effectiveness of injury control programs and public policies. Each of these books fills a niche in the spectrum of needs for knowledge in the field.

What is missing is a book that teaches the novice, or the scientist with little or no experience in injury research, how injury epidemiology is done. The motivation for writing the book was generated by the task of reviewing research proposals for the Centers for Disease Control. Some of the proposals lacked a clear purpose or hypothesis or were deficient in fundamental knowledge of the most relevant data sources and of bias in certain data sources. Study design and statistical power were often problematic as well.

Another reason for writing the book has been the rapid and continuing growth in the number of students enrolled in injury epidemiology courses. Without a comprehensive textbook in injury epidemiology, instructors who are busy with their own research have to devote time to the selection of readings for their courses from a wide variety of journals.

This book is organized around the theme that injury epidemiology should be useful, not just an intellectually fulfilling pursuit. Each chapter suggests research projects that are needed to answer questions that will contribute to more effective or efficient approaches to injury control.

The first chapter traces the background of epidemiology and its use in reducing infectious diseases and the application of concepts from infectious disease epidemiology to injury epidemiology. Better epidemiological research based on what we know about the energy sources that cause injuries is discussed.

Chapter 2 deals with the choice of researchable questions, the logic of classifications of injury, how cases are found by interview or by records of contact with medical care facilities or various agencies, the use of these sources in case identification, and the biases in some of the available data. Several injury severity scoring systems and their uses are compared. The calculation of various rates and ratios is explained and assumptions about the appropriateness of denominators when reporting the rates and ratios are discussed.

Chapter 3 addresses the development and use of injury surveillance systems. The strengths and weaknesses of several surveillance systems are discussed. The chapter also describes a prevention-oriented surveillance system developed by the author for the Indian Health Service and notes some marked reductions in injury that occurred after data on these injuries obtained by surveillance were presented to authorities, who took action.

Chapter 4 discusses the criteria for inferring causation based on epidemiological research. The construction of causal models and the revision of models based on new research findings is illustrated. The importance of logically deduced hypotheses and the strength of a variety of research designs, including statistical power, to test hypotheses are emphasized.

The behavioral theories sometimes applied to injury risk are mentioned in Chapter 5, and their relevance to injury control is discussed. The uses of experimental and other research designs to study the effects of attempts at behavior change are illustrated.

The evaluation of the effects of laws aimed at injury control, and attention to unexpected consequences—favorable and unfavorable—of laws directed at behavior are the subject of Chapter 6. Alternative study designs to address threats to validity and generalizability are discussed.

Chapter 7 deals with the study of characteristics of energy and conveyors of energy in understanding injury incidence and severity. Research methods to estimate the effects on injuries of changes in products, construction, and quality control in production are presented.

The evaluation of emergency response, treatment, and rehabilitation is discussed in Chapter 8. The role of epidemiology in assisting clinical researchers is emphasized.

Chapter 9 addresses the economic concepts that enter into the assumption that injury control should be cost-beneficial. Several examples of cost–benefit analyses of proposed or partially implemented injury control programs are used to illustrate the problems of estimating tangible and intangible costs and benefits. The latter were excerpted from the author's chapter in a report to Congress on cost of injury.

In Chapter 10, an alternative to current piecemeal approaches to injury control is proposed. The proposal is an example of the use of epidemiological and economic data in a "what if" analysis. Prospects for careers in injury epidemiology and control are also discussed.

While the first part of the book is more methodological and the second more topical, the study designs discussed in several of the topical chapters are relevant to the issues and topics in other chapters as well. Rather than attempt to discuss all of the methodological issues in the first few chapters, many are illustrated as they apply to one or another substantitive issue. Therefore, it is recommended that students read the book from beginning to end rather than jumping to a topical chapter without reading the preceding background chapters.

Branford, Conn.   L.S.R.
June 1991

CONTENTS

1. Injury and the Role of Epidemiology, 1

2. The Search for Data and Its Uses, 23

3. Injury Surveillance and Its Uses, 49

4. Causal Analysis and Its Uses, 85

5. Human Factors and Attempts to Change Them, 113

6. Laws and Formal Rules Directed at Individual Behavior, 143

7. Controlling Agents, Vehicles, and Environments, 167

8. Research on Treatment and Rehabilitation, 195

9. Injury Epidemiology and Economics, 215

10. Injury Policy Analysis, 233

Index, 261

INJURY EPIDEMIOLOGY

1

INJURY AND THE ROLE OF EPIDEMIOLOGY

Injury is a neglected public health problem. Although various types of injury deaths—motor vehicles, homicides, suicides, falls, poisonings, drownings—have been listed in mortality statistics for decades, they have been ignored by all but a few epidemiologists and public health researchers. Influential and important discussions of the future direction of epidemiologic and public health research make no mention of injury (Pearce, 1996; Susser & Susser, 1996).

An accurate assessment of deaths, and their relative importance for individual or societal well-being, cannot be made using lists of numbers of deaths by type. Neither preventive measures nor medical treatment "saves lives," as is often claimed. If prevention or treatment is effective, it may delay death for a period of time, but everyone eventually dies. The effects of prevention or treatment on deaths should be measured in potential years of life lost or preserved and years of disability avoided, yet such statistics are rarely seen in medical and public health literature.

In 1985, a committee appointed by the National Research Council/Institute of Medicine (NRC/IOM) published *Injury in America: A Continuing Public Health Problem*. This report concluded: "Each year, more than 140,000 Americans die from injuries, and one person in three suffers a nonfatal injury. . . . Injuries kill more Americans aged 1–34 than all diseases combined, and they are the leading cause of deaths up to the age of 44. Injuries cause the loss of

1

more working years of life than all forms of heart disease and cancer combined. One of every eight hospital beds is occupied by an injured patient. Every year, more than 80,000 people in the United States join the ranks of those with unnecessary, but permanently disabling, injury of the brain or spinal cord" (Committee on Trauma Research, 1985).

Since that time, HIV infection has risen to compete with injury for the lives of the young, but injury remains a major contributor to lost years of life, not only in the United States but in other industrialized countries. In the United States, severe injury rates related to motor vehicles and a few other causes have declined somewhat, but that reduction has been substantially offset by a large increase in injuries from bullets (Sosin et al., 1995).

The NRC/IOM report went on to point to the fact that injuries are highly patterned—subject to study and targeting of interventions, that many interventions are known to be effective but are unused, and that modest increases in funding would have large payoffs in cost savings. Eight years after the report recommended that a Center for Injury Control be established at the Centers for Disease Control (CDC), it was established in 1993. The Center's budget, however, is about a third of the amount allocated to control of tuberculosis, for example, and a pittance (less than 2 percent of CDC's budget) compared to the budgets for numerous other programs.

Should injuries have a higher priority? Reduction of injuries is justifiable on humane grounds, particularly since they disproportionately affect the health of the young. In a time of concern for health care costs, injury reduction is also an economic necessity. Injury control is one of the most promising ways to reduce health care costs in the immediate future. Avoidance of fatty foods, increased exercise, and prevention of smoking among the young is worthwhile, but their health benefits are usually not realized for decades. An injury prevented or reduced in severity has immediate benefits in reduced costs as well as reduced grief, pain, and suffering.

Despite declines, motor vehicle injuries are the leading cause of injury deaths; falls are the leading cause of injury hospitalizations. Firearms, which are the second leading cause of injury deaths in the United States, are less significant in countries where guns are not prevalent. Falls and motor vehicles are the primary contributors to injury hospitalizations.

One aspect of injury addressed in this book is the importance of measuring severity when investigating injuries or considering injury control efforts. In the United States, motor vehicles, firearms, falls, poisonings, fire/burns, and drownings account for about 80 percent of deaths but only 36 percent of nonhospitalized injuries severe enough that their sufferers seek medical treatment (Rice & MacKenzie, 1989).

This chapter introduces some of the important concepts in injury epidemiology and prevention: the distinction between accident and injury, the application of the epidemiologic model for infectious diseases to injuries, the phases of injury in relation to the factors that contribute to incidence and severity, the nature of the agents of injury (the various forms of energy), and strategies to control hazards. The chapter ends with a discussion of the types of data needed to investigate particular research questions regarding injury and injury control.

ACCIDENTS AND INJURIES

The evolution in thought about injuries is reflected in their classification. Injuries often are classified as accidental or intentional. Prior to the 1960s, injury control was primarily focused on "accident prevention" and interpersonal or self-directed violence was largely left to law enforcement, psychiatry, social workers, the clergy, and the like. That is not to say that these professions have not contributed to injury control, or that all attempts to prevent "accidents" have been unsuccessful, but the extent of scientific investigation of the effectiveness of these approaches was very limited.

"Accidents" encompass a very large and fuzzy set of events, only a small proportion of which are injurious. Any unintended, incidental event that interferes in one's daily pursuits is an accident. In writing these few paragraphs, the writer has had several accidents in typing, but he hopes they will be corrected enough so as not to irritate the reader, and thus become irrelevant to exposure of the author to risk of injury.

The word "accident" is intertwined with the notion that some human error or behavior is responsible for most injuries. This focus of attention on the human actors involved tends to detract from an examination of the full range of factors that contribute to injuries and, particularly, their severity.

Although the word "accident" had various meanings historically (Loimer et al., 1996), it is now primarily a euphemism for lack of intent, as though intent were a primary consideration in injury prevention. If two people have an argument that results in a brief exchange of fisticuffs, the incident usually goes unrecorded as an injury. In a similar situation, if one of the persons has a gun and kills the other with it, the case is classified as homicide as though the person intended to kill, which is often not true. Although criminal law has various categories of homicide based on intent, aggregated statistics of the broad category "homicide" are included in "intentional injuries" without any data on the intent of the persons who used the weapon.

Despite numerous criticisms of the misleading implications of the word "accident" and the narrow focus on prevention of events without consideration of severity, the tradition hangs on. In 1989, an international conference billed itself as the "First World Conference on Accident and Injury Prevention." The continued use of the term "accident" was justified in the conference's "Manifesto for

Safe Communities" on the grounds that "we speak many different languages and each country has its own historical and cultural contexts" (*Manifesto for Safe Communities,* 1989). The misleading connotation of unpredictability in the use of the term was recognized in the report, but its continued use was an obvious compromise with the traditionalists, rather than a decision based on the science of injuries.

Here the term *injury* or a specific type of injury—amputations, burns, lacerations, and so on—is used to indicate the phenomenon of interest. Also, when referring to attempts to reduce injury, the term *injury control* is used. While "injury prevention" has been used by respectable scientists, and on occasion even by the author, the term is less precise than "injury control" when severity of injury can be reduced without reducing incidence.

EPIDEMIOLOGY

The word *epidemiology* is derived from the classical Greek word *epidemion,* a verb meaning "to visit," used in connection with human maladies by Hippocrates circa 2400 B.C. The first known published use of the word in modern languages was in 1598, the Spanish *epidemiologia,* in a study of bubonic plague in Spain (Najera, 1988).

There are all sorts of definitions of epidemiology. The scientific study of the visitations of disease and injury on the population is as good as any. The scientific study of the distributions of diseases and injuries in populations, and their causes and "risk factors," is somewhat more descriptive of what epidemiologists do.

Historically, early epidemiologists concentrated their attention on what were later called "infectious diseases." Although the specific organisms that often infected populations were microscopic and unknown, quantification of the numbers of illnesses and deaths by location or exposure to certain environmental conditions led to actions that reduced disease and death in some instances. In nineteenth-century London, John Snow found that cholera occurred largely in people who used one water supply but not people who used another. He didn't know what was in the water that caused the disease, but he knew enough to stop the flow from that supply (Evans, 1993).

Similarly, when there are known effective means of reducing injury or severity, relatively simple studies of when, where, and how people are injured can lead to large reductions by targeting the relevant injury control measures to the circumstances to which they apply (Chapter 3). This approach avoids the question of causation that is a point of both fascination and contention among epidemiologists and other scientists.

Some epidemiologists avoid the word "cause" and use euphemisms such as "risk factor" and "etiology." Often the incidence and severity of disease and injury occur coincident with several factors, some of which may contribute to the incidence or severity and some of which may be correlates of the real causes but play no meaningful role in incidence or severity. For example, if a disease or injury is seasonal, as many are, increase in incidence may be correlated with other seasonal happenings. In northern areas of the United States, the vast majority of injuries to people while riding motorcycles occur during the season that robins are in the environment, but the correlation is known to be spurious. Few, if any, motorcyclists crash when impacting robins. The correlation occurs because both robins and motorcyclists prefer warm weather for their activities.

Since correlations thought to represent causal connections occasionally turn out to be false inferences, the embarrassment to the scientists proved wrong leads other scientists to great caution in claiming causal inference. When dealing with maladies that kill or maim, however, one must sometimes risk embarrassment to contribute to the welfare of fellow human beings. At some point, as evidence accumulates, an attempt to change conditions coincident with the disease that would likely reduce it is appropriate. The amount, type, and quality of the evidence necessary to reach that point is a matter of controversy addressed in this book, particularly in Chapter 4.

A few epidemiologists believe that objective scientific investigation is incompatible with recommendations for changes in policies or practices that epidemiologic research suggests would reduce harm. Some journal editors do not allow discussions of policy implications of research results—much less recommendations for policy changes—in articles reporting the results. Two important points are ignored by those stances: *(1)* The work of the scientist who proposes change based on research is likely to be scrutinized very carefully for bias and error. To the extent that such scrutiny weeds out invalid results, the science is improved. *(2)* Self-imposed or institutional bars to prevent the scientists closest to the data from joining the policy debate increase the probability of misinterpretation or misuse of the data. Therefore, this book is devoted not just to the application of the theory and methods of epidemiology in injury research, but also to the uses and misuses of epidemiologic data relevant to injury control.

Epidemiologic methods are also applied to the study of the effectiveness of policies and practices aimed at the reduction of injury incidence and severity. Although this is called "applied" research and somehow has less prestige than "basic" research, the distinction is false. The study of human activities and other phenomena that increase the risk of injury is no more basic than the study of the human activities that seek to intervene in the causal process to reduce injury. Indeed, reduction of injury (or disease) by deliberately changing a factor inferred as a condition necessary for, or contributing to, specific injuries is additional evidence of causation, particularly if the change is introduced in such a way as to rule out the contribution of other factors to the reduction. Chapters 5–8 of the book discuss the use of scientific methods to evaluate the effects of programs, laws, environmental modifications, medical care, and rehabilitation to reduce injuries or their severity.

Of course, disciplines other than epidemiology also study injury. Clinicians often describe a case or series of cases and scientists in areas ranging from physics to biomechanics contribute to our understanding of the mechanisms of injury. The research methods used by epidemiologists are shared by many disciplines. Statisticians, sociologists, psychologists, and physical and biological scientists use more or less the same methods. Many epidemiologists were originally trained in these disciplines as well as medicine. Nevertheless, the concepts of epidemiology provide a valuable perspective, particularly with respect to reducing disease and injury in the population as a whole or in subsets of the population.

THE EPIDEMIOLOGIC MODEL

Based on the experience of their predecessors in the scientific investigation of infectious diseases, many injury epidemiologists conduct their investigations mindful of a theoretical model developed by infectious disease epidemiologists. The core concepts of this model include the *host* (the person injured), the *agent* that injures, and the *vector* or *vehicle* that may convey the agent, as well as other environmental factors.

Early epidemiologic investigations of what came to be known as infectious diseases showed correlations of the diseases to seasons, water sources, economic status of the populations primarily affected, and the like (Buck et al., 1988). We now know that in some cases these correlates of the diseases were carriers (vehicles or vectors) of infectious agents. In others they were factors that increased or decreased host exposure or susceptibility to the agents, and some were spurious.

Microbiologists subsequently identified tiny biological structures (bacteria, parasites, viruses) that secreted toxins in an invaded host, or removed elements from the host, or caused other changes at the cellular or organ levels, that resulted in sickness and death. Then epidemiologists looked for these agents in the seasons, water, living conditions, and other factors associated with a given disease (Lilienfeld & Lilienfeld, 1980).

In some cases the microorganism was conveyed to the host in inanimate media, such as water and milk, which came to be called *vehicles*. Others were carried to human hosts by insects, by animals, or by direct transmission from human being to human being. These animate carriers came to be called *vectors*. Living conditions, often related to economic status, increased or decreased exposure to the carriers of the agents or increased susceptibility to infection due to nutritional or other factors.

All of these discoveries had implications for control of infectious diseases. The agents could be eliminated from the media in which they reached hosts, such as water and milk. In some cases susceptibility could be reduced by modifying the immune mechanisms of the potential hosts. In others, antibiotic agents could be introduced into the infected hosts to reduce the severity of the illness. Elimination or control of certain carriers, such as rodents and insects, could be tried and, in some cases, accomplished. While diseases sometimes declined as people improved their living conditions, removing harmful agents or carriers in the process, epidemiologic evidence on vehicles or vectors, as well as times, places, and populations involved, was crucial in the deliberate attempts to reduce many infectious diseases.

Although injuries can be characterized using the concepts of infectious disease epidemiology, injury epidemiology lagged in development by decades. The twentieth century was almost two-thirds past before the agents of injury were accurately identified as the various forms of energy—mechanical, thermal, chemical, electrical, ionizing radiation—or too little energy in the case of asphyxiation (Gibson, 1961). And that identification came from a psychologist, not an epidemiologist. Before and since that date, certain authors referred to motor vehicles, guns, and alcohol as agents of injury, but that is inaccurate in the epidemiologic use of the concept of agent. Motor vehicles and guns are vehicles of mechanical energy in epidemiologic parlance, and alcohol contributes to injury by sometimes affecting behavior that places people at greater risk of injurious energy exposure as well as perhaps increasing vulnerability of tissues to energy insults.

Prior to these insights, the research on injury was primarily focused on human characteristics and human behavior correlated with injury incidence and, more rarely, severity—with occasional studies of seasonal and geographical variations and the like. A few isolated researchers looked at human tolerance of mechanical energy as important (DeHaven, 1941; Haddon et al., 1964; Stapp, 1957).

It is not that the characteristics of the energy were unknown. The leading source of injury by far is mechanical energy, the characteristics of which have been known since Sir Isaac Newton's work on the laws of motion in the seventeenth century. Although Newton's laws of motion do not apply near the speed of light, they are applicable to moving motor vehicles and bullets or to falling human beings.

Why did it take so long to recognize energy as the agent of injury? It is more difficult to prove why something does not happen than why it does. After the great decline in death due to infectious diseases in the first half of the twentieth century, many epidemiologists turned their attention to cardiovascular diseases and cancers, at least partly because government support of research on those diseases increased. The popular folklore focused on human behavior or human error as the cause of "accidents" and the small amounts of research funds available were devoted to reinforcement of that view.

Manufacturers of motor vehicles—by the 1920s the leading source of mechanical energy leading to death—deliberately supported the behavioral approach to divert attention from their vehicles (Eastman, 1984), a tradition that continues to this day (Robertson, 1997a, 1997b). The National Rifle Association, the leading opponent of regulation of guns, coined the slogan "Guns don't kill people. People kill people." Mosquitoes don't have lobbyists, but motor vehicles and guns do.

FACTORS AND PHASES OF INJURY

The transfer of energy to human beings at rates and in amounts above or below the tolerance of human tissue is the necessary and specific cause of injury. The amount of the energy concentration outside the bands of tolerance of tissue determines the severity of the injury.

"Injury" usually refers to the damage to cells and organs from energy exposures that have relatively sudden, discernible effects, although some researchers have included damage from chronic low-energy exposures, such as back strain or carpal tunnel syndrome, as injury (Waller, 1985). Chemical and radiation exposures that produce cellular changes resulting in neoplasms are usually called cancerous rather than injurious. A debate regarding the appropriateness of inclusion or exclusion of any harmful condition as injury or disease would be pointless, but at the fuzzy edges of a set of harmful consequences from energy exchanges, a given researcher should make clear the cases that are considered injuries.

Most of the concentrations of energy involved in severe and fatal injuries is the result of modification by human organizations of the energy inherent in matter (Robertson, 1983). Some falls occur from heights unmodified by human construction. A few people are struck by lightning or tornadoes. But motor vehicles and guns, as well as cigarettes, which cause more housefires than any other ignition source, and home swimming pools, which drown more children than other bodies of water, are examples of human inventions that are some of the major sources of serious injuries.

To alert researchers to the factors contributing to injury incidence and severity, and the timing of involvement of those factors, William Haddon Jr. (1972) devised a matrix of broad categories of factors and phases of injury. This matrix, along with some examples of factors known to be important in each cell, is shown in Table 1.1.

Prior to injury, human, vehicle, and environmental factors contribute to the increase or decrease in exposure to potentially damaging energy. For example, alcohol impairs human perceptions, reactions, and judgments and may increase aggressivity. Less efficient brakes on larger vehicles extend stopping distances. Hedges at intersections reduce visibility of oncoming traffic.

During the energy exchange that injures, the susceptibility of the host's tissue to damage may vary. For example, a person with osteoporosis may be disabled by a fall that would hardly bruise a teenager. Sharp points and edges concentrate energy on the host. Flammable building materials increase intensity of heat and smoke in fires.

After the initial energy exchange, the condition of the host, the potential for more energy exposure, and the responses from the environment substantially affect survival and the time and extent of return to preinjury functioning of those who survive. For example, if hemorrhaging is not stopped, the host may die from loss of blood. If a gas tank is ruptured by the initial energy exchange, a spark can result in thermal energy beyond host tolerance. If emergency response is delayed, life that could be preserved by surgery or other intensive treatment may be lost.

Every epidemiological investigation does not have to measure all of the human, vehicle, and environmental factors at various phases to be useful, but in those cases where there is a synergistic effect of particular factors on the outcome being studied, failure to consider them can be misleading. One crucial consideration in the relevance of epidemiology for injury control is the modifiability of the factors measured.

For example, a large number of injury investigations are limited to the distributions of rates of a particular type of injury by age and sex. It is important to know how many potential years of life are affected by injury and whether subsets of the population are disproportionately involved, but other than those

TABLE 1.1. The Haddon Matrix with Examples

| | FACTORS | | |
PHASES	HUMAN	VEHICLE	ENVIRONMENT
Preinjury	1. Alcohol intoxication	4. Braking capacity of motor vehicles	7. Visibility of hazards
Injury	2. Resistance to energy insults	5. Sharp or pointed edges and surfaces	8. Flammable building materials
Postinjury	3. Hemorrhage	6. Rapidity of energy reduction	9. Emergency medical response

considerations, age and sex distributions are uninteresting. We are not going to change the age and sex of individuals in the population.

The major modifiable factors that contribute to injury are energy and the characteristics of vehicles of energy. Human behavior that increases exposure or concentrates energy can be modified under certain conditions (Robertson, 1983), but not by changing immutable factors such as age and sex. Human tolerance to energy exposures varies among individuals by age, sex, and other factors that affect the condition of tissue, such as decalcification of bones and hemophilia. To the extent that diseases that increase susceptibility can be treated, the severity of injury can be reduced by that method, but there are substantial limits to increasing tolerance to energy.

The importance of focus on degree and type of energy exposures was most dramatically illustrated to the writer in a study of worker injuries. In two adjacent buildings of the same company, the injuries to the workers were remarkably different. In Building A, there were virtually no injuries to the workers that were severe enough to be reported on the log required by the Occupational Safety and Health Administration (OSHA) during the eight-year period studied. In Building B, about one in five workers had an OSHA-reportable injury annually. There were some age, sex, and other differences between the work forces in the two buildings, but these accounted for only a small amount of the variation in injuries among the workers in Building B (Robertson & Keeve, 1983), and there was essentially no variation in injuries while at work among people in Building A to investigate.

The major difference between the two buildings was the exposure to energy. In Building B, some of the workers poured molten metal, heated thousands of degrees, from large vats. Others worked adjacent to machines that rolled, shaped, and stamped the metal, forming it into wire, rods, keys, and so on. A fall or a movement of any sort in the wrong direction would place one or another part of a worker's anatomy in contact with thermal or mechanical energy beyond the tolerance of human tissue. The people in Building A also worked with machines—typewriters, photocopying machines, computers—that contained potentially injurious electrical energy. But the manufacturers of those machines had the foresight to shield the energy from the workers so that the potential for contact with the energy was minimal.

THE NATURE OF ENERGY

Injury epidemiologists should have at least a rudimentary understanding of the energy involved in injury and the tolerance of human beings to exposure to that energy. Since incidence and severity of injury are usually classified by vehicles or circumstances rather than by agent, the precise numbers attributable to a given agent in many data sets are not available. In the United States, about 63 percent of fatal injuries and 58 percent of hospitalized injuries are attributed to motor vehicles, falls, and firearms (Rice & MacKenzie, 1989). These, and a proportion of those injuries associated with factors and activities grouped into the "other" category (industrial machines, farm machines, knives, sports, etc.), indicate that mechanical energy accounts for the vast majority of severe injury.

Some energy releases, such as a nuclear explosion, include multiple forms of energy—mechanical, heat, chemical, and ionizing radiation. The acute effects of ionizing radiation have rarely been released and are not discussed in the following brief descriptions of common types of energy that cause the bulk of acute injuries.

Mechanical energy

Any object, animate or inanimate, in motion at velocity substantially less than the speed of light has energy in relation to its mass and speed that is described by a simple formula:

$$F = \frac{mv^2}{2} \qquad (1)$$

where

F = energy in foot-pounds
m = mass
v = velocity in feet per second

Mass can be calculated at the earth's surface by dividing weight in pounds by 32. Velocity in miles per hour can be converted to feet per second by multiplying miles per hour by 1.467. Therefore, a 150 pound motor vehicle occupant traveling at 30 miles per hour has about 4538 foot-pounds of energy, that is, $[(150/32) \times 44^2]/2$. Increase in mass or speed increases the energy, speed obviously more than mass because it is squared in the calculation. At 60 miles per hour, the 150 pound occupant of the vehicle has about 18,150 foot-pounds of energy, twice the speed but about four times the energy at 30 miles per hour.

If the person must stop suddenly, as in a crash of the vehicle, that energy must be dissipated in the vehicle, in the environment, or in the tissues of the individual. When the vehicle stops, the occupant will continue to move at the precrash speed into the interior structures, or into materials in the exterior environment if ejected. The load on the tissue is measured in pounds per square inch. The shape and elasticity of the materials struck will determine the damage to the tissue. Inflexible, protruding, or pointed objects on dashboards, for example, penetrate the heads or other parts of the anatomy of people in crashes.

Devices such as child restraints, lap/shoulder belts, and air bags reduce the severity of injury by reducing contact with less flexible surfaces—the so-called second collision. They also increase the uniformity of deceleration of occupant and vehicle, and they spread the load over dozens of square inches. Energy-absorbing materials, both in the vehicle and in the environment, can also dissipate energy so that the individual's deceleration is less rapid. Helmets used by motorcyclists, by bicyclists, and in certain sports, as well as padding used in certain sports, also may be designed to absorb energy.

The extent of damage to tissue is a function of the structure of the part of the body affected. Contact with an energy source generates forces counter to the load, called *stresses*. These constitute the resistance of the bonds among tissue molecules to deformation. The same tissue may have different capacity for tension stress (pulling molecules apart), compression stress (pushing molecules together), or shear stress (from a tangential force).

Strain refers to the extent of deformation and may be classified as resulting from tension, compression, or shear stress. Tissue varies as to elasticity—the extent to which strain is eliminated when the load is removed—and the regenerative capability of the organism (Stephenson, 1952). Nerves do not regenerate substantially when severed and, therefore, injuries to the brain and spinal cord are especially disabling (Committee on Trauma Research, 1985).

To the extent that the object striking or struck by human tissue is stressed more than the tissue, the energy will be transferred to the inanimate object and the human tissue will be damaged less. DeHaven's classic study of people who survived falls of up to 150 feet found no major injury in some cases where the deformation in the ground, car, or other object struck was as little as a few inches (DeHaven, 1941).

With the exception of persons with diseases such as scurvy, osteoporosis, and hemophilia—which reduce the elasticity of important tissues—human beings are capable of experiencing substantial mechanical force with little or no injury if the load is not concentrated. Stapp conducted experiments with animals in rocket sleds and wind tunnels to test the limits of tissue tolerance and then tested healthy human volunteers, including himself, within the estimated limits. Held in the sled only by 3 inch wide webbed harnesses over the shoulders and legs, and anchored to the sled, the volunteers experienced decelerations up to 35 g with no damage and up to 45 g with little damage (Stapp, 1957). A g is the measurement of gravity at the earth's surface, 32 feet/second^2. The effective weight of a 160 pound person decelerated at 35 g is 5600 pounds. Yet, because the accompanying load was distributed over the surface of the restraining belts to reduce concentration at smaller points, and was partly absorbed by the belts, the test subjects sustained no serious injury.

Biomechanical engineers study the susceptibility of animate tissues to damage from mechanical energy loads. Materials engineers study the properties of matter that increase or decrease their energy-absorbing capability. Experts in these fields should be consulted by epidemiologists who need information on the properties of tissue or other matter involved in a given set of injuries (Nahum & Melvin, 1985).

The velocity of the persons involved in an injury is often not known, but it can be estimated using another formula from elementary physics (Bueche, 1982):

$$v_t^2 = v_0^2 + 2ad \tag{2}$$

where

$$v = \text{velocity in feet per second}$$
$$t = \text{time in seconds}$$
$$a = \text{acceleration}$$
$$d = \text{distance moved in feet}$$

A person in a free fall accelerates at 32 feet per second every second (1 g). If we know the distance fallen, say 5 feet from the top of a sliding board in a playground, the velocity at impact can be calculated as follows from formula 2:

$$v^2 = 0 + 2 \times 32 \times 5 = 320$$

Therefore, the velocity at impact is the square root of 320, which is 17.9 feet per second. If we know the maximum weight of the children who use the sliding board, then we can calculate the energy at impact in the worst-case senario, from formula 1. Let's say the maximum weight of any child likely to climb onto the sliding board is 90 pounds. Then, from formula 1, the energy that should be managed is:

$$F = \frac{(90/32) \times 17.9^2}{2} = 451 \text{ foot-pounds}$$

This, compared to the energy of the mentioned car occupant, should give more than a hint as to why motor vehicle injuries are, on average, more severe than fall injuries.

The surface under the sliding board could be designed to absorb more than 451 foot-pounds of energy over a surface of a few square inches and no damage would occur to children who fall off. If playground builders were to conduct such calculations and compare the results to the energy-absorbing properties of materials, they would find that the concrete or asphalt often placed under playground equipment does not do the job.

Faced with playground managers who do not believe the theoretical formula, an injury epidemiologist might use the basic physics to do a study of injuries in falls from playground equipment. The data to be collected would include severity of injuries, weight of the injured, height of the equipment used, and surfaces under the equipment. Using an appropriate statistical model, the data would be analyzed to examine the extent to which severity of injury is a function of the type of playground surface, controlling for the energy of the falling bodies.

The severity of the second leading cause of fatal injury, gun-related injury, is also substantially a function of the characteristics of the involved vehicles of mechanical energy—guns and bullets. In addition to high velocity applied to less than a square inch of body surface in most cases, which results in frequent deep penetration of vital organs, the extent of fragmentation after penetration increases the damage to organs affected. Muzzle velocities of bullets range widely, from 1200 to 2700 feet per second. They generate energy from 124 to 4440 foot-pounds at close range (DeMuth, 1966).

Bullets used by military forces are required by the Geneva Conventions to be fully jacketed and retain their approximate original shape while moving through human tissue. Bullets sold in the United States for domestic use do not meet such a standard. Their sometimes blunt ends and frequent fragmentation result in wounds that have an average size 27 times those caused by military bullets (DeMuth, 1966). Yet gun-related injuries are often studied by epidemiologists as if all guns and bullets were the same.

Thermal and chemical energy

The deaths and injuries associated with fires, heat, and smoke are the result of use of ignition sources and flammable materials and of the heat and chemical energies generated by burning or heating materials. The most common ignition source in fatal fires is a cigarette dropped in furniture or bedding, often smoldering until the occupants of a household are asleep. The extent to which a cigarette will continue to burn when dropped is a function of type of tobacco, tobacco density, paper porosity, citrate added, circumference, and second paper wrapping (Technical Study Group, 1987). Other fire ignition sources whose variations deserve epidemiologic attention are matches, cigarette lighters, gas stoves, and electrical circuits or appliances. Heat from sources other than ignited fires most often includes heated water and other liquids, heating units on stoves, and space heaters.

The physics and chemistry of combustion vary according to several factors: (1) concentration and type of heat source, (2) shape and size of a combustible, (3) oxygen concentration, (4) vaporization of gasses, and (5) presence or absence of catalysts (National Fire Protection Agency, 1981). Heat is transferred among solids, liquids, and gasses, in proximity to one another, from the medium at higher temperature to the medium at lower temperature. The effect of heat on human tissue is a function of the temperature and the time of exposure (Moritz & Henriques, 1947).

Chemicals may be breathed, as in a fire, or ingested, injected, or absorbed.

The effect is a function of the concentration of the exogenous chemical, its interaction with body chemistry, and the rapidity of elimination relative to individual susceptibility. The dose–response curve may also vary based on genetic susceptibility, physiological development, increased or reduced tolerance resulting from previous exposure, and presence or absence of other chemicals that can have synergistic effects.

Toxicologists divide the process of harm by a chemical into three phases—exposure, toxokinetic, and toxodynamic. Epidemiologists have paid some attention to the first of these in the study of poisonings, but the second and third deserve attention regarding severity. The toxokinetic phase refers to the chemical's absorption through the organism's membranes, usually in the alimentary canal or the lung sacs in the case of common poisonings, as well as the distribution, metabolism, and excretion in the vascular and waste disposal systems. The interaction of the chemical with receptors in target tissues constitutes the toxodynamic phase (Ariens et al., 1976).

Researchers have given some attention to the possibility of reduction of the effects of alcohol and narcotics in the toxodynamic phase based on increased understanding of receptors, but less attention has been given to the toxokinetic phase. For example, suggestion that something could be added to alcohol to reduce absorption in the alimentary canal (Robertson, 1981) is often greeted with the statement that people would just drink more. Perhaps some would, but many people in the process of "partying" likely do not pay attention to the amount consumed. The issue deserves empirical research rather than offhand dismissal.

Electrical energy

Electrical energy is inherent in matter. Atoms are made up of electrons (negatively charged), protons (positively charged), and neutrons (neutrally charged). Gain or loss of electrons in orbit about the nucleus determines whether the atom is positively or negatively charged. The flow of electrons is electrical current. The atoms of different materials, including human tissues, vary in their tendency to hold an electrical charge.

The term *amperes* refers to electrical current flow in a unit of time and varies as a function of the electromotive force (volts) divided by resistance to conductivity (ohms) that characterizes the materials and situation involved. The extent of damage to human tissue in contact with electrical energy increases with amperage. Muscular paralysis occurs at about 0.02 ampere, ventricular fibrillation at 0.10 ampere, and ventricular paralysis at 2.0 or more amperes. The resistivity of skin varies 100-fold as a function of wetness—100,000 ohms when dry but 100 ohms when soaked. The water serves as a low-resistance conductor if the water is in contact with the ground. Thus a 120 volt electrical current in the average home socket will have low amperage (0.001) in contact with dry skin but will be high enough (0.12) to cause ventricular fibrillation if the skin is soaking wet and in contact with the ground. Deaths attributed to heart failure or other causes are sometimes found upon detailed examination to have been caused by electricity (Wright & Davis, 1980).

Asphyxiation

The human organism cannot function with too little energy. The absence of oxygen to sustain endogenous energy conversion, called asphyxiation, causes essential cells in the brain and heart to be damaged within minutes. Asphyxiation can occur from objects or other material blocking the nose and mouth or trachea (e.g., by a plastic bag or balloon fragment), a mechanical blow to the trachea (e.g., by a "karate chop" dashboard tapered toward the occupant in a car crash), constriction of the trachea (e.g., hanging by a rope), or obstruction in the lungs. The most common fatal form of asyphyxia from acute exposure to external sources, counted as injury, is water in the lungs, usually labeled as drowning or near-drowning. Lung congestion from endogenous fluids, as in pneumonia and congestive heart failure, is attributed to diseases.

TECHNICAL STRATEGIES

Similar to cancer epidemiology and control, the varieties of energy sources involved in injury and the differences in populations exposed to the various types of energy mitigate against a single cure for the whole problem. In contrast to cancer, however, one does not have to wait 20 years to find out if a given control strategy is having an effect on the subset of injuries toward which it is targeted.

William Haddon Jr. (1970) defined ten logically distinct technical strategies for injury control. The following is a list of the strategies, with examples relevant to some of the more commonly severe injuries:

1. *Prevent the creation of the hazard in the first place.* Do not allow the manufacture of particularly hazardous vehicles, such as motorcycles, minibikes, and "all-terrain" vehicles. These vehicles are used mainly for recreation, for which there are numerous alternative and less hazardous activities.

2. *Reduce the amount of the hazard brought into being.* Require that passenger vehicles, including utility vehicles, light trucks and vans have lower centers of gravity or wider track width such that track width divided by twice the height of center of gravity ($T/2H$) is not less than 1.2.

Vehicles with lower *T/2H* have 3 to 20 times as many fatal rollover crashes as those 1.2 or greater and the relative risk is strongly correlated to *T/2H*. Require that all motor vehicles operated on a level surface be incapable of speeds greater than 65 miles per hour. (Limitations on maximum speed would also conserve fuel and reduce emissions.) Allow sale of handguns only to police and military units. Reduce the number of pills in a prescription for drugs to a number that would not kill or disable if taken all at once. Reduce flammability of clothing. Reduce maximum temperature capability of water heaters, the source of heat for many scald burns.

3. *Prevent the release of the hazard that already exists.* Improve braking capability of motor vehicles, especially heavy trucks that have longer braking distances than cars and light trucks. Keep guns for target shooting at the shooting range rather than in homes. Provide canes and walkers to the elderly and handrails in their environments. Make matches and lighters less easy for children to ignite.

4. *Modify the rate or spatial distribution of release of the hazard from its source.* Use child restraints and seat belts in motor vehicles. Prohibit automatic and semi-automatic guns. Use lightly woven and smoothly finished fabrics in clothing to reduce burning rates. Install automatic sprinkler systems. Provide systems that replace air rapidly in passenger compartments of motor vehicles to prevent elevated carbon monoxide concentrations.

5. *Separate, in time or space, the hazard and that which is to be protected.* Remove trees and poles from near roadsides. Build pedestrian and bicycle paths separated from roads. Seat children in the back seat of motor vehicles. Prohibit large truck traffic, especially if transporting flammables or toxic chemicals, during periods of congestion. Restrict hunting and target shooting to unpopulated areas. Evacuate coastal areas at times of approaching hurricanes. Use cooking units that children cannot reach or keep children out of the kitchen while cooking.

6. *Separate the hazard and that which is to be protected by interposition of a material barrier.* Increase energy-absorbing capability of vehicle exteriors. Install air bags in passenger vehicles. Require motorcyclists and bicyclists to use helmets. Use energy-absorbing barriers that are compatible with car bumper heights on the fronts and rears of large trucks. Place energy-absorbing barriers between roads and bridge abutments or other necessary rigid structures near roads. Place fences with gates that children cannot open around swimming pools and other small bodies of water in areas where children can reach them. Install guards on boat propellers, industrial machines, and the like, where moving parts can injure those in proximity. Use insulated firewalls in vehicles and build-

ings. Invent an additive to alcoholic beverages and other commonly ingested drugs that reduces absorption through the wall of the digestive
tract into the bloodstream as increasing amounts are ingested.

7. *Modify basic relevant qualities of the hazard.* Eliminate sharp points and
edges on vehicle exteriors. Eliminate protruding knobs and "karate chop"
dashboards in vehicle interiors. Use breakaway designs for utility poles
and light poles along roadsides. Prohibit more than one trailer on tractor-
trailer rigs. Reduce muzzle velocity of guns. Use trigger locks on guns.
Apply to ammunition sold to the public the Geneva Convention regulation that prohibits flattening and fragmenting of bullets used in war. Use
energy-absorbing materials of adequate depth on playground surfaces.

8. *Make what is to be protected more resistant to damage from the hazard.*
Develop treatment for persons with hemophilia and osteoporosis to increase resistance to mechanical energy exchanges. Require physical conditioning before participation in sports that produce condition-related injuries.

9. *Begin to counter the damage already done by the environmental hazard.*
Increase the availability of roadside emergency telephones. Place emergency response teams near areas with relatively high injury rates. Increase use of smoke detectors and carbon monoxide detectors.

10. *Stabilize, repair, and rehabilitate the object of the damage.* Provide prosthetic devices for amputees and wheelchairs, beds, and equipment used
in work and other activities designed to optimize normal living. Provide
job and self-care training.

The adoption of any one strategy is dependent on various aspects of ideology, politics, and costs. Epidemiologists can play a central role in pinpointing
energy exposures, incidence and severity among particular populations, and
evaluation of the effectiveness of strategies to control injury. Costs of injury
control can be minimized by targeting strategies to agents, vehicle or vectors,
hosts, and environments in which the severity of injuries and their associated
costs are most acute.

RESEARCH OBJECTIVES AND DATA NEEDS

To contribute data that are useful in the effort to reduce injury, the researcher
needs a clear understanding of how the data may be used. Too many research
reports describe the cross-tabulations of available data, such as the age and sex
distribution of injury X, without any discernible objective.

Table 1.2 presents a set of research objectives and data that would accelerate
the control of injuries. The International Classification of Diseases has two
types of codes for injury, so-called N codes and E codes. The N codes are

TABLE 1.2. Objectives of Injury Research and Control and Data Needs

OBJECTIVE	DATA NEEDED
1. Select the most important injuries for study or detailed surveillance.	E-coded fatalities and hospitalizations.
2. Efficiently apply known countermeasures.	Surveillance of who, where, when, and how people are severely injured.
3. Find changeable factors that will reduce injury and quantify the reduction expected.	Reliable and valid measures of the factors and research designs to control for confounding factors.
4. Develop causal models of homogeneous subsets of injury.	Measurement of all possible risk factors and specification of sequential time order.
5. Evaluate the effectiveness of an intervention.	Injury rates or risk-related behavior with and without an intervention in a realistic setting, controlling for other factors, preferably with an experimental-control design.
6. Evaluate the cost-effectiveness of alternative interventions.	Cost of each intervention and degree of overlap in effectiveness among them.

diagnosis codes (e.g., type and anatomical location of a fracture) and are usually coded or codable from hospital records. E codes are codes for broad categories of circumstances (motor vehicle, fall, etc.). E codes are available on death certificates, with greater or lesser accuracy depending on type of injury. In hospital records, however, one often cannot tell anything about how an injury occurred. For example, the record of a fracture often does not indicate whether the injury occurred in a motor vehicle crash, a fall, or an assault. Even less often is there information on where the injury occurred (geographic location such as street address or highway milepost). Without such information, specification of the scope of injury problems and the choice of those that need the most attention cannot be adequately done. Clinicians could aid injury control enormously by including in the history when, where, and how an injury occurred.

To apply known countermeasures efficiently, detailed surveillance of to whom and when, where, and how specific types of severe injuries occur is needed (item 2, Table 1.2). There are two reasons for emphasizing only severe injuries, such as hospitalizations and deaths. First, large numbers of minor cuts, bruises, abrasions, and the like, occur in circumstances that are substantially different from severe injuries (Rice & MacKenzie, 1989). Attempts to control the most frequent injuries will misdirect resources from the most severe and costly injuries. Second, the cost of data collection is remarkably reduced by limiting it to only hospitalized and fatal injuries.

Data on location and how the injuries occurred have led to large reductions in fall, pedestrian, and vehicle-occupant injuries in the limited instances in which such data have been collected (Chapter 3). Simple pin maps of types of injury often indicate stretches of roads, intersections, or clusters of housing in which injuries occur. Visits to the sites often reveal obvious remedies such as night lighting, sidewalks, moving or uncovering obscured stop signs, properly timed yellow lights, installation of guardrails, or repair of dilapidated stairs.

In those instances where contributing factors or countermeasures are not obvious, well-designed analytic studies may specify how much a changeable factor would contribute to injury reduction if changed (item 3, Table 1.2). Notice that the emphasis here is on *changeable* factors. Too many research projects are focused on unchangeable factors such as age and sex, or difficult-to-change factors such as some types of behavior.

Suppose, for example, that your community has a high rate of severe injuries to children falling on stairs in households. The research question is the extent that changes in stairs would reduce the injuries. One way to answer the question is to do a case–control study comparing characteristics of stairs where children were injured and stairs in randomly selected households with similar-age children where injuries did not occur. Such a study of stairs in houses of the elderly found substantial differences in levelness, horizontal width, step width, absence of handrails, and lighting (Locklear, 1991). A second aspect of the research would compare the factors relevant to falls of children and the elderly to make sure that any recommended modifications of stairs would reduce injuries in both populations.

The development of elaborate causal models of the sequence of factors that lead to injury is the goal of some researchers, but it is the least productive research activity leading to injury control (item 4, Table 1.2). The point of injury control research is not to specify some original cause in a sequence of factors, but to specify changeable factors that reduce injuries irrespective of other factors. As noted, an injury cannot occur unless there is an energy exchange with the human anatomy beyond the tolerance of human tissue. Any countermeasure that reduces such energy exchanges will reduce injury severity regardless of the factors that increased the probability of the event. The more proximate a risk factor to the energy exchanges, the greater the likelihood that changing the risk factor would have an effect on injuries (Chapter 4).

The effectiveness of interventions, where unknown, can best be studied in controlled experiments (item 5, Table 1.2). That includes medical care interventions, acute care, and rehabilitation (Chapter 8) as well as some types of prevention (Chapter 5). In the case of laws and regulations aimed at prevention, random assignment of treatments is usually not possible, so quasi-experimental designs and other approaches are necessary (Chapters 6–7).

If there is more than one countermeasure that reduces substantially the same types of injuries, the degree in overlap of effectiveness and the relative costs of the countermeasures must be considered (item 6, Table 1.2). The allocation of resources to duplicative efforts consumes the resources available to reduce injuries that are not being addressed (Chapter 9).

SUMMARY

Injury is a public health problem that is neglected relative to its importance in lost life and disability. Injury control has more immediate health and economic benefits than chronic disease control. The infectious model—agent, carrier, host—can be applied to injuries. Interventions can reduce injuries, their severity, or their consequences by modifying these factors at specific phases of the injury—before, during the acute phase, and afterward.

Energy in its various forms—mechanical, thermal, chemical, electrical, and radiation—is the agent of injury. Research that focuses on modification of means of exposure to the agent will contribute most to injury control.

REFERENCES

Ariens J, Simonis AM, and Offermeier J (1976) *Introduction to General Toxicology.* New York: Academic Press.

Buck C, Llopis A, Najera E, and Terris M (eds) (1988) *The Challenge of Epidemiology: Issues and Selected Readings.* Washington, DC: Pan American Health Organization.

Bueche F (1982) *Principles of Physics,* 4th ed. New York: McGraw-Hill.

Committee on Trauma Research (1985) *Injury in America: A Continuing Public Health Problem.* Washington, DC: National Academy Press.

DeHaven H (1941) Mechanical analysis of survival in falls from heights of fifty to one hundred and fifty feet. *War Med* 2:586.

DeMuth WE Jr (1966) Bullet velocity and design as determinants of wounding capability. *J Trauma* 6:222.

Eastman JW (1984) *Styling vs. Safety: The American Automobile and the Development of Automotive Safety, 1900–1966.* New York: University Press of America.

Evans AS (1993) *Causation and Disease: A Chronological Journey.* New York: Plenum Publishing Co.

Gibson JJ (1961) The contribution of experimental psychology to the formulation of the problem of safety. In *Behavioral Approaches to Accident Research.* New York: Association for the Aid of Crippled Children.

Haddon W Jr. (1970) On the escape of tigers: an ecologic note. *Tech Rev* 72:44.

Haddon W Jr. (1972) A logical framework for categorizing highway safety phenomena and activity. *J Trauma* 12:197.

Haddon W Jr, Suchman EA, and Klein D (1964) *Accident Research: Methods and Ap-*

proaches. New York: Harper and Row.

Lilienfeld AM, and Lilienfeld DE (1980) *Foundations of Epidemiology.* New York: Oxford University Press.

Locklear G (1991) A retrospective case-control study of porch step falls occurring on the Fort Apache Indian Reservation, 1987 to 1989. Phoenix: Environmental Health Services Branch, Indian Health Service (mimeo).

Loimer H, Driur M, and Guarnieri M (1996) Accidents and acts of God: a history of the terms. *Am J Public Health* 86:101–107, 1996.

Manifesto for Safe Communities (1989) Stockholm: World Health Organization.

Moritz AR, and Henriques CF Jr. (1947) Studies in thermal injury II: the relative importance of time and surface temperature in the causation of cutaneous burns. *Am J Pathol* 23:695.

Nahum AM, and Melvin J (eds) (1985) *The Biomechanics of Trauma.* Norwalk, CT: Appleton-Century-Crofts.

Najera E (1988) Discussions. In Buck C, et al. (eds), *The Challenge of Epidemiology: Issues and Selected Readings.* Washington, DC: Pan American Health Organization.

National Fire Protection Agency (1981) *Fire Protection Handbook,* 15th ed. Quincy, MA: National Fire Protection Agency.

Pearce N (1996) Traditional epidemiology, modern epidemiology, and public health. *Am J Public Health* 86:678–683.

Rice DP, and MacKenzie EJ (eds) (1989) *Cost of Injury in the United States: A Report to Congress, 1989.* San Francisco: Institute for Health and Aging, University of California, and Baltimore: Injury Prevention Center, Johns Hopkins University.

Robertson LS (1981) Alcohol, behavior and public health strategies. *Abstr Rev Alcohol Driving* 2:1–4.

Robertson LS (1983) *Injuries: Causes, Control Strategies and Public Policy.* Cambridge, MA: D.C. Heath.

Robertson LS (1997a) Health policy and behavior: injury control. In Gochman DS (ed), *Handbook of Health Behavior Research.* New York: Plenum Publishing Co.

Robertson LS (1997b) Mistaken assertions on reducing motor vehicle injuries. *Am J Public Health* 87:295–296.

Robertson LS, and Keeve JP (1983) Worker injuries: the effects of workers' compensation and OSHA inspections. *J Health Polit Policy Law* 8:581.

Sosin DM, Sniezek JE, and Waxweiler RJ (1995) Trends in death associated with traumatic brain injury, 1979 through 1992. Success and failure. *JAMA* 273:1778–1780.

Stapp JP (1957) Human tolerance to deceleration. *Am J Surg* 93:734.

Stephenson RJ (1952) *Mechanics and Properties of Matter.* New York: John Wiley and Sons.

Susser M, and Susser E (1996) Choosing a future for epidemiology: I. Eras and paradigms. *Am J Public Health* 86:668–673.

Technical Study Group (1987) *Toward a Less Fire-Prone Cigarette: Final Report of the Technical Study Group on Cigarette and Little Cigar Fire Safety.* Washington, DC: U.S. Consumer Product Safety Commission.

Waller JA (1985) *Injury Control: A Guide to the Causes and Prevention of Trauma.* Lexington, MA: D.C. Heath.

Wright RK, and Davis JH (1980) The investigation of electrical deaths: a report of 220 fatalities. *J Forensic Sci* 25:514–521.

2

THE SEARCH FOR DATA AND ITS USES

The first step in any research project is to ask a question or state a hypothesis that defines the objective of the study. As noted in Chapter 1, the objective of the study determines the data needed. Even in very limited descriptive studies, one may have the opportunity to examine or collect data on various aspects of an injury: characteristics and behavior of the persons injured or others at the scene, places of occurrence, circumstances, treatment received, and cost of treatment. Many variables are used to describe each of these, and the number of possible combinations of potentially measurable categories of these factors is very large. Data on an enormous number of cases would be necessary to obtain stable statistics if all the possible combinations of classifications of factors were tabulated. Obviously, a coherent and practical research project requires great care in choice of a research question and study design to answer the question.

Students choosing topics for library research papers or data for a thesis often confront an instructor with a vague statement such as "I am interested in children's injuries." The instructer then must lead the student to narrow the topic to a researchable question given the time and resources available. What age range is considered childhood? Since the activities of children vary by age, are there specific activities in a specific age range that you think might be related to certain types of injury? How severe are those types of injuries? Would they occur in a limited number of settings? What are the energy exposures in those settings that might injure? How is the energy conveyed to the hosts? How many would receive treatment and where? Are you more interested in implications for treatment or in reduction of incidence or severity? What do you think is the most important information needed to improve treatment (or reduce incidence or severity)?

To find out what needs to be known, one must first find out what is known. The best way to choose an original research question is to survey the scientific literature on a topic and note questions that come to mind in reading the literature. Literature reviews should not be confined to a computer search of MED-LINE. Such a search will miss important research in the social and policy sciences on injury control. Important epidemiologic research on topics such as behavioral, social, and cultural factors and violence is often found in the behavioral and social science literature not indexed in MEDLINE. If unanswered questions remain at the end of the literature survey, and they are researchable questions, the choices of potential topics for research are evident.

Before embarking on a research project in injury epidemiology, training in scientific methodology and statistics is essential. If one does not understand scientific principles of measurement and classification of phenomena and the use of statistical methods to describe and analyze the data, the production of a publishable or useful study is very unlikely. Indeed, some of the scientific literature is unintelligible to a reader without such understanding, and some of it is easily seen as invalid, or at least highly questionable, when viewed by the informed reader (Riegelman, 1981).

One way of judging the adequacy of a published literature review is the extent to which it is critical of the research being reviewed. A review that just lists and summarizes studies, without indicating which are the most methodologically sound, is not as useful as a critical review. Another criterion is the dates of the studies covered in the review. If the review's bibliography lists no recent or decades-old studies, the review is likely incomplete. Occasionally researchers new to injury epidemiology reinvent the wheel, sometimes in the shape of an octagon, apparently because of the lack of knowledge of previous studies.

Descriptive studies may be devoted to the identification of all injuries in a population, based on some minimum severity criterion, or may be focused on place of occurrence (e.g., roads), particular types of disability (e.g., spinal cord), a subset of the population (e.g., children), injuries associated with a given activity (e.g., swimming), or any number of other categories.

Decisions about what data are needed can be greatly facilitated by thinking at the outset how the data are to be used. Which of the objectives noted in Chapter 1 is a general objective of the study? How can that objective be refined into specific aims? What specific statistical distributions of what variables are needed to reach decisions based on the conclusions? Actually constructing statistical tables that one intends to fill with data will force the identification of variables that must be measured, reveal definitional problems, and identify relevant categorizations.

FINDING USABLE DATA

Often one does not have the resources to collect original data and must find a data set that includes the variables and categories needed to answer a particular question. Many of the classification schemes used by organizations devoted to the compilation of injury statistics were developed before the application of epidemiologic concepts and scientific principles. This does not mean that all of them are useless, but the uses to which the data are put are sometimes illogical and counterproductive to injury control, at least partly due to the classifications.

As noted in Chapter 1, injury classifications are often a mixture of vehicle, host, or circumstantial characteristics. For example, the National Safety Council has for decades attempted to assemble data on "accidents" as well as injuries and has reported its estimates in *Accident Facts,* an annual publication. The broad categories used include work, motor vehicle, public, home, farm, and school. These categories are inconsistent with one of the fundamental principles of classification: classes should be mutually exclusive; that is, a case should be classifiable in one and only one category.

Most farmers would consider their occupational activities as work, and increasing numbers of persons in nonfarm occupations work at home. Some people are injured in or by motor vehicles while engaged in their occupations. The National Safety Council is not alone in use of categories that are not mutually exclusive. In the National Health Interview Survey, conducted by the National Center for Health Statistics, similar categories are used, although in both systems the motor vehicle cases that occur while working or in the home driveway are classed systematically as motor vehicle rather than work or home (National Center for Health Statistics, 1986).

Such categorization problems, along with differences in data sources, can produce remarkable differences in estimates of numbers of injuries, or even deaths, the most easily countable injuries. Total numbers of deaths from injury are probably counted with reasonable accuracy (excepting some electrocutions classified as heart attacks, pneumonia in the elderly, bedridden because of a fall, etc.).

The National Safety Council estimated 11,700 deaths from injury in 1984 compared to 3740 counted by the Bureau of Labor Statistics (BLS) in its annual survey of businesses. Some of this difference arises from the fact that certain small businesses and farms were excluded from the BLS survey, but that cannot possibly account for such a large difference in the estimates (Panel on Occupational Safety and Health Statistics, 1987). In India, the national railway reported 1000 railway-related fatalities compared to more than 10,000 estimated from police reports. The railway reports only cases where a railway employee or equipment was judged at fault (Berger & Mohan, 1996). Obviously, the researcher must be aware of who is doing the counting and the definitions used.

A second principle of classification is that the classes be exhaustive, that is, there should be a category for every case. Again looking at the National Safety Council categories, where would one classify an injury to a child playing touch football in the field of a neighbor's farm? It would be misleading to call it a farm injury, and it didn't happen anywhere in or near the child's or neighbor's home, at school, or in a public place.

Usually the most useful injury categories are those that are relatively homogeneous as to energy source and vehicle or vector of the energy. For example, if one is interested in burns, the place of injury—home, school, restaurant, hotel—may or may not be important. The same energy source may be the major culprit at each of these sites. Burns from heated liquids spilled from unstable cups or other containers may occur in all of these places. To control the damage, knowledge of the extent to which the burns and other injuries (e.g., lung damage from smoke) occur from fires (specified by ignition source and material ignited), tap water, hot drinks spilled from specific types of containers, space heaters by specific types, and so on, is the information that is the most useful (McLoughlin & Crawford, 1985).

The point here is not to censure organizations that employ scientifically inadequate or nonuseful categories. The point is to avoid using categories that are not mutually exclusive, exhaustive, and meaningful relative to the uses to which the data might be put. Injury researchers choose their projects for all sorts of reasons—personal experience with or concern about a particular type of injury, intellectual curiosity, or the need to identify a problem that will attract grant support perhaps being the most common. Whatever the motivation, consideration of the usefulness of the data to be collected would perhaps accelerate the use of categories that enhance the linkage between injury epidemiology and injury control. The definition of what constitutes a case and precision and accuracy of severity measurements are crucial.

CASE FINDING

Once one has decided the set of injuries that are to be investigated and meaningful categories to describe them, a means of finding cases must be identified and implemented. Various people and organizations, public and private, are potential sources for case identification and data on particular sets of injuries—the person injured and witnesses, private physicians and clinics, police, emergency medical responders, hospital emergency rooms, hospital inpatient personnel, rehabilitation facilities, medical examiners, and coroners. Each data source has biases that must be understood and made explicit to avoid misinterpretation of the data.

Figure 2.1 presents the paths through which the vast majority of injury cases flow. Once an individual is exposed to energy sufficient to cause pain or perceptible tissue damage, that person or someone in proximity makes a decision whether to seek medical or other help. Most cases are relatively trivial cuts and bruises and are self-treated or ignored. The person who seeks help may go directly to a private physician or, if police or emergency medical personnel are called, the person may be examined and released or taken to a private physician, hospital emergency room, or the morgue. If admitted to a hospital, the injured person may subsequently be released or sent to another hospital, a rehabilition facility, or, in case of death, to the morgue.

Each of the arrows in Figure 2.1 is a potential path that has a probability of occurrence that is related to several factors, including the circumstances of the injury and its severity. A person may not seek help because of embarrassment, threat from an assailant, knowledge of how to treat an injury, inability to pay for services, geographic remoteness from services, or attitudes regarding the services available. Private physicians and clinics, police, emergency personnel, and hospitals usually have protocols for handling or referring cases, but these are not always followed.

The flow of cases suggests various points at which data may be obtained. An epidemiologist may survey a sample of the population about injuries experienced or may use the records of private physicians, emergency medical services, police, hospitals, rehabilitation facilities, and coroners or medical exam-

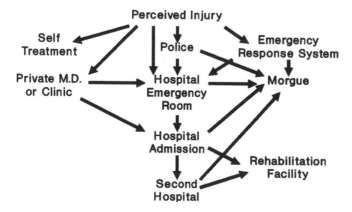

FIGURE 2.1. Flow of injury cases.

iners. Each data source has potential biases that must be considered in using the data. The use of combined data sources sometimes allows an estimate of cases missing from any one and also provides data on several aspects of injury that no one source provides. Since the same injured person may have contact with more than one data source or more than one contact with the same data source, care must be taken not to count the same injury more than once.

The only way to obtain data on injuries that are not brought to medical or official attention is to contact people and question them about injury experience. Such surveys are rife with potential for bias arising from unreliable memory, embarrassment regarding certain types of injury, and differences among people in perceptions of seriousness. The National Health Interview Survey, conducted by the National Center for Health Statistics, includes a few questions about injuries in its ongoing random sample survey of the population. To be included, an injury must have received medical attention or required a day of restricted activity. In one such survey, the rate of these self-reported injuries per population among persons 65 years and older was 19 per 100 compared to 38 per 100 of those less than 45 years old (National Center for Health Statistics, 1986). The elderly may have that many fewer injuries, or their rate could be biased by memory failure or other factors.

A general population survey is an inefficient way to identify severe injuries. The sample size would have to be huge to include significant numbers of deaths or permanently impairing spinal cord or head injuries.

The method of collecting data as well as the perception by the respondent of the persons or organizations soliciting the data may also affect the probability of the respondent's reporting an injury. For example, an annual survey of cervical spine injuries to high school football players was conducted by mailed questionnaire to high school principals and team trainers to identify cases. On the basis of identified cases, the researchers claim that a decline in such injuries occurred from warnings to coaches about teaching players to use the head in blocking and tackling (Torg et al., 1985). These data are inadequate because only a small percentage of the questionnaires are returned and the respondents may withhold information because the researchers were previously active in issuing the warnings about head blocking and tackling. Some respondents may be reluctant to report injuries in which they may perceive themselves or members of their staffs as partially culpable. The researchers have also used newspaper clipping services to identify cases, but these were obtained from a limited and nonrepresentative sample of newspapers. No comparison of cases reported in newspapers to those reported by school officials in the same communities has been reported.

One way of estimating completeness of injury reporting in interviews is to interview more than one person with probable knowledge of the injury. In a study of injuries to football players in Pop Warner leagues, coaches were asked to report injuries that required restricted participation for more than one week. At the end of the season, two players and two coaches, randomly selected from each team, were interviewed and asked to provide the names of anyone on the team who had such an injury. Of the total injuries identified, the coaches were the best source (82 percent of injuries reported), but an additional 18 percent were reported by the other respondents that would not have been found by sole reliance on coaches (Goldberg et al., 1988).

Reporting biases have also been found in official records. A substantial underreporting has been found comparing police reports of certain motor vehicle injuries and hospital records. In the United States, state governments require that motor vehicle injuries be reported to police. Yet in 45 percent of emergency room cases of motor vehicle injuries in five northeastern Ohio counties, no police report could be found (Barancik & Fife, 1985). The cases lost by relying on police records may be even larger in low-income countries, particularly in remote areas where police presence is minimal (Berger & Mohan, 1996).

Furthermore, in Ohio the lack of police reports was correlated with other factors. Police reports were missing for two-thirds to three-quarters of patients less than 16 years old, those who were passengers of vehicles other than passenger cars, and Medicaid recipients.

Medical records, augmented by death certificates and coroner or medical examiner records of the fatally injured, are the best sources for case identification for most studies (e.g., Kraus et al., 1975, 1984). Although many such records do not contain data on the circumstances of injury and other variables (to be discussed in Chapter 3), they usually provide information on characteristics of the injury and its severity. If the injury can be disabling, the disability may not be recorded in the data from acute care hospitals. For example, some cases of spinal cord injury not identified in acute care records in one surveillance system were found in records of rehabilitation facilities (Thurman et al., 1994).

Once the case has been identified, other data can be obtained by matching to other records, if available, or by contacting the person injured or witnesses to the incident. Injuries that were not brought to medical attention will not be included, but as noted in the next section, the more severe injuries that are the primary targets for injury control are unlikely to be excluded.

SEVERITY OF INJURY

The specification of injury severity is an essential element of the use of injury epidemiology for injury control. In any given year, virtually everyone experiences minor injuries, such as small scratches, bruises, and burns. Most of these heal with little or no treatment and do not interfere with one's activities. The energy sources, vehicles and vectors, and other circumstances of injuries, are often not the same for those that are relatively severe and those with trivial consequences (Chapter 1). Since trivial injuries are so common, priority in the devotion of resources to control of injuries based on total numbers in a given category can result in substantial misallocation of resources with respect to reducing the cost of injuries and the improvement of the quality of life of the severely injured or their families.

The measurement of injury severity is based on numerous clinical signs and symptoms such as respiration rate, consciousness, blood pressure, heart rate, number and types of organ and system damage (area and depths of burn, ruptured spleen, site-specified severance of the spinal cord, etc.). Researchers are engaged in attempts to develop summary scores of these factors that are meaningful in terms of decisions related to severity reduction, acute care, and rehabilitation. Several competing scoring systems have been developed and no single one is likely to emerge that would be acceptable to everyone for the variety of potential uses.

Severity scores are used in acute and follow-up medical care to triage patients (decide where and by whom patients should be treated), to plan for the different levels of care needed according to severity distributions, and to evaluate the effectiveness of treatment. Epidemiologists use severity scores to establish minimal criteria for surveillance of injury, to measure the effects of energy and other factors on injury severity (including the effects of attempts at injury control), and to estimate injury effects on mortality, disability, and costs (Baker, 1983).

The elements of one severity scoring system, the Trauma Score, are shown in Table 2.1 (Champion et al., 1981). The signs and symptoms in this system are widely used by emergency medical personnel for triage and by emergency care physicians for initial evaluation of patients, such that records for use in research are often available. The originators of the score have revised it and the version in Table 2.1 is used in research (Champion et al., 1989).

Examples from another severity rating system, the Abbreviated Injury Scale (AIS), are shown in Table 2.2. It is based on a dictionary constructed from expert judgment of the severity of particular injuries (Committee on Injury Scaling, 1980). The AIS is seldom used for triage, but it is used in epidemiologic studies as well as in the evaluation of medical care outcomes and costs. The scoring procedure has been simplified into a standardized instrument that can be used in case abstraction from medical records (Barancik & Chatterjee, 1981). Also, comparison of AIS scores from hospital record reviews and those obtained using a computer program to compute AIS scores from computerized hospital discharge records found agreement in 48 to 75 percent of cases depending on the type of injury (MacKenzie, 1997; MacKenzie et al., 1989).

A derivative of the Abbreviated Injury Scale is the Injury Severity Score

TABLE 2.1. The Revised Trauma Score

COMPONENT	RATE	POINTS	SCORE
A. Respiratory rate (RR): number in 15 seconds times 4	10–29	4	
	>29	3	
	6–9	2	
	1–5	1	
	0	0	A. _____
B. Systolic blood pressure (SBP): cuff pressure, either arm— auscultate or palpate	>89	4	
	76–89	3	
	50–75	2	
	1–49	1	
	0	0	B. _____
C. Glasgow Coma Scale (GCS)			
1. Eye opening	Total		
Spontaneous 4	GCS		
To voice 3	points		
To pain 2	13–15	5	
None 1	9–12	4	
2. Verbal response	6–8	3	
Oriented 5	4–5	2	
Confused 4	3	1	C. _____
Inappropriate words 3			
Incomprehensible words 2			
None 1			
3. Motor response			
Obeys commands 6			
Purposeful movement (pain) 5			
Withdrawal (pain) 4			
Flexion (pain) 3			
Extension (pain) 2			
None 1			

Total GCS points $(1+2+3)$ _____

$$\text{Score} = -3.5718 + 0.9368(C) + 0.7326(B) + 0.2908(A)$$

Sources: Champion et al., 1981, 1989.

TABLE 2.2. The Abbreviated Injury Scale—Examples

CODE	DESCRIPTOR	EXAMPLES
0	No injury	
1	Minor	Superficial abrasion or laceration of skin; digit sprain; first-degree burn; head trauma with headache or dizziness but no other neurological signs
2	Moderate	Major abrasion or laceration of skin; unconscious <15 minutes; finger or toe crush/amputation; closed pelvic fracture
3	Serious	Major nerve laceration; multiple rib fracture without flail chest; abdominal organ contusion; hand, foot, or arm crush/amputation
4	Severe	Ruptured spleen; leg crush; chest wall perforation; unconscious <24 hours
5	Critical	Spinal cord transection; extensive/deep laceration of kidney or liver; extensive second- or third-degree burns; unconscious 24+ hours
6	Unsurvivable	Decapitation; torso transection

The Injury Severity Score (ISS) is the sum of the squared AIS in the three most severely injured parts of the anatomy.

Source: Hartunian et al., 1981.

(ISS), the sum of the squared AIS in each of the three most severely injured of seven defined regions of the anatomy. These regions are head, neck, thorax, abdomen and pelvic contents, spine, extremities and bony pelvis, and external skin and muscles. The ISS was developed by researchers concerned with refining the prediction of injury outcome, particularly in the case of multiple trauma (Baker et al., 1974). They noted that the probability of survival in a series of hospitalized trauma patients increased exponentially as a function of the AIS score of the most severe injury. Cross-tabulation of the three most severe injuries in different areas of the anatomy indicated that the square of these AIS scores was a strong predictor of probability of survival.

These scoring systems are attempts to quantify a mixture of quantitative and qualitative elements of the extent of injury. Notice that the quantitative elements of the Trauma Score such as respiration rate and blood pressure are given a low (adverse) score when higher or lower than normal. Although each of these measurements could be used quantitatively without categorization in segments, mathematical modeling of them in combination to obtain a useful score would be very complex and difficult to use in emergency situations without a specially designed calculator with the logic built into it.

An index combining the Trauma Score and the Injury Severity Score, as well as patient age, has been developed using logistic regression, with probability of survival as the outcome (Boyd et al., 1987). Logistic regression is a technique that

assigns weights to different factors regarding their relative power to predict probability of a discrete outcome such as death versus survival (e.g., Selvin, 1991).
Cases in which the patient dies despite a high probability of survival or survives
despite a low probability of survival are suggested as worthy of peer review by the
American College of Surgeons (Committee on Trauma of the American College
of Surgeons, 1987). The validity of this approach has been verified for children's
injuries as well (Kaufmann et al., 1991). Modifications of the measurements improve prediction of death from penetrating injuries (Champion et al., 1990).

Since the ISS leaves out some injuries, a system called the Anatomic Profile
(AP) was developed to summarize the AIS of all injuries. A committee of clinical
experts defined sets of injuries to comprise components of a score (Table 2.3). The
square root of the sum of the squares of the AIS of each injury in each component
was related to probability of survival and the weights in the equation at the bottom
of Table 2.3 were obtained by logistic regression. The D component (nonserious

TABLE 2.3. Injury Assignments to Anatomic Profile Components

COMPONENT	INJURY	AIS SEVERITY	ISS BODY REGIONS	ICD-9-CM CODES
A	Head/brain	3–5	1	800, 801, 803, 850-854
	Spinal cord	3–5	1,3,4	806, 950, 952, 953
B	Thoracic	3–5	3	807, 839.61/.71, 860-862, 901
	Neck front	3–5	1	807.5/.6, 874, 900
C	Abdomen/pelvis	3–5	4	863–868, 902
	Spine w/o cord	3	1,3,4	805, 839
	Pelvic fracture	4–5	5	808, 839.42/.52/.69/.79
	Femoral artery	4–5	4–5	904.0/.1
	Crush above knee	4–5	4–5	928.00/.01, 928.8
	Amputation above knee	4–5	5	897.2/.3/.6/.7
	Popliteal artery	4	5	904.41
D	Face	1–4	2	802, 830
	All others	1–2	1–6	Other than above

Score $= 4.0801 - 0.4914(A) - 0.2066(B) - 0.0161 (B^2) - 0.0351 (C^2)$
where A, B, or C is, in each case, the square root of the sum of the squares of the AIS
of the injuries in the component.

Source: Copes, et al., 1990.

ICD-9-CM Codes are the diagnosis (N) codes discussed in Chapter 1 (Health Care Financing Administration, 1980).

injuries) was dropped because it did not explain any additional variation in survival. Comparison of the AP scores and ISS scores indicated an improvement in the prediction of survival by using the AP (Copes et al., 1990).

Physicians who treat trauma in children have been critical of the use of indices based on measurement of trauma and outcomes for adult patients. A Pediatric Trauma Score, the elements of which are shown in Table 2.4, has been shown to have excellent correlation to the probability of survival of traumatized children (Tepas, 1989).

The AIS, ISS, and AP are indices of trauma mainly from mechanical energy. One interesting question is the feasibility and usefulness of scoring that would include heat, electrical or chemical injuries, and asphyxiations. Mortality from burns is an exponential function of surface area burned and age of the patient (Rutowski et al., 1976). Comparison of the predictability of the Trauma Score or Pediatric Trauma Score, as currently used, and statistically adjusting the weights of components, in studies of mortality and disability from burns, electricity, poisonings, and asphyxiations would be a useful research project. Since survival from both mechanical and thermal energy insults to human tissue are exponential functions of the injury severity to areas of the organism, there may be common biological processes at work that could be identified and targeted in treatment.

Study of nonfatal outcomes in relation to injury severity scoring has been limited. Length of hospital stays and disability from motor vehicle injuries are substantially predicted by the Injury Severity Score (Bull, 1975), but other scoring systems might improve predictability. It has been noted, for example, that a lesion to the eye that would be minor in another body area can cause blindness (Jorgensen, 1981), and that head and spinal cord injuries with low AIS scores can result in substantial impairment (Conboy et al., 1986; MacKenzie et al., 1986).

TABLE 2.4. Pediatric Trauma Score

| | POINTS | | |
COMPONENT	+2	+1	−1
Size	>20 kg	10–20 kg	<10 kg
Airway	Normal	Maintainable	Unmaintainable
Systolic blood pressure	>90 mm Hg	50–90 mm Hg	<50 mm Hg
Central nervous system	Awake	Obtunded/loss of consciousness	Coma/decerebrate
Open wound	None	Minor	Major/penetrating
Skeletal	None	Closed fracture	Open/multiple fracture

The score is the sum of the points for each component.
Source: Tepas, 1989.

The severity and persistence of disabling impairments from injury have not been extensively investigated. The National Health Interview Survey periodically notes prevalence (the proportion of the population with a condition at a given point in time) of certain impairments—vision, hearing, speech, absence and deformities of extremities, and paralysis—and percentage that occurred in the year of the survey (National Center for Health Statistics, 1986). However, the severity and prognosis of these impairments would require more detailed data.

Special studies of certain types of long-term disability have indicated the substantial excess of particular circumstances for certain types of injury. For example, the Utah Health Department's 1989–91 surveillance of spinal cord injury found that 65 percent of nonfatal spinal injuries to vehicle occupants occurred in rollovers (Thurman et al., 1995), about twice what would be expected from the proportion of occupant deaths occurring in rollovers.

Attempts have been made to develop impairment and disability scales analogous to the Abbreviated Injury Scale (MacKenzie et al., 1996; States & Viano, 1990). Those engaged in this activity adopted a seven point scale, like the AIS, despite the fact that they couldn't identify seven points on some dimensions. One effort includes several dimensions of impairment (mobility/dexterity, cognitive/psychological, cosmetic/disfigurement, sensory, pain, sexual/reproductive) and disability (employment, daily living, life expectancy), including severity and duration (States & Viano, 1990). The descriptors of these scores are presented in Table 2.5. As was the case with the Trauma Score and the Abbreviated Injury Scale, the categories were formed based on clinical experience, but they must be studied in terms of reliability and validity and revised accordingly before widespread use.

Reliability (sometimes called precision) refers to the repeatability of a measurement. For example, do different people interviewing the same patient or reviewing the same medical record produce the same score? *Validity* (sometimes called accuracy) refers to whether the dimension that one is attempting to measure is actually being measured. Reliability of data is often easily assessed by comparing independent recording of the data, but the determination of validity is much more difficult. If a scale is to measure injury severity relevant to survival, and it is strongly predictive of survival, it satisfies a major criterion for validity. A major validity test of an impairment scale is the extent to which it predicts degree and permanance of disability.

One problem evident in the proposed impairment and disability scales (Table 2.5) is the presence of the same or similar criteria in both scales. Notice that ability to perform tasks such as typing, hand tool use, and work are included in the mobility/dexterity and pain impairment scales; self-support, which may require these activities, is in the disability scale. Similarly, "usually requires institutional care" is in the cognitive/psychological impairment scale and "insti-

TABLE 2.5. Proposed Impairment and Disability Scales

Mobility/dexterity impairment

1. *Minor.* Mobility or dexterity is detectably impaired but functional ability is intact; i.e., minor limp due to knee with degenerative arthritis, mild tremor, limitation of motion in some but not all digits, thumb normal, detectable weakness in hands.

2. *Moderate.* Walking distance is limited to less than $\frac{1}{4}$ mile. Uses cane occasionally. Can use stairs; difficulty in balance. Hands weak, or usefulness impaired by tremor or spasticity. Typing and driving difficult.

3. *Serious.* Cane, crutches, prosthesis, and/or walker is necessary for walking except in dwelling. Stairs are difficult, railing essential. Motor deficit of hands or extremities. Cannot type or use hand tools. Unilateral hand amputee.

4. *Severe.* Wheelchair is used by choice, but patient can stand and walk with apparatus; i.e., crutches or walker. Severe motor weakness, incoordination or spasticity, self-feeding slow or uncertain.

5. *Very severe.* Wheelchair is required for ambulation although patient can stand and walk short distances with assistance. Virtually complete motor paralysis. Virtually no hand function. Bilateral hand amputee.

6. *Totally immobile and dependent.* Hoist is required for transfer; patient cannot stand, requires aide for activities of daily living. Has no useful function in upper extremities.

Cognitive/psychological impairment

1. *Minor.* Mild inappropriate behavior; occasional errors in language and arithmetic.

2. *Moderate.* Noticeable memory loss, difficulties with simple arithmetic, difficulty in self-expression, infrequent disorientation and dizziness. Mild mental retardation.

3. *Serious.* Occasional disorientation, significant memory loss or language impairment, and occasional signs of psychosis. Moderate mental retardation.

4. *Severe.* No memory for recent events; disoriented, psychotic, requires sheltered home, speech unintelligible. Severe mental retardation.

5. *Very severe.* No memory, total loss of speech, psychotic, usually requires institutional care. Profound mental retardation.

6. *Coma.* Vegetative, no purposeful response to stimuli, brain dead.

Cosmetic/disfigurement impairment

1. *Minor.* Normally covered, amenable to cosmetic makeup, readily covered orthosis.

2. *Moderate.* Can be covered by cosmetics and/or forces change in dress, may require orthesis but not prosthesis.

3. *Serious.* Prothesis or cover-up required.

4. *Severe.* Readily observable, not amenable to cosmetic, prosthetic, or clothing cover-up.

Sensory impairment

	VISION	HEARING	SENSATION	TASTE AND SMELL
1. *Minor.*	Minor loss but does not interfere with usual activities, correctable with readily available aids such as glasses or hearing aids.			
2. *Moderate.*	Correctable to 20/100 in best eye.	Hearing loss not fully correctable.	26% to 50% loss to special senses or limbs.	Complete loss of taste or smell.

(continued)

TABLE 2.5. Continued

	VISION	HEARING	SENSATION	TASTE AND SMELL
3. *Serious.*	Complete loss of vision in one eye, partial in other eye.	Total hearing loss.	Greater than 50% loss.	Complete loss of both taste smell.
4. *Severe.*	Total vision loss.			

Pain impairment

1. *Minor.* Occasional pain, analgesics not required or used, no interference with sleep.

2. *Moderate.* Occasional pain, more frequent or occasional use of nonnarcotic analgesics.

3. *Serious.* Constant or occasional severe pain, nonnarcotic analgesics required for sleep, work. Narcotic analgesics occasionally required.

4. *Severe.* Constant or severe occasional pain requiring narcotics or invasive therapy. Sleep poor, unable to work. Recreation and socialization severely limited.

5. *Very severe.* Constant or severe pain requiring narcotics or invasive therapy. Sleep poor, unable to work. No recreation or socialization.

6. *Uniformly causes total impairment.* Constant and/or occasional pain uncontrolled except with large doses of narcotics, which affect the central nervous system. Incomplete control with invasive therapy.

Sexual/reproduction impairment

1. *Minor.* Decreases frequency of intercourse because of occasional pain or decreased libido.

2. *Moderate.* Inability to have satisfactory erection, loss of libido. Pain with intercourse. Reduced fecundity.

3. *Serious.* Complete loss of capability for an erection, loss of libido. Pain precluding intercourse. Complete absence of fecundity.

Disability scale

0. *No disability.* Self-support (full-time work and full recreational activity compatible with patient's age).

1. *Minor.* Self-support with reduced recreational activity.

2. *Moderate.* Self-support with no recreational activity.

3. *Serious.* Independent living (limited or no assistance with activities of daily living), may be capable of part-time work.

4. *Severe.* Living at home but with assistance of aide less than four hours per day and/ or assistance with shopping, meal preparation, and medications.

5. *Very severe.* Full care at home with aide more than four hours per day or institutional care but with ability to perform some activities of daily living.

6. *Extreme.* Institutional care with external life-support systems such as mechanical respiratory assistance or tube feeding.

Source: States and Viano, 1990.

tutional care" is included in the disability scale. Thus the scales are not independently determined and will by definition be correlated. Also, the disability scale does not have exhaustive categories; in the "extreme" group, persons may be institutionalized who do not require life support systems or tube feeding.

These scales need revision before being studied empirically, as recognized by the proponents who suggested that they be examined by expert consensus panels (States & Viano, 1990). Field tests to assess potential problems and establish weights for the effects of impairment on disability are also recommended before use in a full-scale research project. One obviously shouldn't just add up scales that may not be additive in effect, and double counting of particular elements should be eliminated.

The Functional Capacity Index (FCI) is a somewhat simpler attempt to measure limitations of normal function and has been subjected to limited field testing. Also designed to mirror the AIS, it has three to seven levels of indication of ability to perform ten activities: eating, excreting, sex, ambulation, use of hands and arms, bending/lifting, seeing, hearing, talking, and thinking. To assess interrater reliability, weights were assigned by raters from convenience samples of experts and white- and blue-collar workers. Although raters assigned similar weights within dimensions, clinical experts tended to underestimate the importance of various activities relative to the other raters. There was also large variation in intrarater reliability among some scales when the ratings were repeated after a two week period (MacKenzie et al., 1996).

Studies of disability in activities of daily living among the elderly indicate a hierarchy of factors (Dunlop et al., 1997). One type of scale worth investigating is a scale where a number indicates a cumulative effect (Guttman, 1946). For example, if the data so indicated, a 1 would indicate "cannot walk," a 2 would indicate "cannot walk" and "cannot transfer from chair to bed," and so on.

The researcher should not adopt any injury or disability scoring system without careful consideration of what is being measured relative to the hypotheses and possible uses of the research. The injury severity scales mainly indicate probability of death and are not very useful as measures of probability of impairments and disabilities among those who survive (MacKenzie et al., 1996). Some disability measures may be distorted because they are related to eligibility for insurance or government benefits (Aarts & DeJong, 1992; Bloch, 1982).

The extent to which a particular limitation is disabling depends on an individual's desires for specific activities and the environment in which they are pursued. There are three stages prior to disability that offer the opportunity for prevention: *(1)* pathology (e.g., traumatic denervation of an arm), *(2)* impairment (e.g., atrophy of muscle), and *(3)* functional limitation (no pulling strength). The effect on the persons's life depends on the extent that pulling strength is necessary for work, recreation, and the like (Pope & Tarlov, 1991).

INJURY DISTRIBUTIONS

The first step in describing injuries statistically is to count the numbers in the categories or on the scale of interest, called a *distribution*. For example, injury severity has been described as distributed in the shape of a pyramid with deaths at the top, hospitalizations in the middle, and others at the base (Guyer & Gallagher, 1985). More refined categories of injuries by type and severity scales, however, are not pyramid-shaped by severity. For example, there are substantially more deaths from motor vehicles than nonfatal, critical (AIS-5) injuries. Drownings and near drownings tend to result in death or a much lower number of severely brain damaged and impairment cases from oxygen deficits, or persons survive without injury.

Among the most commonly reported distributions of injury is by age. While an age distribution of injuries of a given type may be of use in targeting age groups for prevention, another important way of looking at age of the fatally injured is by years of potential life lost. This is calculated by multiplying the number of deaths at a given age times the years that persons of that age would be expected to live (from a life table) and summing the total number of years lost. The calculations for the "leading causes of deaths"—cardiovascular diseases, cancers, and injuries—are presented in Table 2.6 for the United States in 1991. Cardiovascular disease deaths are more than six times injury deaths but less than twice injuries in years of life lost before age 85. Some researchers subtract age of death from 65 to obtain "productive years of life lost," but that practice implies that the only value of life is economic. The years lost prior to age 65 from injury (5.1 million in 1991) exceeded those lost from cardiovascular diseases (4.0 million) or cancers (4.3 million). Cardiovascular diseases and cancers mainly kill the elderly, whereas injuries mainly kill the young.

Such comparison of potential years of life lost has resulted in more attention to injuries but is seldom used in detailed research. Potential years of life lost by type of injury would also be suggestive of the importance of concentrating on certain types of injury that take more years than the total numbers of fatal injuries in a given category would indicate.

INJURY RATES

Injuries are often reported as rates per population, or some other denominator such as per miles driven for motor vehicle injuries or per hours flown for injuries in aircraft. The population rate is calculated by dividing the number of people injured by the number of people in the population:

$$\text{Rate} = \frac{\text{Number of injuries in a year in the population}}{\text{Number of people in the population}}$$

TABLE 2.6. Deaths and Years of Potential Life Lost from Cardiovascular Diseases, Cancer, and Injuries—United States, 1991

AGE	MEDIAN YEARS EXPECTED	DEATHS			YEARS OF LIFE LOST		
		CARDIO-VASCULAR	CANCERS	INJURY	CARDIO-VASCULAR	CANCERS	INJURY
0–4	74.5	1,278	603	4,434	95,211	44,924	330,333
5–9	69.6	168	580	1,878	11,693	40,368	130,709
10–14	64.6	216	526	2,567	13,954	33,980	165,828
15–19	59.8	466	741	12,199	27,867	44,312	729,500
20–24	55.1	820	1,073	15,989	45,182	59,122	880,994
25–29	50.4	1,547	1,806	14,573	77,969	91,022	734,479
30–34	45.7	2,971	3,511	13,886	135,775	160,453	634,590
35–39	41.0	5,561	6,223	12,130	228,001	255,143	497,330
40–44	36.5	10,018	10,686	9,960	365,657	390,039	363,540
45–49	32.0	15,106	16,013	7,478	483,392	512,416	239,296
50–54	27.6	21,366	23,909	5,754	589,702	659,888	158,510
55–59	23.5	33,423	36,901	5,316	785,441	867,174	124,926
60–64	19.7	55,410	57,294	5,637	1,091,577	1,128,692	111,049
65–69	16.1	84,047	76,507	4,286	1,353,157	1,231,763	69,005
70–74	12.9	112,291	82,806	6,058	1,448,554	1,068,197	78,148
75–79	10.0	139,677	78,439	6,610	1,396,770	784,390	66,100
80–84	7.5	155,560	60,962	6,396	1,166,700	457,215	47,970
85+		276,291	56,054	9,052			
Total		916,218	514,636	144,203	9,316,602	7,829,098	5,362,307

Source: National Center for Health Statistics, 1995, 1996.

This rate is usually multiplied by 100,000 to get the rate per 100,000 population, or by 10,000 or 1000 if the injuries of interest occur in larger numbers.

To be accurate, the people injured in the numerator must have come from the population in the denominator and both must be counted accurately. Most such calculations are approximations based on estimates of the population from the census or some other source. Some of the injured during the year, or whatever time period chosen, may be visitors from outside the population and some of the population may have been outside the area all or part of the year.

These potential biases may not be important in total population estimates when the visitors' injuries or the numbers of the population that are outside the area are small relative to the total numbers involved. Estimates of injury rates per population for smaller areas such as cities, counties, or even states may be substantially affected by seasonal influxes of tourists or students, roads carrying large amounts of nonlocal traffic, and the like.

The basic principle in calculating population rates is that cases in the numerator should only come from the population in the denominator. This is a major

problem in hospital trauma registries where the population from which the injuries come is often difficult or impossible to define (Waller, 1988). To calculate
rates for segments of the population, or using some other denominator such as
miles driven in the case of motor vehicle injuries, one must be able to place
cases in the numerator and denominator into the same mutually exclusive and
exhaustive categories. For example, if the injury cases are classified by age as
0–4, 5–9, 10–14, and so on, and the population data are classified by age as 0–
3, 3–6, 7–10, the rates for each age group cannot be calculated without reclassi-
fying one or the other.

Use of denominators other than population is an attempt to obtain a more
refined estimate of rate per exposure. For example, the Federal Aviation Administration reports injuries in aircraft crashes per hours flown. Obviously a person
who doesn't travel in airplanes will not crash in one, although occasionally
people on the ground are injured by crashing aircraft. Aircraft usually crash
during attempts to take off or land. In the same make and model of airplane, a
person who flies the same number of hours over shorter distances is at greater
risk per hour flown than when flying the same number of hours over longer
distances. Therefore, rate per hours flown can be a misleading indicator of risk.

Hours of exposure becomes even more problematic when considering numerous activities. For example, drownings of young children often occur in home
swimming pools. How does one estimate hours of exposure of young children
to home swimming pools? Hours in or by the pool are inadequate because
many wander into the pool from the house or yard at times when use of the
pool is unintended by their adult supervisors. Some wander into a neighbor's
pool. Do we count the number of hours the children are awake? Do we multiply
the number of hours awake times the number of pools in the neighborhood?
What constitutes the neighborhood in defining the likelihood of home pool exposure?

Trends in rates of motor vehicle fatalities are sometimes based on total
deaths per million total miles driven, the latter based on self-reports, periodic
odometer monitoring, road use surveys, or sales of fuel. The deaths per mile
are often decreasing even in periods when the population rate is steady or increasing. This occurs, for example, when use of vehicles in urban areas is increasing faster than use in rural areas. In urban areas, the speed limits are lower
and congestion of traffic during the misnamed "rush hours" also reduces
speeds, thus lowering the energy exchange in crashes. Crashes in urban areas
are more frequent per mile but they are less severe, and vehicle occupant death
rates are lower than in rural areas.

An auto industry analysis of occupant fatalities in cars and light trucks by
hour of day and day of week noted that 32 percent of such fatalities occurred
between 11:00 p.m. and 5:00 a.m., although diaries of personal vehicle use
indicate that only 4.5 percent of total mileage was accumulated during those

hours (Schwing & Kamerud, 1988). Unfortunately, the authors went on to speculate about "risk-taking behavior," which they did not measure, as the explanation. It is difficult to believe that behavior during those hours is so radically different from behavior during the remainder of the day. As will be further noted in Chapter 3, lighting roads at sites where severe crashes clustered at night virtually eliminated the problem, which suggests that visibility at night may explain a substantial proportion of the diurnal variation in fatalities per mile. Nevertheless, the point that using mileage as exposure does not necessarily indicate quality of exposure is a valid one.

When considering separately other road users struck by motor vehicles, such as pedestrians and bicyclists, rates per mile of motor vehicle use in urban areas are higher than in rural areas. This is probably because more people walk or use bicycles in urban areas, but miles walked or bicycled are difficult to estimate accurately and are rarely used.

The point here is that there is no absolutely right or wrong measure of exposure. The choice should be justified by the issue to be researched and what can be learned about injury reduction from the results. The use of one or another measure of exposure has various implications for interpretation that may not be obvious.

RELEVANCE AND IRRELEVANCE OF RATES

One focus in the collection of data on incidence, severity, and other aspects of injury is to quantify the risk of the injury in question. *Risk* is the probability that the injury, or a specific level of severity, will occur in use of a given product or participation in a given activity. Risk is an estimate of what will happen in the future, whereas *rate* is an indication of relative frequency in the past. Risk is usually derivable from rates based on the assumption that the previous relative frequency will continue, adjusted for the deaths that eliminate future participation (Kelsey et al., 1986), but interpretation is sometimes difficult depending on how accurately the denominator reflects quality of exposure. For very rare events, such as meltdowns at nuclear power plants, estimates of risk are based on probability of various combinations of failures in the technology rather than the previous frequency (Gould et al., 1988).

The scientist who calculates injury rates using whatever denominators should be aware of poor methodology and tricky interpretations that have been applied to the data. Particularly in regulatory and product liability forums, the word risk is often preceded by adjectives such as "reasonable" or "acceptable." From a technical standpoint, an injury rate is the occurrence per specified unit of exposure and merely reflects the occurrence per exposure during the specified period of time. Standing alone, the rate does not indicate anything about whether it was reducible by the manufacturer of an involved product (short of not manufacturing the product) or by the user of the product.

The risk of a product is the expected number of injuries per product during its use. If a given make and model of motor vehicle has an occupant death rate of 20 per 100,000 vehicles per year and it will be in use an average of 10 years per vehicle, its occupant fatality risk is $(10 \times 20)/100,000$, or 0.002 or, stated in the inverse, 1 occupant death per 500 vehicles. Too many "risk analyses" fail to account for the lifetime risks of products or practices. Failure to understand the difference between annual risk and cumulative risk over the life of products has resulted in grotesque errors in estimating the effects of potential preventive measures (Chapter 10).

Manufacturers and others opposed to regulation, or "experts" and attorneys involved in product liability lawsuits, often cite the injury rate from the product in question relative to injury rates from other products as indicative of reasonableness or acceptability. Given the variety of denominators available to calculate rates and the difficulty in measuring exposure, the placement of a given rate in an array of rates of injury by products or users can be very different, depending on the denominator used and the comparability of the research methods in case finding and exposure measurement.

An interesting case of such arguments about rates and risk occurred regarding the consideration of regulation of "all-terrain vehicles" by the U.S. Consumer Products Safety Commission (CPSC). These vehicles are propelled by modified motorcycle-type engines at speeds up to 60 miles per hour. They have three or four balloon tires and are steered by handlebars similar to those on a motorcycle. The steering is not as easy as it looks, however, requiring weight shifts by the rider different from those on a bicycle or motorcycle. The vehicles are unstable when in motion and will roll over at low speeds, sometimes onto the rider, if the rider does not apply the weight shift at the moment needed (Deppa, 1986).

Sales of all-terrain vehicles, which are marketed in the United States as a recreational vehicle for families (including children), increased rapidly in the early 1980s to the point that about 2.5 million were in the hands of consumers by 1986. CPSC estimates of deaths on the vehicles increased from 26 in 1982 to 268 in 1986, and estimates of injuries from a survey of those treated in hospital emergency rooms increased from about 8600 in 1982 to 86,400 in 1986. The CPSC was pressured by the Congress and consumer groups to ban the vehicles or issue safety standards for them.

Arguments ensued among the staff and commissioners of the CPSC as to whether or not the rate of injuries to occupants of all-terrain vehicles should be compared to those of occupants of other motorized, off-road vehicles such as snowmobiles and mini/trail bikes. Initial comparisons indicated that the rate of injury per vehicle of all-terrain vehicles was two times that of mini/trail bikes and four to five times that of snowmobiles. Based on a few anecdotal reports of hours of use per vehicle in public hearings, however, the rates per hours of use for all-terrain vehicles were said to be less than those of the other vehicles (Verhalen, 1986). A majority of the commissioners voted that the comparison was irrelevant to the issue of whether all-terrain vehicles should be regulated (General Acounting Office, 1986), but the industry commissioned research on injuries per hours of participation in other recreational activities in an attempt to justify the risk of all-terrain vehicles.

An economist formerly employed at the CPSC was hired by the industry to conduct a survey of hours of use of mini/trail bikes and snowmobiles. Based on these data and CPSC counts of injuries, he argued that the injury rate per hours of use were no different among the three types of vehicles (Heiden, 1986). In subsequent congressional hearings (Heiden, 1990) and in lawsuits against manufacturers, comparisons were also made to injuries per hour of people engaged in other activities such as organized football, use of motorcycles and other on-road vehicles, general aviation, snow skiing, and swimming. With the exception of organized football games and general aviation, the estimates of hours of participation were extrapolated from surveys that used categories for time of participation such as "daily or almost daily," "about once or twice a week," "about once or twice a month," and "less than once per month." These are useless for estimation of hours of participation and, given the problems of remembering hours of participation, questions regarding more specific hours of participation in most activities are likely to be unreliable or invalid.

Aside from methodological issues, this case illustrates some of the uses or misuses of epidemiologic data of which the researcher should be aware. While it may be useful to present the public with information about risks of engaging in activities that are substitutable one for the other per hour, per person, per vehicle, or product, or whatever, the comparison of descriptive injury rates per whatever exposure unit among various activities or products does not tell us whether the risks are "reasonable" or "acceptable" or whether products involved are defective.

Two products may have the same injury rate, one of which could have been reduced by product modifications at less cost, no cost, or little cost, whereas the cost of modification of the other may be very large. The calculation of cost-savings, cost-effectiveness, risk-benefit, or cost-benefit of injury reduction modifications to products, or injury control programs generally, is not based on risk per hour or risk per product or activity. These calculations are based on total costs of the injuries relative to the total costs of product modifications or programs to reduce them (Chapter 9).

If a product or activity were considered "reasonable" or "acceptable" as long as its injury rate was less than that of the most risky products and activities, manufacturers and promotors of products and activities would be free to add one new risk after another with impunity. The fact that more risky products are for sale does not indicate user acceptability of a less risky product when the vast majority of purchasers have no way to assemble the data on relative rates.

One methodology that has been used to assess public acceptability of risk is to compare perception of current restrictions or regulations to desired restrictions or standards for motor vehicles, guns, commercial aviation, industrial chemicals, nuclear power generation, and nuclear weapons. In random sample surveys of the population in Connecticut and the Phoenix metropolitan area, the respondents rated desired restrictions and standards far above restrictions and standards prevalent in 1982–83, a period of severe economic recession and strong antiregulation political sentiment (Gould et al., 1988).

Epidemiologic data on injury rates are relevant to the issue of modifiability of products and activities when and if the specific characteristics of the products and activities that increase or decrease the rates are delineated using sound epidemiologic research. The methods for such analytical epidemiologic studies are discussed in Chapter 4. Chapter 3 deals with injury surveillance—a special case of descriptive epidemiology that is useful for problem identification and targeting control strategies.

SUMMARY

Research questions should focus on homogeneous subsets of injuries and changeable factors possibly related to incidence and severity. Certain available data sources emphasize nonchangeable factors such as age and sex and include classifications that are not useful. Data without valid indicators of severity may be misleading because the factors relevant to reducing severe injuries are often not involved as frequently in nonsevere injuries. Improved means of quantifying severity of injury and disability are under investigation. Case identification requires a knowledge of the flow of cases among treatment facilities.

Injury rates are calculated by dividing numbers of injuries by population at risk or measures of exposure. Rates are useful for inferring relative risk in relation to factors that can be changed to reduce risk. Rates are misleading when they are high but are based on relatively rare exposures or do not reflect the future exposures inherent in the lifetime exposure to a product or activity.

REFERENCES

Aarts LJM, and DeJong PR (1992) *Economic Aspects of Disability Behavior.* Amsterdam: North Holland.

Baker SP (1983) Panel: current status of trauma severity indices. *J Trauma* 23:193–196.

Baker SP, O'Neill B, Haddon W Jr, and Long WB (1974) The injury severity score: a method for describing patients with multiple injuries and evaluating emergency care. *J Trauma* 14:187–196.

Barancik JI, and Chatterjee BF (1981) Methodological considerations in the use of the Abbreviated Injury Scale in trauma epidemiology. *J Trauma* 21:627.

Barancik JI, and Fife D (1985) Discrepancies in vehicular crash injury reporting: Northeastern Ohio Trauma Study IV. *Accident Anal Prev* 17:147–154.

Berger LR, and Mohan D (1996) *Injury Control: A Global View.* Delhi: Oxford University Press.

Bloch FS (1982) *Disability Determination: The Administrative Process and the Role of Medical Personnel.* Westport, CT; Greenwood Press.

Boyd CR, Tolson MA, and Copes WS (1987) Evaluating trauma care: the TRISS method. *J Trauma* 27:370–378.

Bull JP (1975) The Injury Severity Score of road traffic casualties in relation to mortality, time of death, hospital treatment time and disability. *Accident Anal Prev* 7:249–255.

Champion HR, Sacco WJ, Carnazzo AJ, Copes WS, and Fouty WJ (1981) Trauma score. *Crit Care Med* 9:672–676.

Champion HR, Sacco WJ, Copes WS, Gann DS, Gennarelli TA, and Flanagan ME (1989) A revision of the trauma score. *J Trauma* 29:623–629.

Champion HR, Copes WS, Sacco WJ, Lawnick MM, Bain LW, Gann DS, Gennarelli T, MacKenzie E, and Schwaitzberg S (1990) A new characterization of injury severity. *J Trauma* 30:539–544.

Committee on Injury Scaling (1980) The Abbreviated Injury Scale, 1980 Revision. Park Ridge, IL: American Association for Automotive Medicine.

Committee on Trauma of the American College of Surgeons (1987) Appendix G. Quality assurance in trauma care. In *Hospital and Prehospital Resources for Optimal Care of the Injured Patient.* Chicago: American College of Surgeons.

Conboy T, Barth J, and Boll T (1986) Treatment and rehabilitation of mild and moderate head trauma. *Rehabil Psychol* 31:202–215.

Copes WS, Champion HR, Sacco WJ, Lawnick MM, Gann DS, Gennarelli T, MacKenzie E, and Schwaitzberg S (1990) Progress in characterizing anatomic injury. *J Trauma* 30:1200–1207.

Deppa RW (1986) Report on the engineering evaluation of all-terrain vehicles. Washington, DC: U.S. Consumer Product Safety Commission.

Dunlop DD, Hughes SL, and Manheim LM (1997) Disability in activities of daily living: patterns of change and a hierarchy of disability. *Am J Public Health* 87:378–383.

General Accounting Office (1986) Consumer Product Safety Commission: concerns about staff memorandum relating to all-terrain vehicles. Washington, DC: U.S. Congress.

Goldberg B, Rosenthal PP, Robertson LS, and Nicholas JA (1988) Injuries in youth football. *Pediatrics* 81:255–261.

Gould LC, Gardner GT, DeLuca DR, Tiemann AR, Doob LW, and Stolwijk JAJ (1988) *Perceptions of Technological Risks and Benefits.* New York: Russell Sage Foundation.

Guttman L (1946) An approach for quantifying paired comparisons and rank order. *Ann Math Stat* 17:144–163.

Guyer B, and Gallagher SS (1985) An approach to the epidemiology of childhood injuries. *Pediatr Clin North Am* 32:5–15.

Hartunian NS, Smart CN, and Thompson MS (1981) *The Incidence and Economic Costs of Major Health Impairments.* Lexington, MA: D.C. Heath.

Health Care Financing Administration (1980) *International Classification of Diseases. 9th revision. Clinical Modification: ICD-9-CM. 2nd ed. Vol. 1. Diseases; Tabular List.* Washington, DC: U.S. Department of Health and Human Services.

Heiden EJ (1986) Some additional evidence on comparative safety for ATVs and related vehicles. Washington, DC: Heiden Associates.

Heiden EJ (1990) Statement. Washington, DC: Commerce, Consumer, and Monetary Affairs Subcommittee of the House Government Operations Committee, U.S. House of Representatives.

Jorgensen K (1981) Use of the Abbreviated Injury Scale in a hospital emergency room. *Acta Orthop Scand* 52:273–277.

Kaufmann CR, Maier RV, Kaufmann EJ, Rivara FP, and Carrico CJ (1991) Validity of applying adult TRISS analysis to injured children. *J. Trauma* 31:691–697.

Kelsey JL, Thompson WD, and Evans AS (1986) *Methods in Observational Epidemiology.* New York: Oxford University Press.

Kraus JF, Franti CE, Riggins D, and Borhani NO (1975) Incidence of traumatic spinal cord injury. *J Chronic Dis* 28:471–492.

Kraus JF, Black MA, Hessol N, Ley P, Rokaw W, Sullivan C, Bowers S, Knowlton S, and Marshall L (1984) The incidence of acute brain injury and serious impairment in a defined population. *Am J Epide*miol 119:186–201.

MacKenzie EJ (1997) ICDMAP-90 computer software. Bel Air, MD: Tri-Analytics, Inc.

MacKenzie EJ, Shapiro S, Moody M, Siegel JH, and Smith RT (1986) Predicting post-trauma functional disability for individuals without severe brain injury. *Med Care* 24:377–387.

MacKenzie EJ, Steinwachs DM, and Shankar B (1989) Classifying trauma severity based on hospital discharge diagnoses: validation of an ICD-9CM to AIS-85 Conversion Table. *Med Care* 27:412–422.

MacKenzie EJ, Damiano A, Miller T, and Luchter S (1996) The development of the Functional Capacity Index. *J Trauma* 41: 799–806.

McLoughlin E, and Crawford JD (1985) Burns. *Pediatr Clin North Am.* 32:61–76.

National Center for Health Statistics (1986) *Types of Injuries and Impairments Due to Injuries, United States.* Hyattsville, MD: U.S. Department of Health and Human Services.

National Center for Health Statistics (1995) *Vital Statistics of the United States, 1991. Volume 2: Mortality, Part B.* Hyattsville, MD: U.S. Department of Health and Human Services, pp. 180–199.

National Center for Health Statistics (1996) *Vital Statistics of the United States, 1992: Life Tables.* Hyattsville, MD: U.S. Department of Health and Human Services, p. 12.

Panel on Occupational Safety and Health Statistics (1987) *Counting Injuries and Illnesses in the Workplace: Proposals for a Better System.* Washington, DC: National Academy Press.

Pope AM, and Tarlov AR (1991) *Disability in America: Toward a National Agenda for Prevention.* Washington, DC: National Academy Press.

Riegelman RK (1981) *Studying a Study and Testing a Test.* Boston: Little, Brown.

Robertson LS (1981) Patterns of teenaged driver involvement in fatal motor vehicle crashes: implications for policy choices. *J Health Polit Policy Law* 6:303–314.

Rutowski W, Nasilowski W, Zietkiewicz W, and Zienkiewicz K (1976) *Burn Therapy and Research.* Baltimore: Johns Hopkins Press.

Schwing RC, and Kamerud DB (1988) The distribution of risks: vehicle occupant fatalities and time of week. *Risk Anal* 8:127–133.

Selvin S (1991) *Statistical Analysis of Epidemiologic Data.* New York: Oxford University Press.

States JD, and Viano DC (1990) Injury impairment and disability scales to assess the permanent consequences of trauma. *Accident Anal Prev* 22:151–160.

Tepas JJ III (1989). Update on pediatric trauma-severity scores. In Haller JA Jr (ed), *Emergency Medical Services for Children.* Columbus, OH: Ross Laboratories.

Thurman DJ, Burnett CL, Jeppson L, Beaudoin MD, and Sniezek JE (1994) Surveillance of spinal cord injuries in Utah, USA. *Paraplegia* 32:665–669.

Thurman DJ, Burnett CL, Beaudoin DE, Jeppson L, and Sniezek JE (1995) Risk factors and mechanisms of occurrence in motor vehicle-related spinal injuries: Utah. *Accident Anal Prev* 27:411–415.

Torg JS, Vegso JJ, Sennett B, and Das M (1985) The national football head and neck injury registry: 14 year report on cervical quadraplegia, 1971 through 1984. *JAMA* 254:3439–3443.

Verhalen RD (1986) ATV project: comparative injury tables. Washington, DC: U.S. Consumer Product Safety Commission.

Waller J (1988) Methodologic issues in hospital-based injury research. *J Trauma* 28:1632–1636.

3

INJURY SURVEILLANCE AND ITS USES

The word "surveillance," with its connotation of unkempt police watching the residences of suspects, or someone's phone being tapped, may not be the best way to describe an epidemiologic activity. The epidemiologic use of the term refers to collection of data on who, when, where, and sometimes how people become diseased or injured. The data are purged of individual identifiers so that the individuals involved are anonymous.

The purpose of injury surveillance usually is to monitor trends in particular types of injuries. More detailed data on the who, when, where, and how of injuries can be used to target injury control measures to relevant circumstances and populations and increase cost-effectiveness of resource allocation. Identification of relatively homogeneous subsets of injuries in defined locations and populations coupled with a systematic review of Haddon's technical options for injury control (Chapter 1) can lead to substantial reductions if implemented. Some examples of the power of surveillance data in injury control are reserved for the end of this chapter. First, a description of some important surveillance systems is in order.

Several governmental and private agencies in the United States maintain surveillance systems that continually or periodically collect data on injuries. Some of these systems include data useful for more detailed study than simply following trends. The purpose of this chapter is to identify major injury surveillance systems, note some of their strengths and weaknesses, and suggest improvements for usefulness in injury control, particularly prevention-oriented surveillance in local areas.

The criteria for judging the adequacy of a surveillance system depend on its intended use and other possible uses (Klaucke, 1992). The measurement of trends in injuries of a given type requires that the definition of the type does not change during the time period studied and, where all injuries of the type are not counted, the sampling method does not change in such a way as to alter the comparability of the count during segments of the time period. For example, the International Classification of Diseases includes two types of codes for injury, diagnosis codes—sometimes called N codes—and codes for "external causes," called E codes. The 1968 addition to the E codes of a category for "injuries undetermined whether accidental or purposely afflicted" resulted in discontinuity in the trend in infant homicides. Apparently, a number of cases that would have been called homicide before the new category was added were placed in the undetermined category thereafter (Jason et al., 1983).

As noted in Chapter 2, using surveillance or any data to correlate injuries to other factors requires attention to issues of classification and relevance to injury control. If rates are calculated, changes in the population exposed or changes in measurement of exposure during the period examined must be considered. For example, trends in injury per population are sometimes adjusted for changes in the age distribution of the population but not for other factors that may also have changed. Even population age adjustments can be misleading. In the case of motor vehicle injuries, for instance, the proportion of the population that is licensed in an age group may change such that population age adjustment is inadequate to account for changes in exposure by age.

Finding clusters by geographic areas is of major importance in targeting certain injury control efforts. Distributions of injuries in certain regions may suggest very different priorities from those indicated by national or other larger areas. For example, during 1988–92 drowning was the second leading cause of injury mortality in Alaska (Lincoln et al., 1996). In one hospital in rural Ghana, burns were the second leading cause of admissions (Mock et al., 1995). Complete counts of severe injuries during a period of time, rather than samples, are required to reveal clusters, particularly if the areas are small. Usually the smaller the area, the longer the time period required for stable numbers. The Centers for Disease Control has produced a review of statistical methods for dealing with clusters (Centers for Disease Control, 1990).

A number of sources of injury surveillance data have been evaluated on a variety of criteria including importance to public health, usefulness in comparison to cost, acceptability to the persons who must record the data, timeliness of reporting, representativeness of injuries in a defined population, sensitivity (identification of all cases), specificity (misclassification of noncases as cases), simplicity of data collection and management, and flexibility in inclusion of injuries not originally included (Graitcer, 1987). That evaluation is not repeated here, but each of those attributes of a surveillance system affects its use or usefulness.

GENERAL SURVEILLANCE

The National Center for Health Statistics assembles mortality records that provide information on trends and clusters of fatal injuries by age, sex, state, city, and county (Baker et al., 1992). The data are based on death certificates that are usually filled out by physicians at the time of pronouncement of death or soon thereafter. They are coded by nosologists for the clinical nature of injury and area of the body injured (N codes) and "external cause" (E codes).

The accuracy of reporting of certain types of injury on death certificates has been questioned by researchers who investigated cases in detail. In one state, about one in four cases of child deaths coded as intentional homicides were of questionable validity. It is unlikely that the death was intended in a variety of circumstances, for example, in the cases of pedestrians killed by hit-and-run drivers and children killed while playing with guns (Lapidus et al., 1990). Fatal motorcycle injuries were underestimated by 38 percent on death certificates when checked against police reports (Lapidus et al., 1994). In another state, a study of asphyxiation by food found that data on the death certificates were substantially incomplete, apparently due to the rush to complete the certificate so that the body could be released to the family (Salmi et al., 1990).

The advantage of death certificate data is that they are available nationally on computer databases, and counts can be generated for local areas, but detailed examination of medical examiner and coroner records are often more useful in areas where a thorough investigation is routine. In some cities or counties, an autopsy by a qualified forensic pathologist is required in cases of violent death, intentional or unintentional, but the results are usually in narrative form with no computerized coding of detailed circumstances of the death (Raasch, 1985). The data, if coded and computerized, would be very useful for increased understanding of injury circumstances. In many jurisdictions, however, a coroner, sometimes with no medical or other qualifications, is in charge of the investigation, which may be no more thorough than acceptance of the information on the death certificate. The wise researcher will examine the records in detail and conduct an independent investigation of their reliability and validity before assuming that they are coded accurately.

Hospital records are an important source of identification of severe, nonfatal injuries. The extent of use of International Classification of Diseases codes on hospital discharge records varies widely among hospitals. The National Hospital Discharge Survey provides computerized data on a national probability sample of 200,000 hospital discharges annually, including all discharges, not just those associated with injury. Data on hospitalized injuries at the local level are available in hospitals that maintain a trauma registry, but in communities with more than one hospital, one or more may not have a registry, and the patients in those that do may not be representative of all injured patients from the area of interest.

Even in hospitals where the injury coding is done systematically, the E codes are often missing, particularly in cases with so many N codes that there is no room for E codes on computer files, as the data are currently structured (Marganitt et al., 1990). In many cases, the medical history and notes by physicians and nurses in hospital records do not contain enough detail about the circumstances of an injury to classify it by E code or specific geographic location.

Universal E coding of hospital discharge records has been advocated by the Council of State and Territorial Epidemiologists and several states now require them. The Indian Health Service routinely requires such coding in its hospitals, and E codes for injuries were found on 99.3 percent of its injury case records, although 25 percent lacked sufficient information for validity of detailed three-digit codes. Comparison of the codes and detailed examination of a sample of hospital records indicated excellent reliability in general categories (motor vehicle, fall, etc.), but discrepancies increased in the more refined subcategories (Smith, Colwell, & Sniezek, 1990).

Although universal E coding would provide much better information on trends and clusters of injuries by type, severity, and a few demographic characteristics, it would mainly serve as a source to identify cases of particular types of injury for more detailed investigation. Cases without E codes are identifiable as injuries by N codes, which are much more complete.

Since the codes are revised periodically, the researcher must be careful in examining trends in data that bridge a revision. The codes are relatively specific for some causes of injury, but in other cases, the aggregation of causes is frustrating to the researcher when more refined categories are needed. Also, new products and activities that are introduced after the latest revision will not have specific E codes.

The available general surveillance systems of injuries that do not require hospitalization are valuable only for indication of frequency and overall cost estimates. The problems of categorizations, and self-reporting based on time away from usual activities in the National Health Interview Survey, were noted in Chapter 2. The National Medical Care Utilization and Expenditure Survey, based on a separate sample of households interviewed regarding use of medical care, gives some indication of clinical symptoms and costs of medical care related to injury, but no information on circumstances (Rice & MacKenzie,

1989). Given the priority to reduce death and severe injury, and the often differing circumstances that contribute to severe and nonsevere injuries, devotion of resources to collection of more detailed data on less severe injuries would be difficult to justify. Exceptions may occur in work or other settings where very severe injuries are rare but musculoskeletal injuries result in inability to work or drawn-out pain and suffering.

SPECIAL SURVEILLANCE SYSTEMS

Governmental agencies with statutory responsibility for monitoring certain types of injuries, or regulating products and activities that are associated with injuries, maintain special surveillance systems. Some of these provide sufficient detail for analytic as well as descriptive epidemiologic studies.

Motor vehicles

Among the best surveillance system in terms of detailed data on vehicles and vectors as well as environmental circumstances is the Fatal Accident Reporting System (FARS) of the National Highway Traffic Safety Administration (NHTSA). Begun in 1975, this system collects data on virtually all fatalities related to motor vehicles that occur on public roads in the United States for cases in which the fatally injured person died within 30 days. Most of the data are from police reports, but additional information is included from motor vehicle licensing agencies, hospitals, and coroners or medical examiners. Data tapes can be purchased from NHTSA and all but the most recent years are available on CD-ROM disks at no cost from the Bureau of Transportation Statistics of the U.S. Department of Transportation. Subsets of specific variables on specific cases can be downloaded or cross-tabulated by modem from the University of Michigan's Transportation Research Institute at modest cost.

The completeness and accuracy of FARS data are specific to each variable and vary among states and over time for some variables. For example, measurement of blood alcohol concentration of fatally injured drivers increased in the 1980s and was completed for more than 80 percent of such drivers in more than half of the states since 1984 (National Highway Traffic Safety Administration, 1988). In years and states where blood alcohol is not tested as systematically, the possibility of bias in selection of those tested is of concern.

Speed of vehicles in crashes is missing in more than half of FARS cases and, where it is found, the reliability is questionable. Fault-finding by police is also questionable since such judgments are made after the fact of the crash and may be based on reports by biased or unreliable eyewitnesses or lack of knowledge of vehicle factors and conditions. For example, the driver may be blamed for a rollover that would not have happened if the vehicle were more stable, or a mechanical failure may be obscured by the destruction of evidence by crash forces.

An unusual attribute of the NHTSA files, FARS and others, is the specificity of vehicle information. Codes for vehicle make and model, as well as vehicle identification numbers that can be decoded as to make and model for verification, are included in the data. This allows characteristics of specific vehicles, coded in the vehicle identification number or obtained from other sources, to be examined in relation to fatal injuries.

A system with data similar to that in FARS, but based on a randomized area sample of motor vehicle crashes on public roads reported to police, is the National Accident Sampling System (NASS). This system was pilot tested in 1978 and has collected data representative of the defined crashes in the United States since that year. Since many motor vehicle injuries are not reported to police (Chapter 2), the numbers of injuries estimated from the NASS is an underestimate. The data include more detail on injuries than FARS, including injuries by area of the anatomy as well as AIS and ISS scores. These can be used for analytic studies as well as giving some indication of national trends in nonfatal injuries.

Since NASS is based on a sample of a limited number of counties or clusters of counties around the country (about 8400 crashes per year are in the sample), it is obviously not useful for local injury surveillance unless the area of interest is in one of the sampling areas. Most states and many smaller jurisdictions have computerized files of motor vehicle cases investigated by police. Injury codes in these state and local files are not considered refined enough for adequate indication of injury severity other than death. There are too many cases in which a bloody but superficial cut is coded as severe, whereas in other cases a person with a severe internal injury is coded at the scene as suffering a nonsevere injury. In a comparison of police rating of injury and hospital records of children struck as pedestrians or bicyclists, for example, the ISS score ranged from 0 to 30 in the least severe police code and 1 to 40 in the most severe nonfatal code (Agran et al., 1990).

The police in most states use A, B, and C as codes for more to less serious injury in addition to K for persons killed. Figure 3.1 shows the distribution of fatal and A ("incapacitating") injury by the clinically based maximum abbreviated injury score of passenger car and light truck drivers in the National Accident Sampling System. The deaths increase with injury severity but the police judgments of incapacitating injury are not reflective of injury severity.

A few researchers combine fatal and A injuries in state police files in their studies, for example, in the assessment of seat belt effectiveness (e.g., Reinfurt & Chi, 1981; Streff, 1994). Because A injuries are far more frequent than

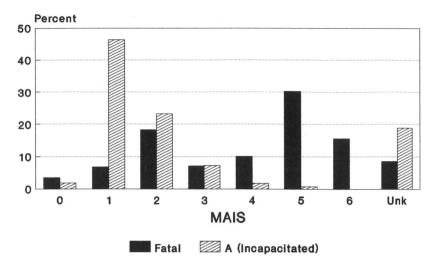

1993 NASS Light Vehicle Drivers

FIGURE 3.1. Maximum Abbreviated Injury Score (MAIS) of police, in percent, K (fatal) and A (incapacitated) codes.

fatalities and nearly half the A injuries are nonserious injuries that occur to belted drivers, estimates of belt effectiveness or other factors in such studies are not valid.

Police files are used in some areas for identification of clusters of crashes on sections of roads, but the clusters of all reported crashes do not necessarily reflect the sites of the more severe injuries. A system still used in several states weights a fatal crash as only 9.1 times as important as a crash that only involved property damage (Federal Highway Administration, 1981). Site modifications based on such systems are too often directed to sites where crashes without injury are frequent, neglecting sites where severe injuries are clustered.

Beginning in 1988, the National Highway Traffic Safety Administration initiated a program to sample a larger number of police-reported crashes among the states. The crashes included in this General Estimates System are an area probability sample of those reported to police throughout the country (National Highway Traffic Safety Administration, 1990). The data are exclusively those recorded by police. The advantage of the sample is the larger number of cases compared to the National Accident Sampling System (about 48,000 per year). The disadvantage is that the data on injury have not been augmented from other sources, as was the case in the NASS, and suffer from the poor indicators of injury severity in all police data. The vehicle identification number is missing in a third of the cases.

Assaults and homicides

The Federal Bureau of Investigation (FBI) collects data from local police on several crimes, including assaults reported to police and homicides that are deemed criminal, in its uniform crime reporting system. Comparison of death certificates and deaths attributed to homicide in the FBI system indicate about 9 percent fewer homicides in the FBI files, at least partly because presumed noncriminal homicides, such as a felon killed by a law enforcement officer, are not included, and 4 percent of local jurisdictions do not report to the FBI (Rokaw et al., n.d.).

The FBI data include valuable information on trends in weapons used, demographic characteristics of victims, and relationship to assailants where known, but no data on the nature of the injuries. Medical examiner or coroner files can be used to identify homicide cases at the local level and are usually adequate for indicating trends, or clusters in certain neighborhoods, bars, and the like.

Since nonfatal assaults are often not reported to police, ongoing interview surveys of the population—the National Crime Surveys—are sometimes used as sources of data on trends and some of the correlates. The trends in assault rates per population from the FBI reports and the Crime Surveys moved in opposite directions during 1974–88, apparently because of increased reporting of assaults to police (Jencks, 1991). Data on nature and severity of injury are inadequate in the Crime Surveys and children younger than 12 years are not interviewed. Computerized files of these surveys are available from the National Criminal Justice Reference Service. The sampling system is complex, with households interviewed seven times and then replaced in the sample. Before using the data, consultation with experts familiar with the files is recommended.

Hospital records are the best source of data on serious nonfatal assault cases at the local level, although assaults are probably underestimated from these sources, and the inaccuracy spills over into other categories. Assaults are sometimes reported to hospital personnel as falls or gun "accidents."

Suicides and attempts

Surveillance of suicides is based on death certificates (Centers for Disease Control, 1986). Since there may be doubt as to intent in some cases and pressure to protect families in others, the numbers recorded as suicides are thought to be an undercount. Nonfatal suicide attempts in hospital records are subject to substantial misidentification as accidents for the same reasons. Because suicides can also cluster, apparently from imitative behavior, the Centers for Disease

Control urges local communities to establish means of monitoring suicides and attempts, but the extent to which this is done is unknown.

Occupational injuries

The Bureau of Labor Statistics (BLS) conducts an annual survey of employer summaries of injuries that are recordable according to standards of the Occupational Safety and Health Administration (OSHA). The evidence of underreporting in some cases and overreporting in others, as well as the lack of detail on machines, work practices, or worker characteristics, severely limits the usefulness of the data (Panel on Occupational Safety and Health Statistics, 1987).

Users of these data should be aware that some of the categories do not make sense clinically. For example, repetitive motion injuries are classified as illness, unless they result in back strain, which is always called injury.

More detailed data on worker injuries in industries subject to worker compensation laws are collected by BLS from the workers' compensation records of about 30 states. Important variables such as nature of injury, body part affected, occupation, and aspects of circumstances are included routinely, but others such as age, time of injury relative to time work began, and extent of disability are optional. Lost work time is a misleading indication of severity because it is strongly related to maximum compensation in a given state for certain injuries (Robertson & Keeve, 1983). Also, industries and even plants within the same company vary in the practice of assigning workers to other duties that can be performed after certain injuries, as opposed to having the worker take time off until he or she can return to regular duties.

The National Institute for Occupational Safety and Health (NIOSH) attempts to estimate fatal occupational injuries in its National Traumatic Occupational Fatality database (Centers for Disease Control, 1987), but the case identification is dependent on accurate coding of occurrence at work. Whether or not a death is work-related is supposed to be recorded on the death certificate, but the information is often missing. Fatal injuries in agriculture, for example, were undercounted by 20 percent when compared to independent sources (Murphy et al., 1990). One study that identified cases of fatal farm injuries from both death certificates and newspaper clippings found 14 percent in newspaper clippings that were not identified in death certificates (Hayden et al., 1995), and newspaper clippings are undoubtedly incomplete.

Investigation of adequacy of death certificates at the local level is recommended before they are used. Similarly, hospital records often do not contain data on the place of injury. Also, nonhospitalized emergency room records are inadequate for case-finding because larger industries have their own clinics to treat less serious injuries.

Consumer products

The U.S. Consumer Product Safety Commission (CPSC) uses a sample of hospital emergency rooms and also uses death certificates to identify trends in product-related injuries and emerging problems. Major products—alcohol, most forms of transportation, and firearms—are excluded. Occasional special studies are conducted, such as the all-terrain–vehicle case discussed in Chapter 2. In the general survey and specific studies, brand names and models of the products are not identified, precluding the comparison of injury incidence and severity by product characteristics. The sample of hospitals is small relative to the number in the country and cannot be used for identification of local injury clusters.

Fire-related injuries

About 40 states report data on fire incidence to the National Fire Data Center, based on reports from local fire marshalls. Several important aspects of these data are computerized, including location, date, response time of the fire department, type of construction, and type of injury. A detailed comparison of these records and death certificates, coroner or medical examiner records, and hospital records is needed to determine the completeness and reliability of reporting.

Boat-related injuries

The Coast Guard maintains records of deaths and some injuries related to use of boats. Probably no more than 10 percent of nonfatal injuries related to boat use are reported to the Coast Guard. The data include boat type, cause of accident, and alleged alcohol use as well as demographic variables. The data on causes may not be reliable and alcohol use is usually not confirmed by toxicological tests. A study of completeness of reporting of deaths, and reliability of other codes, should be undertaken before using these data.

Addresses and telephone numbers of the agencies that control distribution of data may change and new data systems may be added from time to time. The internet can be searched by agency names for current information.

Outcome conditions

Some states and other entities have established systems of surveillance for particular types of injury outcome, such as spinal cord or brain injuries. Focus on such injuries may be useful because of the effects on lives of the injured and those who must care for them as well as the costs.

When a complete census of such conditions is problematic, as in low-income countries or where hospitals are not cooperative, *capture–recapture* analysis, the sampling method originally used for estimating animal, bird, and insect populations, can be employed. In this method, the number of cases that turn up repeatedly in different samples indicates the incidence (or prevalence, depending on the sampling methods) of the outcome conditions (Chiu et al., 1993).

HOSPITAL-BASED SURVEILLANCE

Certain hospitals have increased the recording of data on injuries in trauma registries, partly for use in monitoring quality of care and partly as a database for research (Scheib et al., 1989). The use of hospital data for surveillance is limited by the differential case mix among hospitals and the lack of specification of the source population (Payne & Waller, 1989). If the population served uses more than one hospital and the preference for a given hospital or the criteria of the emergency response system for using a given hospital change over time, the trends in injuries in the registry can be misleading. Epidemiologists call this *selection bias*. Hospitals in the same community or region sometimes refuse to share data because they do not want the competition to have information about their "market."

In at least one state, Pennsylvania, an attempt to adopt uniform data recording among hospitals designated as trauma centers resulted in substantial compliance—81.5 percent (Gillott et al., 1989). While this system allows for a larger sample size for studies to increase quality assurance, the lack of inclusion of hospitals that are not trauma centers limits the usefulness of the data for surveillance and other epidemiologic studies.

Several states contracted with the National Highway Traffic Safety Administration to match hospital and police records in a system called the Crash Outcome Data Evaluation System (CODES). Data from this system have thus far been used to mislead the United States Congress regarding the effectiveness of seat belts because of invalid reporting of belt use to police. One report claimed 85 percent belt effectiveness in reducing motor vehicle occupant injuries, which is absurd (Chapter 7). NHTSA has refused requests under the Freedom of Information Act by outside researchers to gain access to the data, despite the fact that it was collected with taxpayer money. Matched hospital, police, and other data are potentially useful for targeting countermeasures and analytic studies, but if the data are not available to the research community, the uses are limited and the results are not subject to independent study.

There is a fundamental issue that people collecting surveillance data must address: How are the data being used? Taxpayers, the medically insured, or patients are paying for what is often a formidable effort in data collection. Are they getting anything for their money? What changes in emergency response or treatment have been made based on the data? How many road sections have been modified or lights installed or other changes made based on concentrations of cases at specific road sites at specific times? What changes in police deployment, arrest policies, and so on, have occurred based on data regarding concentrations of assaults in space, time, public places, or recidivism of spouse and child abuse? What changes in laws regarding alcohol, guns, or use of personal protection have been considered or enacted based on the data? Indeed, have the data been given to anyone in a position do do something to reduce injury incidence and severity? If so, were they presented in a form that suggested specific changes?

RISK FACTOR SURVEILLANCE

The Centers for Disease Control and Prevention coordinates a telephone survey in numerous states which attempts to measure behavioral risk factors, including several related to injury such as smoking, alcohol use, and seat belt use (Anda et al., 1990). Despite research indicating that self-reports of these behaviors are invalid, articles based on them are prevalent in the literature with no caveats regarding validity (e.g., Escobedo et al., 1995; Wechsler et al., 1995). A comparison of self-reported belt use from that survey and observed seat belt use from the annual observational survey of the National Highway Traffic Safety Administration illustrates the importance of not relying on self-reports of behavior. As displayed in Figure 3.2, self-reported belt use is substantially higher than that observed in the vicinity of large cities from each state from which data were available—an average difference of 21.5 percentage points in 1988. Belt use is less in rural areas than in and around cities, so the actual difference could be larger (Robertson, 1992).

Self-reported driving while intoxicated and other claims of heavy alcohol use in the behavioral risk factor survey also were not predictive of alcohol in fatally injured drivers. As shown in Figure 3.3, there was a sixfold variation among states regarding claimed driving after drinking but less than a twofold variation in actual percentage of alcohol measured by toxicologists in fatally injured drivers. Alcohol in fatally injured drivers was used for this comparison because it is objectively measured in more than 80 percent of fatally injured drivers in the states indicated. It does not include those who survived while killing other road users because alcohol is not measured objectively in such drivers often enough to avoid selection bias, but there is no reason to believe that the ratio of dead to surviving drunk drivers varies among states.

A high correlation between self-reported alcohol use in the behavioral risk factor survey and alcohol sales in 21 states has been reported, but the correlation of alcohol sales and self-reported drinking and driving was poor (Smith,

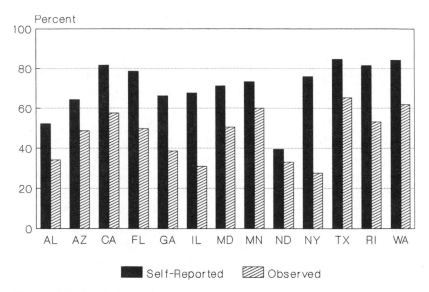

FIGURE 3.2. Seat belt use, in percent.

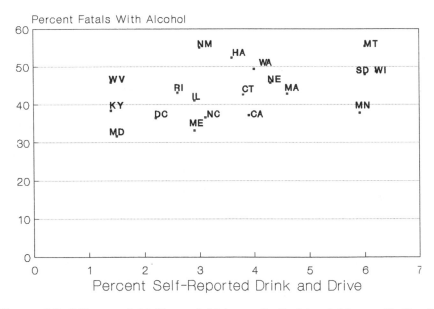

FIGURE 3.3. Self-reported drinking and driving vs fatally injured drivers with illegal alcohol, in percent.

Remington, et al., 1990). The funds used for collecting data on self-reported behavior would be better used to improve surveillance of objectively measured risk factors. For example, belt use, child restraint use, and motorcycle and bicycle helmet use are easily observable, and an estimate of use in a given area can be obtained by observations at randomly selected sites and times.

PREVENTION-ORIENTED SURVEILLANCE

Previous successful efforts in injury control based on surveillance have included the following steps:

1. Surveillance of injury incidence and severity to identify clusters of similar injuries and the hazards that increase incidence and severity.
2. Identification of one or more technical strategies to eliminate or reduce the hazard.
3. Implementation of the technical strategy among the populations at high risk.
4. Continued surveillance to monitor the trend in the injuries.

An outstanding example of the application of this approach occurred in the study and subsequent reduction of fatal falls to children in New York City. Epidemiologists from the health department devised a surveillance system of the circumstances of the falls and found that 66 percent of injuries in fatal falls to children up to five years of age occurred when the children crawled out of windows in high-rise buildings. The research also identified the areas of the city where these deaths most frequently occurred (Bergner et al., 1971).

A barrier that could be placed over windows, preventing children from crawling out, was the technical approach identified as most feasible under the circumstances. A campaign was launched in high-risk neighborhoods to persuade the parents or landlords to install the barriers (Spiegel & Lindaman, 1977). Eventually, the health department required landlords to install such barriers when requested by tenants. In association with these efforts, the deaths from childrens' falls from high-rise windows declined from about 30–50 per year in the 1960s to 4 in 1980. Total reported falls declined proportionately during the same period (Bergner, 1982). Subsequently, as attention to the issue declined, the falls and fatalities increased somewhat. In July 1986, the city changed the regulation to require barriers in buildings where there were children less than 11 years old.

In addition to illustration of the steps necessary for efficient injury control, the New York experience with childrens' falls from heights suggests the local nature of certain hazards. In cities and towns with few or no high-rise buildings (indeed in the boroughs of Queens and Staten Island, as the researchers found in New York), a campaign to install barriers in windows would be inappropriate because the problem is rare relative to other types of injury. Therefore, local injury surveillance is necessary to identify major injury problems that vary widely among local areas, and their circumstances and specific locations within the areas. The local health department is an appropriate agency for such an activity, but hospitals and other agencies could also do the work.

Numerous technical strategies are available for injury control, but efficient use requires data on the extent to which they are needed where the problem is most acute (Chapter 1). For example, certain road modifications, signaling systems, and lighting reduce relevant injuries by more than 50 percent (Federal Highway Administration, 1982). Yet modifying every mile of road with every possible modification would be very expensive.

By conducting detailed surveillance of the circumstances, frequency, and locations of serious injuries, the health department or other organization can recommend action to agencies or organizations in a position to implement, require, or distribute technology or other approaches. For example, if particular road intersections were found to have high rates of severe injury crashes, the data and suggestions for changes, such as extension of the yellow phase of traffic control lights at the specified intersections, would be forwarded to the road or police department that has jurisdiction. If skid strips on stairs, handrails, or other approaches were identified as likely ameliorative strategies for specific types of falls found among the elderly, the recommendations for specific modifications could be made to vulnerable community residents by visiting nurses or other persons who provide services to the elderly.

Investigation of the circumstances of drownings of young children in one state revealed that all of the drownings in bathtubs occurred with young siblings but no adults present. All drownings in pools and larger bodies of water were from falls into the water, not swimming or wading. These results indicate the need for adult supervision of young children's baths and the lack of barriers to prevent children from falling into larger bodies of water (Jensen et al., 1992).

Geographic distributions of injuries have been used to designate the placement and staffing of emergency medical services and trauma treatment centers. For example, one emergency medical service that covered a metropolitan area of 600 square miles found that 25 percent of the calls occurred in two 3 by 4.5 mile areas. The severe injuries were distributed similarly (Pepe et al., 1990). Geographic clusters of child pedestrian injuries combined with information about the children and the neighborhoods suggest modifications to reduce the problem (Braddock et al., 1994)

As indicated in the discussion of extant surveillance systems, few include data in sufficient detail to identify specific types of injury by specific locations, and none directly identify environmental modifications that could have reduced incidence and severity. To provide such information, a supplementary data collection system was developed for the Indian Health Service (Robertson, 1985).

The data to be gathered are indicated on the forms in Appendices 3.1 through 3.7, one form each for injury from motor vehicles, burn or smoke, drowning or near drowning, a fall, assault, suicide attempt, and others. The forms include not only the circumstances of the injury, but also a list of possible actions that might have prevented the injury or reduced its severity. The surveillance is not oriented simply to the collection of data; it is prevention-oriented.

Confining the initial effort to the more severe cases was deemed appropriate to avoid excessive effort expended on relatively trivial injuries that may occur in large numbers but are relatively unimportant in terms of long-term consequences for the persons injured and use of community resources. The definition of "serious" is somewhat arbitrary and can be changed as progress is made in prevention of the more severe cases. Fatalities and hospitalized injuries should receive first priority in most instances.

Since the Indian Health Service (IHS) provides outpatient as well as inpatient and preventive services in many Native American communities, access to cases by injury prevention specialists is no doubt easier than it would be in communities with more fragmented services. Nevertheless, the potential cost savings to be obtained by targeted injury control efforts informed by data should be appealing to hospitals. Reimbursement systems based on average costs for diagnosis-related groups have resulted in insufficient payments to hospitals for certain severe injuries because of the skewed distributions of costs (e.g., Jacobs, 1985).

Initial experience with the use of the IHS system indicated that lack of expertise in identifying potentially effective environmental modifications was a problem. A fellowship program to train injury control specialists and a series of seminars for other users of the system were instituted (Smith, 1988), and many successful injury control projects have been implemented by the graduates and others in their communities.

Technical assistance to state and local communities not served by the Indian Health Service is available from the injury prevention centers funded by the Centers for Disease Control (CDC) or from CDC. A current list of injury prevention centers is available from CDC.

Computer software has been developed by the Indian Health Service that provides for easy entry of the data from the surveillance system. The program can be edited for use in any community. As sufficient numbers accumulate, a summary of the circumstances cross-tabulated by the suggested actions that might have had a preventive effect provides a priority list for action.

Development of detailed computerized codes for injury locations to identify geographic clusters may be cumbersome, but good database management systems, such as EPIINFO used by IHS, allow listing of case identifiers by other variables. Once high-priority actions have been identified, cases that would have been reduced by a given action can be listed and the locations marked on detailed maps of local areas by referring to the location information on the original forms.

Location can be a powerful factor in concentrating resources. In Stockholm, Sweden, 47 percent of assaults on public streets occurred on 3 percent of all streets in a single year and street homicides in a 40 year period were highly concentrated on the same streets as those identified in the assault study. The assaults were near places of "entertainment" (bars, theaters, etc.) and one or more of those involved was often an intoxicated male (Wikstrom, 1995). In one city, 45 percent of child pedestrian injuries were located in 16 percent of the census tracts (Lapidus et al., 1991).

Numerous projects have been undertaken by the Indian Health Service based on surveillance data (Smith & Robertson, in press). Injury control specialists on the White River Apache Reservation in Arizona found a cluster of severe pedestrian injuries that occurred at night on a 1.2 mile section of road in a two year period. The tribal government and IHS collaborated in the installation of lights that illuminated the road section at night (Aikin & Rothfus, 1989). Comparison of the installation site and adjacent sites during the five years before and five years after the installation, controlling for average daily traffic and the removal of a liquor store in the area, indicates that about six fewer pedestrian injuries than expected occurred after the installation (A Dellapena & J Peabody, personal communication, 1997).

In Browning, Montana, 59 severe motor vehicle injuries, including 13 fatalities, occurred in a two mile stretch of road during a seven year period. Overhead lighting and curbs that channeled parking lot traffic to controlled entry points were installed. In the two year period year after lighting and curbs were installed, only two severe injuries occurred in that stretch of road (J Lee & L Beck, personal communication, 1991).

After being shown data on a cluster of 22 fatal pedestrian injuries at night on a two mile section of the road between Gallup, New Mexico, and the Navajo Nation, state authorities agreed to put night lighting of the road section in their five year plan for road modifications. No fatalities occurred in the lighted section in the two years after installation (N Bill, personal communication, 1995).

The Hoopa Health Association Emergency Medical Services gathered data on motor vehicle fatalities that occurred on the 100 miles of road through and adjacent to the Hoopa, Yurock, and Karok reservations in northern California.

The primary cause of death was vehicles plunging over steep embankments. Comparison of the sites where the state installed guardrails ten years before and ten years after the installation to noninstallation sites, corrected for average daily traffic, indicated some 21 fewer deaths than expected in the period after installation (Short & Robertson, 1997).

A visit to the site of each severe injury to consider environmental modifications that might have reduced the injuries is strongly recommended. For example, visits to the sites of child pedestrian injuries on the Pine Ridge Reservation in South Dakota indicated that the surfaces and equipment on nearby playgrounds were in such poor condition that the children apparently preferred to play in the streets or driveways of homes (Price, 1990).

The choice of recommended ameliorative actions should not necessarily be confined to the more obvious ones that can be fitted on a one page form. The narratives and comments may suggest others. Those included on the forms are oriented to actions that can be initiated at the local level and do not include actions delegated to federal regulatory agencies. A review of the literature on the technical strategies for specific injuries provides expertise in the identification of additional options (e.g., Federal Highway Administration, 1982; Haddon, 1970; Robertson, 1983).

Ideally, every community would have an injury surveillance system analogous to that of IHS. If the numbers in a given community were too limited for generalization, small communities in similar areas could pool the data to assess patterns for their environment. A system for accumulating data from the local systems at the state (or provincial) and national levels would give each level of government, or private entity, information on injury patterns relevant to agencies or organizations under its purview. Since national systems may be long in coming, local communities that are concerned about their injury problems can take the initiative.

Use of the IHS or similar forms could be required of medical examiners, coroners, and hospitals. The mechanism of enforcement of quality of data from medical examiners and coroners is not evident, but hospitals could be required to obtain the data to qualify for reimbursement by Medicare, Medicaid, or private insurance.

If and when a national system is developed, the information gathered in local surveillance systems must be made uniform on certain variables. For use by national regulatory agencies and independent researchers, the specific identification of product brand names and other identifiers such as serial numbers should be included. Where structures or other facilities that are, or could be, subject to local codes and ordinances are involved, the builders or maintainers should be identified. The mere fact that the data are being collected could serve as motivation for some organizations to undertake injury control actions. The data would give them better information on actions to take.

SUMMARY

Surveillance of who, when, where, and how people are injured has proved to be a powerful tool for targeting injury control measures of known effectiveness. Some extant surveillance systems have quirks in the data that can mislead the user. Missing data elements are a major problem in many. Certain data, such as police codes of injury severity and self-reported injuries and behaviors (e.g., seat belt and alcohol use), are invalid.

REFERENCES

Agran PF, Castillo DN, and Winn DG (1990) Limitations of data compiled from police reports on pediatric pedestrian and bicycle motor vehicle events. *Accident Anal Prev* 22:361–370.

Aiken D, and Rothfus G. (1989) Personal communication.

Anda RF, Waller MN, Wooten KG, Mast EE, Escobedo LG, and Sanderson LM (1990) Behavioral risk factor surveillance, 1988. *Morb Mortal Wkly Rep* 39:1–21.

Baker SP, O'Neill B, Ginsburg M, and Li G (1992) *The Injury Fact Book* 2nd ed. New York: Oxford University Press.

Bergner L (1982) Environmental factors in injury control: preventing falls from heights. In Bergman AB (ed), *Preventing Childhood Injuries*. Columbus, OH: Ross Laboratories.

Bergner L, Mayer S, and Harris D (1971) Falls from heights: a childhood epidemic in an urban area. *Am J Public Health* 61:90

Braddock M, Lapidus G, Cromley E, Cromley R, Burke G, and Banco L (1994) Using a geographic information system to understand child pedestrian injury. *Am. J. Public Health* 84:1158–1161.

Centers for Disease Control (1986) *Youth Suicide Surveillance*. Atlanta: Department of Health and Human Services.

Centers for Disease Control (1987) Traumatic occupational fatalities—United States, 1980–1984. *Morb Mortal Wkly Rep* 36:461–470.

Centers for Disease Control (1990) Summary of methods for statistically assessing clusters of health events. *Morb Mortal Wkly Rep* 39:17–23.

Chiu W, Dearwater SR, McCarty DJ, Songer TJ, and LaPorte RE (1993) Establishment of accurate incidence rates for head and spinal cord injuries in developing and developed countries: a capture-recapture approach. *J Trauma* 35:206–211.

Escobedo LG, Chorba TL, and Waxweiler R (1995) Patterns of alcohol use and the risk of drinking and driving among U.S. high school students. *Am J Public Health* 85:976–978.

Federal Highway Administration (1981) *Highway Safety Engineering Studies: Participant Notebook*. Washington, DC: U.S. Department of Transportation.

Federal Highway Administration (1982) *Synthesis of Safety Research Related to Traffic Control and Roadway Elements* (2 vol). Washington, DC: U.S. Department of Transportation.

Gillott AR, Thomas JM, and Forrester C (1989) Development of a statewide trauma registry. *J Trauma* 29:1667–1672.

Graitcer PL (1987) The development of state and local injury surveillance systems. *J Safety Res* 18:191–198.

Haddon W Jr (1970) On the escape of tigers: an ecologic note. *Technol Rev.* 72:44.

Hayden GJ, Gerberich SG, and Maldanado G (1995) Fatal farm injuries: a five-year study utilizing a unique surveillance approach to investigate the concordance of reporting between two data sources. *J Occup Environ Med* 37:571–577.

Health Care Financing Administration (1980) *International Classification of Diseases. 9th revision. Clinical Modification: ICD-9-CM. 2nd ed. Vol. 1. Diseases; Tabular List. Vol. 2. Diseases; Alphabetic Index. Vol. 3. Procedures; Tabular List and Alphabetic Index.* Washington, DC: U.S. Department of Health and Human Services.

Jacobs LM (1985) The effect of prospective reimbursement on trauma patients. *Am Coll Surg Bull* 70:17–22.

Jason J, Carpenter MM, and Tyler CW (1983) Underrecording of infant homicide in the United States. *Am J Public Health* 73:195–197.

Jencks C (1991) Is violent crime increasing? *Am Prospect* 1 (Winter):98–109.

Jensen LR, Williams SD, Thurman DJ, and Keller PA (1992) Submersion injuries in children younger than 5 years in urban Utah. *West J Med* 157:641–644.

Klaucke DN (1992) Evaluating public health surveillance systems. In Halperin W and Baker EL Jr, *Public Health Surveillance.* New York: Van Nostrand Reinhold.

Lapidus GD, Gregorio DI, and Hansen H (1990) Misclassification of childhood homicide on death certificates. *Am J Public Health* 80:213–214.

Lapidus GD, Braddock M, Banco L, Montenegro L, Hight D, and Eanniello V (1991) Child pedestrian injury: a population-based collision and injury severity profile. *J Trauma* 31:1110–1115.

Lapidus GD, Braddock M, Schwartz R, Banco L, and Jacobs, L (1994) Accuracy of fatal motorcycle-injury reporting on death certificates. *Accident Anal Prev* 26:535–542.

Lincoln JM, Perkins R, Melton F, and Conway GA (1996) Drowning in Alaska waters. *Public Health Rep* 111:531–535.

Marganitt B, MacKenzie EJ, Smith GS, and Damiano AM (1990) Coding external causes of injury (E-codes) in Maryland Hospital Discharges 1979–88: a statewide study to explore the uncoded population. *Am J Public Health* 80:1463–1466.

Mock CN, Adzotor E, Denno D, Conklin E, and Rivara F (1995) Admissions for injury at a rural hospital in Ghana: implications for prevention in the developing world. *Am J Public Health* 85:927–931.

Murphy DJ, Seltzer BL, and Yesalis CE (1990) Comparison of two methodologies to measure agricultural occupational fatalities. *Am J Public Health* 80:198–200.

National Committee for Injury Prevention and Control (1989) Appendix A. Injury prevention: meeting the challenge. *Am J Prev Med (Supplement).* New York: Oxford University Press.

National Highway Traffic Safety Administration (1988) *Fatal Accident Reporting System 1987.* Washington, DC: U.S. Department of Transportation.

National Highway Traffic Safety Administration (1990) *General Estimates System 1988.* Washington, DC: U.S. Department of Transportation.

Panel on Occupational Safety and Health Statistics (1987) *Counting Injuries and Illnesses in the Workplace: Proposals for a Better System.* Washington, DC: National Academy Press.

Payne SR, and Waller JA (1989) Trauma registry and trauma center biases in injury research. *J Trauma* 29:424–429.

Pepe PE, Mattox KL, Fischer RP, and Matsumoto CM (1990) Geographic patterns of urban trauma according to mechanism and severity of injury. *J Trauma* 30:1125–1132.

Price D. (1990) Motor-vehicle related pedestrian injuries on the Pine Ridge Indian Reservation. Unpublished MPH thesis. New Haven, CT: Yale University.

Raasch FO Jr (1985) Forensic analysis of trauma. In Nahum AM and Melvin J (eds), *The Biomechanics of Trauma.* Norwalk, CT: Appleton-Century-Crofts.

Reinfurt DW, and Chi GYH (1981) Automatic vs manual safety belt systems: a comparison using state accident data involving 1975–1979 model VW Rabbits. In Green RN and Petrucelli E (eds), *Proceedings: International Symposium on Occupant Restraints.* Morton Grove, IL: American Association for Automotive Medicine.

Rice DP, and MacKenzie EJ (eds) (1989) *Cost of Injury in the United States: A Report to Congress.* San Francisco: University of California Institute for Health and Aging, and Baltimore: Johns Hopkins University Injury Prevention Center.

Robertson LS (1983) *Injuries: Causes, Control Strategies and Public Policy.* Lexington, MA: D.C. Heath.

Robertson LS (1985) *Epidemiological Assessment of the Contributing Factors of Injury Mortality and Morbidity among Native Americans.* Springfield, VA: National Technical Information Service.

Robertson LS (1992) The validity of self-reported behavioral risk factors. *J Trauma* 32:58–59.

Robertson LS, and Keeve JP (1983) Worker injuries: the effects of workers' compensation and OSHA inspections. *J Health Polit Policy Law* 8:581–597.

Rokaw WM, Mercy JA, and Smith JC (no date) Comparability and utility of national homicide data from death certificates and police records. Washington, DC: Centers for Disease Control.

Salmi LR, Dabis F, Rogier C, and McKinley T (1990) Quality of death certificates: studying or burying? *Am J Public Health* 80:751.

Scheib BT, Thompson ME, and Kerns TJ (1989) Federal influences on the development of trauma registries. *J Trauma* 29:835–841.

Short D, and Robertson, LS (1997) Motor vehicle death reductions from guardrail installation (mimeo).

Smith PF, Remington PL, Williamson DF, and Anda RF (1990) A comparison of alcohol sales data with survey data on self-reported alcohol use in 21 states. *Am J Public Health* 80:309–312.

Smith RJ (1988) IHS fellows program aimed at lowering injuries, death of Indians, Alaska natives. *Public Health Rep* 103:204.

Smith RJ, and Robertson LS (in press) Unintentional injuries and trauma. In Rhoades ER (ed), *The Health of American Indians and Alaska Natives.* Baltimore: Johns Hopkins University Press.

Smith SM, Colwell LS, and Sniezek JE (1990) An evaluation of external cause-of-injury codes using hospital records from the Indian Health Service, 1985. *Am J Public Health* 80:279–281.

Spiegel CN, and Lindaman FC (1977) Children can't fly: a program to prevent childhood morbidity and mortality from window falls. *Am J Public Health* 67:1143.

Streff FM (1994) Field effectiveness of two restraint systems: the 3-point manual belt versus the 2-point-motorized-shoulder, manual lap belt. *38th Annual Proceedings, Association for the Advancement of Automotive Medicine.*

Wechsler H, Dowdall GW, Davenport A, and Castillo S (1995) Correlates of college student binge drinking. *Am J Public Health* 85:921–926.

Wikstrom PH (1995) Preventing city-center street crimes. In Tonry M, and Farrington DP (eds), *Building a Safer Society: Strategic Approaches to Crime Prevention.* Chicago: University of Chicago Press.

Appendix 3–1
Motor Vehicle Injury Form

Community _____ Census tract _____
Location of the incident (specify road, street, or intersection and
distance to an identifiable reference point such as an intersection,
business, or milepost number)

_____

_____

_____

_____

Severity: _____ Fatal _____ Hospitalized _____ Ambulatory (fracture,
loss of consciousness only—exclude others)

Age _____   Gender: M _____ F _____
Single vehicle occupant

_____ Fixed object   If fixed object: _____ Tree _____ Utility pole

_____ Rollover   _____ Bridge abutment

_____ Both   _____ Light pole

_____ Animal on the road   _____ Sign pole _____ Other

                                    (What? _____)

Multiple vehicle occupant _____ Frontal _____ Side _____ Rear

Motorcyclist _____ Single vehicle _____ Multiple vehicle

Pedestrian _____ Cross intersection _____ Crossing elsewhere

            _____ Walking along road _____ Vehicle came off road

            _____ Laying in road _____ Other (What? _____)

Bicyclist   _____ Crossing intersection _____ Crossing elsewhere

            _____ On road parallel to traffic _____ On road

            against traffic _____ Motor vehicle came off road

            _____ Other (What? _____)

Lighting: _____ Daylight _____ Dark _____ Dark but lighted

_____ Dawn or dusk

Signals: _____ None _____ Flashing warnings

_____ Red-yellow-green _____ Stop sign

_____ Yield sign _____ Other (What? _____)

Crash protection: _____ Seat belt _____ Child restraint

_____ Crash helmet

Roadway jurisdiction: _____ City or town _____ County _____ State

_____ Federal

Modification that might have prevented the injury or reduced severity (check all that apply):

_____ No pass stripe   _____ Roadside hazard removal

_____ Rumble strips   _____ Signal or sign at intersection

_____ Lengthen yellow phase at signalized intersection

_____ Install or lengthen pedestrian walk signal

_____ Median barrier   _____ Reflectors on curve

_____ Snow removal   _____ Improve road skid resistance

_____ Separate pedestrian walkway from road

_____ Reflectors on vehicles or clothing

_____ Lighted roadway   _____ Curb to limit road access

_____ Other (What? _____)

_____ Additional observations

Appendix 3–2
Burn or Smoke Injury

Community _____ Census tract _____

Address _____

Severity: _____ Fatal _____ Hospitalized _____ Ambulatory (loss of
        consciousness and/or immobilization only—exclude others)

Age _____   Gender: M _____ F _____

Victim sleeping when fire began? _____ Yes _____ No

Place of fire: _____ Home _____ Car _____ Other (Where? _____)

If home, number of door exits to the home? _____

Location of the victim _____ Bedroom _____ Living room

                            _____ Bathroom _____ Kitchen

                            _____ Other (Where? _____)

Ignition or

heat origin: _____ Cigarette _____ Cooking unit

        _____ Woodburning space heater

        _____ Kerosene space heater

        _____ Other space heater _____ Chimney

        _____ Electrical wiring _____ Arson

        _____ Household water _____ Food or drink

        _____ Other (What? _____)

Material first ignited: _____ Chair or sofa _____ Bed

                _____ Loose papers

                _____ Clothing on person _____ Other clothing

                _____ House framing _____ Cooking grease

                _____ Other (What? _____)

If in a building, smoke detector installed? _____ Yes _____ No

      If yes, did detector give alarm? _____ Yes _____ No _____ NA

     Was a fire extinguisher available? _____ Yes _____ No

        If yes, was it used? _____ Yes _____ No _____ NA

Modification that might have reduced injury or severity: (check as many as apply)

_____ Additional exit   _____ Fire ladder

_____ Smoke detector   _____ Batteries in detector

_____ Fire extinguisher   _____ Sleeping nearer exits

_____ Fire-resistant clothing   _____ Fire-resistant furniture

_____ Fire-resistant mattress or sheets

_____ Automatic sprinkler system

_____ Properly installed cooking unit

_____ Properly installed wood stove

_____ Properly installed kerosene heater

_____ Cleaned chimney   _____ Reduced hot water temperature

_____ Less tip-prone food or drink container

_____ Other (What? _____)

_____ Additional observations

Appendix 3–3
Drowning or Near Drowning

Community _____ Census tract _____

Directions to location _____

_____

_____

Severity: _____ Fatal _____ Hospitalized _____ Ambulatory (loss of
consciousness only—exclude others)

Age _____ Gender: M _____ F _____

Victim know how to swim? _____ Yes _____ No

Water temperature at time of the incident? _____

Body of water involved: _____ Bathtub _____ Supervised beach

_____ Unsupervised beach _____ River nonbeach

_____ Lake nonbeach _____ Ocean nonbeach

_____ Irrigation ditch _____ Drainage ditch _____ Swimming pool

_____ Flood _____ Other (What? _____)

Watercraft involved: _____ None _____ Motorboat _____ Sailboat

_____ Surfsail _____ Rowboat _____ Canoe _____ Motorized raft

_____ Nonmotorized raft _____ Other (What? _____)

Preventive gear available: _____ Lifeline _____ Life jacket

_____ Floating cushion _____ Nonsinkable boat _____ Fenced area

_____ Flares _____ Boat-to-shore communication

_____ Other (What? _____)

Modifications that might have prevented the incident or reduced severity:

_____ Fenced swimming pool _____ Other fencing

_____ Lifeline _____ Life jacket _____ Floating cushion

_____ Nonsinkable boat _____ Supervised swimming area

_____ Flood warning and evacuation _____ Flare

_____ Boat-to-shore communication

_____ Other (What? _____)

_____ Additional observations

_____

Appendix 3-4
Injury From a Fall

Community _____ Census tract _____

Directions to the site _____

_____

_____

Severity: _____ Fatal _____ Hospitalized _____ Ambulatory (fracture, loss of consciousness only—exclude others)

Age _____   Gender: M _____ F _____

Type of fall: _____ Same level _____ Different level (approximate

number of feet _____)

Same level location: _____ Bathtub _____ Other bathroom

_____ Bedroom _____ Kitchen _____ Living room

_____ Basement _____ Attic _____ Home yard _____ Sidewalk

_____ Street _____ Public building _____ Private building

_____ Sports field _____ Other (Where? _____)

_____ Not applicable

Different level location: _____ Exterior stairs to house entrance

_____ Stairs to upper floors _____ Stairs to attic

_____ Stairs to basement _____ Stairs in public building

_____ Stairs in nonresidential private building

_____ Home porch or landing _____ Window _____ Roof

_____ Tree _____ Cliff or other dropoff _____ Ladder

_____ Horse

_____ Other (Explain _____

Modification that might have prevented injury or reduced severity:

_____ Skid strips in tub _____ Skid strips on stairs

_____ Nonskid rug _____ Nonskid shoes _____ Handrail

_____ Snow or ice clearance _____ Soft carpet

_____ Stair repairs _____ Fence or other barrier

_____ Sports equipment (What? _____)

_____ Other (What? _____)

_____ Additional observations

Appendix 3–5
Assault Injury

Community _____ Census tract _____

Directions to the site _____

_____

_____

Severity: _____ Fatal _____ Hospitalized _____ Ambulatory (fracture, loss of consciousness only—exclude others)

Age _____   Gender: M _____ F _____

Where did the assault occur? _____ Home _____ Other house

_____ Bar _____ Other business _____ Elsewhere

Assailant relation to the injured? _____ Spouse _____ Father

_____ Mother _____ Child _____ Sibling _____ Other relative

_____ Other family _____ Acquaintance _____ Stranger

_____ Unknown

Weapon used in the assault? _____ Body (fists, feet, etc.) _____ Gun

_____ Knife _____ Other sharp object _____ Blunt object

_____ Fire or heat _____ Poison

_____ Other (What? _____)

Apparent reason for the assault? _____ Rage _____ Robbery

_____ Mental illness _____ Other (What? _____)

Modification that might have prevented injury or reduced severity:

_____ Limit number of drinks purchasable in bars

_____ Metal detector at door of bar and refuse service to those armed with gun or knife

_____ Do not allow bottles that shatter as containers for alcoholic beverages

_____ Provide lighting in high-risk area

_____ Arrest of the assailant involved in previous incident

_____ Remove assailant from the home

_____ Remove person assaulted from the home

_____ Other (What? _____)

_____ Additional observations

Appendix 3–6
Self-inflicted Injury

Community _____ Census tract _____

Directions to site _____

_____

_____

Severity: _____ Fatal _____ Hospitalized _____ Ambulatory (fracture, loss of consciousness only—exclude others)

Age _____   Gender: M _____ F _____

Where did the attempt occur? _____ Home _____ Relative's home

_____ Other home _____ Jail _____ Other public building or business

_____ Out of doors _____ Other (Explain _____)

Weapon used: _____ Gun _____ Knife

_____ Other sharp instrument _____ Carbon monoxide

_____ Prescription drug _____ Other drug _____ Other poison

_____ Rope _____ Jump _____ Other (What? _____)

Circumstances: _____ Physical illness _____ Mental illness

_____ Copying recent real event _____ Copying television event

_____ Copying other fictional event _____ Financial loss

_____ Reaction to rejection by spouse or lover

_____ Reaction to difficulty with other family member

_____ Other (What? _____)

Modification that might have prevented injury or reduced

severity: _____ Encourage seeking of treatment for depression

_____ Increase awareness of depression symptoms in families and sources of help especially if friend or popular figure recently attempted suicide

_____ Encourage families with depressed members to limit access to guns, drugs, etc.

_____ Encourage families not to leave depressed members alone in circumstances or areas where previous suicide attempts occurred

_____ Reduce incarceration for nonserious offenses that result in jailhouse suicide attempts

_____ Increase surveillance of incarcerated persons

_____ Other (What? _____)

_____ Additional observations

Appendix 3–7
Other Severe Injury

(Use specified form for motor vehicles, drowning, fire, falls, assaults, and suicide attempts; this form is for other injuries that were hospitalizations, fatalities, and ambulatory cases that involved loss of consciousness, fractures, and worse conditions)

Community _____ Census tract _____

Directions to the site _____

_____

_____

Severity: _____ Fatal _____ Hospitalized _____ Ambulatory fracture
         or loss of consciousness

Age _____   Gender: M _____ F _____

Type of energy that caused the damage to the person:

_____ Mechanical _____ Heat or lack of heat _____ Chemical

_____ Electrical

What conveyed the energy to the person (be specific: e.g., if farm tractor, machine, or other product, give make, model, moving part that caused injury):

_____

_____

_____

_____

List as many strategies you can think of that could be employed to reduce the incidence or severity of this type of injury in the future:

_____

_____

_____ Additional observations

_____

4

CAUSAL ANALYSIS AND ITS USES

In a course on the use of epidemiology for injury control, the author asked the students, as part of an examination, what is wrong with this statement: "Alcohol is consistently associated with unintentional injury deaths, therefore alcohol abuse must be reduced to lower rates of death and disability due to injury." Only one in twenty came close to writing a correct answer, even though numerous instances to the contrary were noted throughout the course. Motor vehicle injuries, for example, have been reduced by improved vehicle crashworthiness, lighting dark sections of road, channelling traffic—without reducing alcohol or otherwise changing drivers.

In explaining the answer to the students, the statement was rewritten: "Gender is consistently related to injury, therefore gender must be changed to reduce injury." The nervous laughter, particularly from the gender often at higher risk (males), suggests that some might have understood the point.

The statement about alcohol on the exam was not original. It was published by prominent leaders in public health (Brown et al., 1990). It is part of the larger problem inherent in the assumption in much public health literature that specification of complex interaction of factors—sometimes called causal webs—is key to injury and disease reduction (Krieger, 1994). To the contrary, while the notion of the causal web may be useful to call attention to the complexities of multiple causation, it may disable our minds in thinking about prevention (Renwick, 1973).

The "public health model" is usually presented as follows: *(1)* identify the problem (surveillance); *(2)* identify risk factors; *(3)* develop and test interventions; *(4)* implement interventions and measure effectiveness (e.g., Powell et al., 1996). In fact, many interventions and therapies have been successful without the second step. One does not need to know the "risk factors" for a headache to use an analgesic. Focusing on multiple risk factors in causal webs may lead astray rather than toward injury control. When the New York Health Department did its study of children's fatal falls, what would have happened if the researchers had attempted an analysis of numerous risk factors that could contribute to children falling from windows, such as no adult present, intoxicated adults, numerous factors that distracted adults, and inquisitiveness, hyperactivity, or numerous other characteristics of children? Would there have been attempts to change those factors rather than install window barriers? If so, it is unlikely that the falls would have declined nearly to the extent produced by the window barriers.

Multiple causation of disease and injury, for which the causal web is the most common metaphor, is repeatedly demonstrated. It does not logically follow, however, that multifactorial theories or analyses lead to rational prevention policy. This was recognized in the original conceptualization of the "causal web" (McMahon et al., 1960), but it is commonly forgotten. Those of us who study injuries in the United States are not fond of metaphors regarding guns, but there were instances in which "magic bullets" were found despite multiple causation of infectious diseases (Evans, 1993).

If we have to deal with causal webs, perhaps we need a metaphor for something more effective than bullets against webs and spiders—like brooms. To Krieger's (1994) provocative question regarding causal webs: "Has anyone seen the spider?" should be added, "Has anyone seen the housekeepers with the preventive brooms?"

Proponents of the search for complex causes before consideration of preventive action argue that without understanding of causes, prevention may fail because of confounding factors or may have unintended consequences. *Confounding* refers to the attribution of risk to a factor that has little or no effect but is mistakenly thought to have an effect because it is correlated to a factor that is important.

In rare instances, confounding has misled preventive efforts and adverse "side effects" have also occurred, but the nature of certain types of causes is such that the potential for unintended consequences is minimized. Complete understanding is an elusive goal that is yet to be accomplished for most phenomena. How much, then, do we need to know for injury control?

To eliminate an injury, one need only find a controllable necessary condition for the injury, and control that condition. Even the least resilient of human anatomies can tolerate some mechanical energy load (commonly measured in pounds per square inch, kilograms per centimeter, etc.). In the road environment, any combination of energy management by vehicle components or the surrounding environment that keeps loads below that tolerance will eliminate injury. While energy management to that extent has not been accomplished, and may not be feasible in the extreme for economic or other reasons, substantial reduction in motor vehicle death rates occurred due to increased vehicle crashworthiness. There are claims of unintended consequences in increased risky driving by those protected, but these claims are not supported by the better research (Chapters 6 and 7).

Causal analysis of injury can inform preventive approaches when it specifies factors that are substantially changeable and that account for a proportion of a given type of injury and rules out factors that are spuriously correlated to injury. Attention to the nature of types of causes gives guidance to the extent that a given injury might be reduced if a given factor were changed.

In examining data on potential causes of injuries, it is useful to bear in mind the types of distributions that are found when conditions are necessary, sufficient, or contributing factors. Examples are shown in Tables 4.1 through 4.3 where the designation of 0 and "some" cases refers to a proportion of all cases in the table.

If A is a necessary condition for B, then B will not occur in the absence of A, and the joint distribution of A and B will look like that in Table 4.1 when the measurement of both is accurate. As noted in Chapter 1, keeping the height of playground equipment below the level that can produce enough energy in a fall to injure the heaviest users will eliminate such injury.

If A is sufficient for B, then B will always occur in the presence of A, but the absence of A does not imply the absence of B unless A is also necessary for B (Table 4.2). A competently used guillotine will behead anyone placed under it, but all beheadings are not by guillotine. Occupants of cars that run under trailers of tractor-trailer rigs are sometimes beheaded.

In Table 4.3, if the lower left and upper right cells were both zero, factor A would be both necessary and sufficient for B, but such effects are very rare. In Table 4.3 as shown, A increases the probability of B, and more cases of B are found in the presence of A, but A is neither necessary nor sufficient for B. Some people who drink and drive are not in crashes and many drivers in crashes have

TABLE 4.1. Distribution of Observations when A Is a Necessary Condition for B

	B	NOT B
A	Some	Some
Not A	0	Some

TABLE 4.2. Distribution of Observations when A Is a
Sufficient Condition for B

	B	NOT B
A	Some	0
Not A	Some	Some

not consumed alcohol, so alcohol is a contributing factor, neither necessary nor sufficient to cause a crash.

Since prevention of a necesary condition for harm completely reduces the harm, the more closely the distribution of injuries of a given type and severity (B) in relation to the presence of some factor (A) resembles the distribution in Table 4.1, the greater the number of such injuries that will be prevented if A is eliminated.

CRITERIA FOR CAUSATION

The old Henle–Koch criteria for attributing causes to infectious diseases required that a microorganism or other factor be found both necessary and sufficient to produce a given infectious disease, but clearly those criteria were too stringent. Many microorganisms were found necessary but not sufficient for the infection to occur (Kelsey et al., 1986). Nevertheless, by controlling the microorganism, its access to the host, or host resistance, the disease could be controlled. Similarly, as noted in Chapter 1, an energy exchange with the human organism is a necessary and specific condition for injury, but the degree of the energy exchange necessary in individual cases may vary by the nature of the tissues affected, which makes them more or less tolerant of energy insults. Nevertheless, if the energy exchange can be kept below the tolerance of the most vulnerable tissue, injury will not occur. Where it is not possible to reduce energy exchanges to that degree, it is nevertheless possible to greatly reduce severity by reducing energy exchanges.

Several criteria must be met for a strong inference of causation. First, the cause must precede the effect in time. For example, a study of alcohol mea-

TABLE 4.3. Distribution of Observations when A Increases the
Probability of B

	B	NOT B
A	More	Some
Not A	Some	More

sured in the breath of emergency room patients found that some claimed to have consumed alcohol after the injury (Wechsler et al., 1969). In those cases, if true, alcohol could have not contributed to the incidence, although it might affect recovery.

Second, the hypothesized cause must be correlated to the effect, that is, they must have joint distributions similar to one of those in Tables 4.1 through 4.4, or in the case of noncategorical variables such as blood alcohol concentration, there should be a dose–response covariation. The cliché among some scientists that "correlation doesn't mean causation" is not precise. Correlation is a necessary but not sufficient condition for inference of causation.

The absence of correlation does not totally rule out causation if measurement is unreliable, biased, or invalid or if other factors intervene in such a way as to mask the correlation. Occasionally claims of lack of correlation are disproved when better research designs controlling for other factors are used (e.g., Zador et al., 1984). In other cases, the effect may be under- or overestimated for lack of control of relevant factors. For example, the National Highway Traffic Safety Administration estimated that placement of fuel tanks in front of rear axles of passenger cars reduced fatal rear impact fires by 29 percent (Tessmer, 1994). The analysis did not account for the fact that cars were being reduced in size during the period that gas tanks were being relocated. When vehicle size and tank location were considered simultaneously in a multivariate analysis, forward-located tanks were found to reduce rear fire fatalities by more than half (Robertson, 1993).

Third, the correlation must be demonstrated as large enough, given the numbers of observations in the sample, that it is unlikely to have occurred from random fluctuations in drawing samples of that size. If the sample size is too small, however, a causal connection may be falsely rejected. Statistical power is a function of sample size. Studies often lack a large enough sample to detect magnitudes of covariation that would have practical use if detected. Textbooks in statistics contain criteria for sampling and tests for random fluctuation in samples (e.g., Armitage, 1971; Selvin, 1991). Certain computer programs used for data entry and statistical calculations include features for estimating statistical power before a study is undertaken (e.g., Dean et al., 1994).

Fourth, the research design must be adequate to rule out covariation between the hypothesized cause and other factors that could explain the same variation or to specify how such covariation represents a causal sequence. This is the previously mentioned problem of confounding. Many research projects that demonstrate a nonrandom correlation between A and B are criticized by saying: "You didn't control for X." The criticism may be legitimate if X could reasonably be expected to affect both A and B strongly enough to account for their correlation, but some such criticisms have no basis in terms of plausible causal mechanisms or potential magnitude of the effect.

Fifth, the mechanism of the causation should be plausible in terms of what is known about the phenomena in the relevant discipline. Occasionally the theories of physics, chemistry, biology, or behavior are revolutionized by some seemingly implausible research finding, but far more often such a finding is subsequently shown to be the result of faulty research methodology.

CAUSAL MODELS

The more plausible hypotheses are those that are deduced from what is known. Some important discoveries occur as a result of hypotheses based on hunches, observations of a few cases in a clinic or morgue, and the like, but the odds of finding something useful are greater when the hypothesis to be tested provides a link in a causal model.

In the case of injury, a hypothesis is more plausible if the proposed cause has a likely connection to the concentration of energy, an energy exchange with tissue, or the vulnerability of tissue. If the hypothesized cause could not directly affect one or more of these factors, it is likely to be a relatively weak and indirect contributor to the incidence or severity of injury. To aid thinking about the research that is needed to fill gaps in knowledge, a diagram of the hypothesized causal paths of a given set of injuries is often useful.

For example, it is well known that age is correlated to severe motor vehicle injuries, but age is merely a measure of how often one has circled the sun. While age indicates differential risk that can be used to target injury control efforts, it is not a cause of injury. Age is an inexact proxy measure of human limitations and behaviors, including exposure to more or less risky energy sources (knowingly or unknowingly) that result in concentration of energy or energy exchanges, and physical conditions that affect tissue vulnerability.

Correlating such factors as age and sex to injury rates has been called "black box" epidemiology (Susser and Susser, 1996). Without precise knowledge of the exposures to energy and behaviors in the presence of those exposures, by age and sex, the causal mechanisms involved are lumped in a box, the contents of which are unknown.

Figure 4.1 illustrates some possible paths of causation whereby correlates of age may contribute to the necessary and specific causes of motor vehicle–occupant injury or severity. The direction of the arrows represents the known or hypothesized direction of effect of a given factor on another.

An energy exchange with vulnerable tissue results from energy generated by speed and mass necessary for the damage of vulnerable tissue and insufficient room for vehicle occupants to decelerate as indicated by vehicle size. The power of an engine, measured as horsepower in given increments, is necessary for given increments in speed. Vehicle size and horsepower account for about

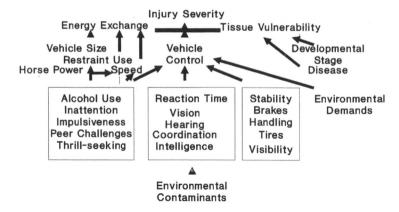

FIGURE 4.1. A model of motor vehicle injury.

55 percent of the variation in occupant fatalities per 100,000 passenger cars of particular makes and models (Robertson, 1991). Observations of age, sex, and speed of drivers at sites where vehicles rolled over indicated that younger drivers were driving faster than the average speed at the sites, but there was no correlation of speed and sex. Age, however, was not correlated with rollover and speed was not correlated to vehicle stability. Therefore, the effect of vehicle stability on rollover cannot be confounded by speeding or young drivers (Robertson & Maloney, 1997).

Loss of control of one or more vehicles usually precedes a crash. Loss of control is affected by vehicle stability, steering characteristics, braking capacity, and tire characteristics in interaction with inputs from the driver—speed, steering, braking. Vehicle stability accounts for about 62 percent of the variation in fatal rollover crashes per 100,000 utility vehicles, independent of other major known risk factors. These vehicles have stability less than the vast majority of cars (Robertson, 1989).

Inputs to the vehicle by the driver are modified by impairment or other effects of alcohol and other drugs as well as variations in human limitations such as reaction times (time from signal of need to change inputs to actual behavior), vision, hearing, intelligence, and coordination of senses and motor function. The effect of each is not known precisely and is more or less contingent on the demands of the driving environment. Therefore, the extent of reductions in injuries that could be achieved by changing the factors that are changeable is in more or less doubt for each one. The other listed behavioral factors may affect speed, reaction time, steering or braking, and degree of vehicle use, but how often is largely unknown. Factors related to age may also affect tissue vulnerability including developmental stages, alcohol or other drugs, and certain diseases.

As depicted in Figure 4.1, the effects of given variables are in straightforward causal chains, but some of the links among factors may be more complicated. Although the effect of alcohol is usually referred to as impairment, there are several aspects of the correlation of alcohol and injuries that suggest a more complex causal pattern. Alcohol in drivers in motor vehicle crashes is more highly correlated to injury severity than to incidence (Haddon et al., 1968). Alcohol is found more often in the victims of assault and homicide than in drivers killed in motor vehicle crashes (Baker et al., 1971; Wechsler et al., 1969). Therefore, it is unlikely that the effect of alcohol is just to impair performance or make tissue more vulnerable. Based on these and other findings, a more elaborate model of alcohol use and its effects has been suggested (Robertson, 1983), as displayed in Figure 4.2.

In biological systems, the system goes out of control when there is positive feedback, that is, factor a increases factor b, which in turn increases factor a directly or through its effect on other factors. In the model, alcohol use is hypothesized as partly a consequence of inherited biological factors that affect emotions that may then contribute to increased drinking in an uncontrolled feedback. If such feedback occurs, the individual effects in the loop do not have to be large to have an enormous effect in a few iterations. For example, if $b = 1.02a$, $c = 1.03b$, and $a = 1.02c$, the three factors will about double in 10 cycles and about quadruple in 20 cycles.

If the alcohol model is supported by research evidence, then elimination of alcohol might not eliminate all of the injuries with which it is associated. The emotions that contributed to drinking may also contribute to the behaviors leading to injuries and would be present in the absence of alcohol, albeit to a lesser degree (McClelland, 1984). Chapter 7 includes an analysis that indicates that removal of all alcohol from drivers would reduce fatal crashes about half the

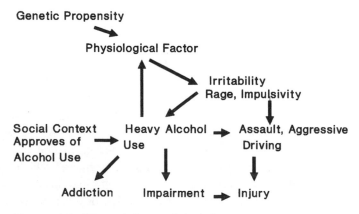

FIGURE 4.2. A general theory of alcohol.

amount presumed from data on alcohol "involvement." Too often, the human mind converts "involved" to "caused."

This dynamic model of the causes and consequences of alcohol use is more comprehensive regarding the possible reasons for the involvement of alcohol in assaults as well as other injuries, and for eventual alcohol addiction. It suggests that if the physiological factor possibly intervening between the genes and increased use can be identified and controlled, a variety of problems would be alleviated.

These are relatively simple examples of causal models. Numerous variations have been suggested just for driver factors in motor vehicle injury (Michon, 1985). The value of a model is not necessarily its complexity or completeness, but whether it suggests testable hypotheses regarding variables that have a major influence, particularly variables that are controllable for injury prevention or severity reduction.

STUDY DESIGNS

The choice of study designs to investigate a given set of factors is affected by numerous considerations. What is the unit of analysis (people, vehicles, environments)? In what population should the study be conducted? To what population of people, vehicles, or environments will the results be generalizable? What measurements of the factors are available or could be obtained? How reliable and valid are the measurements? Can the data be collected without violating ethical guidelines? How can the study isolate the effects of given factors independent of, or in combination with, other relevant factors? How much time will be needed to complete the study? How much will the study cost?

No single study will specify degree of effect of all the factors in a causal model. The goal of a prevention-oriented research project is to specify the extent to which injury or injury severity would be reduced by changing a given factor hypothesized to contribute to the injury or severity, other things being equal. A study design should be chosen that eliminates or minimizes the probability that factors other than the changeable factor of interest somehow bias that estimate.

Students of epidemiology are familiar with the general descriptive terms that are used to describe study designs, but they are noted here for readers unfamiliar with them. A *cohort* is a sample or population of units of analysis on which the researcher collects data continuously or periodically over a period of time. In a *retrospective study,* the researcher attempts to obtain data on a cohort accumulated in the past. In a *prospective study,* the data are gathered for a period of time after the fact of the generation of hypotheses and identification of the cohort to be studied.

Controlled experiments

The most definitive results of research are produced by data gathered prospectively in controlled experiments. That design requires that the researcher has control of one or more hypothesized causal factors, at least to the extent of being able to assign units of analysis (people, vehicles, environments) to experimental and control groups. The assignment is randomized such that effects of other factors on injury or other relevant outcomes are random.

The controlled experiment is appealing not only because it maximizes the confidence that other factors are equalized by random assignment; it also illustrates that the causal factor in question is controllable, although control in an experiment does not necessarily imply that control is possible to the same degree in the natural occurrence of the factor of interest.

If the experimental manipulation of a given variable has more than an extremely remote possibility of increasing injury, ethics dictate that the experiment should not be conducted. For example, most researchers would not consider an experiment in which drivers in the experimental group would be given alcohol and then sent out to drive in traffic, although a few such studies have been conducted on environmentally benign driving ranges or roads without other traffic.

The effects of alcohol on various behaviors, including driving in environments simulated by motion pictures and other devices, have been studied by controlled experimental designs. These studies have specified the effects of alcohol on impairment of various behaviors—reaction time and steering, for instance—and on certain emotions (e.g., Loomis & West, 1958). Apparently no experiment has yet been undertaken to disaggregate the effects of alcohol and emotions, separately and in combination, on behaviors highly predictive of injury.

The generalizability of laboratory experiments to the "real world" can always be questioned. Use of experimental and control groups stratified on other factors (e.g., age, sex, impulsiveness) not only allows the researcher to test for effects of combinations of factors, but also addresses the issue of generalizability to segments of the population. Such more complicated experimental designs increase both the numbers of persons (or other units of analysis) needed for statistical power and the associated costs of the research. A textbook on experimental designs should be consulted regarding varieties of designs for efficiency and statistical power.

Case–control studies

A study design that can approximate the conditions of a controlled experiment is the case–control design. A case may be an injured person, a vehicle that rolled over, a section of road where a vehicle hit a tree, and so on. The analogous controls would be persons not injured, vehicles that did not roll over, sections of road that the vehicle traversed without hitting trees. The research question is how relevant individual, vehicle, or environmental factors differ between cases and controls. The controls may be matched on certain factors (age, sex, time, place, etc.) or unmatched.

For example, the important role of alcohol in motor vehicle injuries was demonstrated by case–control studies (e.g., Haddon et al., 1961). Alcohol was measured in fatally injured pedestrians and in randomly selected persons at the same places, walking at the same time of day, same day of week, and moving in the same direction as the fatally injured. Therefore, these environmental factors were the same for the cases and controls and could not account for the large differences in alcohol found in the cases and controls. The same design was also used with drivers as the unit of analysis (McCarroll & Haddon, 1962).

One way of studying the alcohol issues in Figure 4.2 would be to replicate these case–control studies and measure hypothesized biological factors that might contribute to alcohol use, other behaviors, or both jointly. Two major problems would be encountered in such a study. First, while measurement of alcohol in breath samples of controls may be allowed by sufficient numbers of persons selected as controls, requests for blood or other biological specimens might not be acceptable. Second, good evidence that trauma does not change the hypothesized biological factor is necessary before assuming that a difference between cases and controls is indicative of causation.

Selection of people engaged in the same activity at the same site, time of day, day of week, and so on, may not be possible for activities that occur at the case sites infrequently, such as use of all-terrain vehicles or snowmobiles. A child injured in a home may have no siblings close enough in age to serve as controls within the household, although children in reasonable proximity in the same neighborhoods may serve as controls depending on the factors of interest. For example, children who were killed in a cluster of unsolved child homicides were compared to children from the same neighborhood regarding potential risk factors. Several factors indicative of greater exposure (time and specific hours away from home alone, running errands for money) were identified as placing the killed children at greater risk (Goodman et al., 1988).

Within-household controls are inappropriate if the hypothesized hazard is common to all members of the household. A study of risk of having a gun in a household, for example, used households in the surrounding neighborhood of those with a fatal shooting as controls, and statistically controlled for such factors as illicit drug use and a history of physical fights. The study documented that gun ownership increased the risk of homicide, given the same history of drug use and fighting (Kellerman et al., 1993).

The selection of controls in case–control studies requires careful thought, and measurement of certain factors retrospectively can be quite problematic. In clinical situations, it is tempting to select controls from patients who have arrived at the same clinic or hospital for reasons other than injury. If the hypothesized causal factor contributes in some way to problems other than injury that lead people to seek medical care, however, the comparison of cases and controls will underestimate the contribution of that factor to injury. If the hypothesized causal factor is reduced by factors that also led to the seeking of medical care, the effect of that factor would be overestimated.

For example, a study of alcohol in emergency room patients compared those injured to those who appeared for illnesses (Wechsler et al., 1969). Since we do not know the effect of the mix of illnesses seen in such clinics on alcohol use or the effect of alcohol use on seeking medical care for injury or illness, the extent of over- or underestimation of alcohol's effect on injury is uncertain from such a comparison. If alcohol contributes to the problem presented by the control patients or to the probability of seeking medical attention, the difference in alcohol measured between cases and controls could be less than if persons exposed to the circumstances of injury who had no reason to seek medical attention were chosen as controls. If the medical condition is such that the control patient would not have been engaged in activities similar to that of the injured person, the effect of aspects of those activities would be overestimated.

One study used people who died of other causes as controls to emphasize the overinvolvement of people in certain occupations in motor vehicle deaths (Loomis, 1991). Since the controls are just as dead as the cases, the usefulness of such a study for preventing death is ephemeral.

Even worse is a survey of people who were involved in motor vehicle crashes and a random sample of licensed drivers not involved in crashes as to frequency of use of cellular phones (Violenti & Marshall, 1996). No determination was made of whether the phone was in use when the driver crashed, much less cellular phone use at the same times and places. A later study that more precisely specified phone use in proximity to the time of the crash from records of phone calls suggested an increased risk of motor vehicle crashes related to phone use in cars (Redelmeier & Tibslirani, 1997).

The fundamental issue in selection of cases and controls is: What should be allowed to vary as the hypothesized cause, or causes in stratified samples, and what should be held constant? If the variables to be held constant can be other than randomly distributed between cases and controls, the purpose of the design is defeated. If the factor or factors allowed to vary as causes are not directly connected to injury or are unchangeable, the study is a waste of limited resources for research.

Collection of retrospective data on cases and controls also presents numerous problems. In assault cases, it may not be possible to identify the assailant or, if identified, the assailant may not cooperate or may falsify information. If a person is injured in a neighborhood, controls who have knowledge of the injury may give misleading information because of denial of personal vulnerability or other psychological factors. Even if data can be obtained by observation, such as by watching children engaging in the activity involved in the case, knowledge of the injury may have resulted in changes in participation in the activity.

The human host or vector (assaulted person, driver) has been the unit of analysis in most case–control studies, to the neglect of factors that may be more subject to change for injury control. Case–control designs can also provide strong evidence regarding vehicle and environmental factors.

For example, advocates of the use of tractor-trailer trucks with more than one trailer argued that their use presented less risk because the crash rates per vehicle were similar, but fewer trucks were used because each carried more cargo per trip. A case–control study of trucks in crashes and trucks observed at the same time of day, on the same roads, moving in the same direction, revealed that two-trailered trucks were two to three times more likely to crash in the same environment, more than offsetting the advantage of carrying increased cargo (Stein & Jones, 1988).

In a study of environmental factors in motor vehicle crashes, the driver and vehicle can serve as their own controls. For example, the characteristics of crash sites where occupants of vehicles died striking fixed objects along the roadside were compared to sites one mile away in the direction from which the vehicle traveled. Since the driver and vehicle factors presumably did not change in a mile, those factors were virtually constant at the case and comparison sites. The substantial differences in road curvature and gradient of the road, coupled with no difference in number of potential objects along the road, indicated that environmental modifications would greatly reduce the severity of fixed-object crashes at sites with the identified characteristics (Wright & Robertson, 1976).

Subsequent research using this study design found excess involvement of similar road characteristics in off-road rollover fatalities (e.g., Wright & Zador, 1981), vehicles running into water leading to occupant drownings (Wintemute et al., 1990), and multiple-vehicle crashes at other than intersections (Fulgham et al., 1989). Since two vehicles were involved in the latter study, two control sites were studied for each case, one each a mile in the direction from which the vehicle traveled.

The power of case–control designs is sometimes poorly understood by those in a position to disseminate the results. For example, the specification of curvature and grade characteristics as road conditions that can be used to target sites for modification is ignored by federal road authorities. *Public Roads* is a Federal Highway Administration publication that circulates to the officials who decide where, when, and how roads are to be built or modified. Articles on a decision-making system called the "Interactive Highway Safety Design Model" (Lum & Reagan, 1995; Reagan, 1994) contained no information on curvature and grade criteria established by the mentioned case–control studies. When the editor of *Public Roads* was informed of this in 1996, he refused to publish material on the issue.

Retrospective cohort studies

The more removed in time of data gathered retrospectively, the greater the problems in measurement. Occasionally one may be able to use extant records, such as school records, arrest records, or motor vehicle records, to obtain direct or proxy measures of certain variables. The most common source of data in retrospective studies is interview or questionnaire, but the steepness of the for-get curve and the tendency for people to recreate their histories to foster a more favorable image severely limit the validity of recalled information. For example, in a study of people in motor vehicle crashes involving injury that was reported to police, persons involved were interviewed at different time periods following the incident. The percentage of interviewees who reported the injury declined from 97 percent in the first 3 months to 73 percent 9–12 months after the crash (National Center for Health Statistics, 1972). More frequent but less severe injuries may be thought too trivial to mention or may be forgotten. Comparison of weekly fall reports among the elderly and recall at the end of the year indicated significant underreporting at year's end (Cummings et al., 1988).

Where specific measures of variables worthy of study have been obtained in a cohort in the past, and it is possible to obtain data on subsequent injury, a retrospective cohort study may be less costly than a prospective study. For example, a cohort of children was studied at the time they were shedding their baby teeth. Concentration of lead in the teeth was measured as well as academic achievement, reaction times, and several other aspects of psychomotor performance. Also, teachers' behavioral ratings of various behaviors (distractable, hyperactive, impulsive) that might increase risk of injury were obtained (Needleman et al., 1979). If the subsequent clinical records of these children could be identified, the extent of the correlation of relevant factors to subsequent injuries might be studied. Such a study would require tracing those that had moved and checking reliability of reported clinical facilities used.

Prospective cohort studies

The likelihood of collecting reliable and valid data is much better when data are collected prospectively in a cohort of relevant units of analysis and the cohort is followed to measure the incidence and severity of the outcomes of interest. A major disadvantage of this design is that very large samples and a long period of data collection are required to obtain statistical power when the outcome is relatively rare.

For example, in the United States, the annual hospitalized or fatal injury rate from motor vehicles is about 300 per 100,000 population for males and less than 200 per 100,000 population for females. If one could obtain data on hypothesized causes in a cohort of 100,000 people representative of the population, it would take nearly four years of data collection to obtain data on 1000 injury cases. Controlling statistically for several factors would spread the cases very thinly among the various combinations of factors. The numbers of cases identified would be increased if less severe injuries were included but, as noted previously, the causes of less severe injuries are often different from causes of more severe injuries. In the case of motor vehicles, for example, the causes of low-speed "fenderbenders," which occur more often during the day in congested traffic, are often different from the causes of severe and fatal injuries which occur disproportionately at night, at higher speeds, and in little—often no—traffic.

A prospective cohort design may be efficient for study of certain age groups with higher injury rates. For example, about one in five newly licensed 16-year-old drivers will have a motor vehicle crash resulting in injury or more than $400 in property damage within two years. If reliable and valid data on the behavioral factors and abilities in Figure 4.1 could be obtained from 16 year olds in several high schools, and their licensure, vehicle use, and crash experience could be measured in a subsequent two year period, the data might provide better specification of the magnitude of the hypothesized paths in the model for that age group. In communities with a substantial dropout rate before age 16, however, the generalizability of the findings would be limited. Also, follow-up of those students who leave home or whose families move would be difficult.

An interesting example of a prospective cohort study involves the extent to which people who used tranquilizers (benzodiazepines) were treated for injury. Using claims from a health insurance plan, researchers compared the injury claims for 4554 persons less than 65 years old who had a pharmacy claim for tranquilizers during a nine month period, but not during the preceding three months, to a sample of persons who did not have a claim for tranquilizer use and were unrelated to the users. Three nonusers were matched to each user by age, sex, and calendar month when tranquilizer use began.

One obvious question is whether any difference in injury rates is the result of factors that precipitated the perceived need for tranquilizers rather than the possible effect of the drugs. Also, the use of the drugs could at least partly be the result of postinjury anxiety. The researchers found that injury claims were substantially higher in the user group in the three months prior to prescription of the drug. Therefore, comparison of the rate of injury while the users were using the drug was controlled statistically for preuse injury rate, as well as general care-seeking and use of mental health services. The relative risk of hospitalization for injury to those who had no injury in the three months prior to prescription of the drug was higher than for the total study group (Oster et al., 1990). Apparently, neither prior injury nor discretionary use of medical services totally accounted for the higher injury rates of tranquilizer users.

Cross-sectional studies

A cross-sectional study involves measurement of relevant variables in a sample of appropriate units of analysis during a specified time period. The effect of a given factor is estimated by the direction and degree of its correlation to the outcome of interest. The validity of the inference of causation depends on assumptions about the time order of the variables and the extent and pattern of covariation among the factor of interest and other factors.

Suppose that a researcher obtained measures of some or all of the behavioral factors in Figure 4.1 in a series of drivers hospitalized for injury and correlated them to relevant circumstances of the injury. The data indicate that attention spans are shorter and impulsiveness is more frequent among drivers who ran off the road and hit fixed objects than in drivers who were struck from behind. Since the presence of subclinical brain injuries may be different in the two sets of drivers, and such injuries could affect attention spans or impulsiveness, the inference that these factors were present in the degree measured prior to the crashes would be questionable.

Cross-sectional studies also do not provide definitive evidence of causation when there is covariation among hypothesized causal factors. If A is correlated to B, but X is also correlated to A and B, there are several possibilities. A could cause X, which causes B. X could cause A, which causes B. The three variables could be intertwined in a feedback system. Also, the correlation could be spurious. This happens when X causes A and B independently, and there is no causal relationship between A and B. Again, that is what epidemiologists call "confounding."

Some of these possibilities can be ruled out by reasonable assumptions about the time sequence of the factors, or whether the X factor can reasonably be expected to play a causal role. For example, when researchers examined the rollover rates of certain utility vehicles (Jeeps, Broncos, Blazers), they inferred from physics that the higher rollover rates of these vehicles relative to cars was the result of differences in stability—the g force to overturn the vehicle—calculated by the width between the center of the tires divided by twice the height of center of gravity (Snyder et al., 1980). Road tests of the least stable vehicle, the Jeep CJ-5 driven by remote control, indicated that it would roll over in low-speed turns (Insurance Institute for Highway Safety, 1980). A critic of the research claimed that the higher rollover rates of lower stability vehicles could have occurred because of differences in mileage or use by higher risk drivers or in higher risk environments (Joksch, 1983).

Since the rollover rates of the least stable utility vehicles were 3–20 times those of cars, the argument that mileage could account for the difference was unreasonable. The least stable vehicles would have to have been driven more miles in a year than most vehicles are driven in their average ten years of use for their rates to be the result of more miles of use (Robertson & Kelley, 1989). Also, other risk factors would contribute to all types of crashes—hitting trees and poles, hitting other vehicles—yet the stability factor was strongly correlated to rollover rates, but hardly at all to nonrollover rates.

Since miles of use by particular drivers in particular environments was unknown, it was not possible to correlate rates of rollover and other types of crashes in relation to use of the vehicles by particular drivers in particular environments. By using a mathematical model of the potential relationship of proportional mortality of higher and lower risk drivers and environments, however, it was possible to rule out other factors as an explanation of the correlation of stability and rollover.

If stability were correlated to different use of the vehicles by low- and high-risk drivers or in low- and high-risk environments, the ratio of rollover crashes under low-risk conditions to those under high-risk conditions would be a function of the ratio of mileage in low- and high-risk conditions and therefore should be correlated to stability. Stated mathematically:

$$c \frac{L}{H} = \frac{RL}{RH} = b(S)$$

where

$$L = \text{low exposure to a risk factor}$$
$$H = \text{high exposure to a risk factor}$$
$$c = \text{constant ratio of risk from low- to high-risk factor}$$
$$RL = \text{fatal rollovers in low-risk–factor situations}$$
$$RH = \text{fatal rollovers in high-risk–factor situations}$$
$$b = \text{slope of the correlation}$$
$$S = \text{stability value for a given vehicle}$$

Using data from the Fatal Accident Reporting System (FARS) for several years, RL/RH was not significantly correlated to vehicle stability for any of the major driver or environmental risk factors, except whether or not the vehicle rolled over on or off the road. The ratio of on-road to off-road rollovers was higher the less stable the vehicle. This suggests that the side force of turning contributed more often to those rollovers, since ramping or going over embankments would usually occur off the road (Robertson, 1989).

Although data on every possible risk factor are not included in FARS, there are none excluded that could be correlated to stability, and exclusively to rollover crashes, strongly enough to render the strong correlation of stability and rollover as spurious. Furthermore, the correlation of stability and rollover has causal plausibility. It is predicted from well-known physics.

Where major variables are unmeasured or are intercorrelated without a clear indication of time sequence, a cross-sectional study cannot be definitive in specifying causal chains. One useful function of cross-sectional studies is to indicate maximum magnitude of a given correlation. If the correlation of a hypothesized causal factor and the type, severity, or risk of injury is weak or nonexistent in a cross-sectional study, it is unlikely to be found a major factor in a study with a more powerful design unless the cross-sectional study includes invalid or biased measurement.

Using logical assumptions about the time sequence of variables in a causal model, it may be possible to analyze cross-sectional data in ways that enhance confidence in the degree of contribution of particular hypothesized causal chains. Social scientists have developed methods for such analyses of what they call causal paths using regression for quantitative variables (Blalock, 1964) and comparison of proportions and loglinear techniques for categorical data (Hellevik, 1984). These models are highly sensitive to assumptions of direction of causation and variable specification, however.

An example of misuse of "causal path analysis" is an attempt to discredit the studies of vehicle stability and rollover using police reports from Michigan and Florida. Unable to find behavioral and environmental factors that explained the variance attributable to stability, the authors of the study included "single-vehicle accident" as a "cause" in the model (Donelson et al., 1994). Since the majority of rollovers of lower stability vehicles occur when the vehicle rolls rather than slides to the side, collisions with other vehicles are less frequent than in nonrollovers. Also, "single-vehicle accident" does not mean that no other vehicle was involved. In some instances, the driver is making a sharp turn to avoid a collision with another vehicle. In multiple-vehicle crashes, it is not possible to specify which vehicle rolled in the Florida data. Therefore, the vehicles may have been misclassified as well.

Attribution of lack of collision with another vehicle as a cause of the rollover should have been obviously absurd to the authors and those who reviewed the paper prior to publication. The lack of reference in the paper to any of the previous research on rollover should have been a signal of ethical lapse and bias as well.

Ecological studies

Frequently one can easily obtain data on injuries in geographical areas and correlate the rates to other characteristics of those geographical areas obtained from other sources. For example, one might correlate injury rates per population in states or counties to census data on incomes, housing characteristics, and the like, in those counties. The correlations obtained are called ecological correlations.

A major problem with causal inferences from ecological correlations is that the hypothesized causal factor, or the factors that are controlled statistically, may not have occurred in the same unit of analysis as the effect (Robinson, 1950). Under certain conditions, inference to individual behavior can be estimated from aggregated data, but the range of potential error in the estimates is quite variable (King, 1997). If motor vehicle occupant injuries were found higher in low-income areas, that doesn't necessarily mean that persons with low income are any more likely to be the persons in severe crashes in those areas. The roads in low-income areas could be more hazardous because of lack of funds to maintain them, upgrade them, or remove hazards. They may be equally hazardous to all vehicle occupants irrespective of individual income.

The usefulness of ecological correlations depends on the interpretation. If the correlation were used as justification to modify the roads in the lower income areas, the injury rate may be reduced if the modifications chosen are effective. If the data are used to argue against action on the grounds that poverty is intractable, they are a hindrance to action.

Almost as silly as correlating motorcycle crash rates over time with number of robins in the environment over time is work on correlations of unemployment and fatal crash rates by statisticians at the National Highway Traffic Safety Administration (NHTSA). Fluctuations in total number of deaths are almost perfectly correlated inversely with fluctuations in unemployment, corrected for the 1974 oil boycott (e.g., Hedlund, 1984). Stress theories would predict greater risk per mile driven among the unemployed. Indeed, when rural mileage is entered into a multivariate equation with unemployment and fatalities per population, the inverse correlation between unemployment and the fatal rate reverses, that is, there is a higher fatality rate per population when the unemployment rate is high (Leigh & Waldon, 1991). Even if the NHTSA study held up under scrutiny, at the individual level unemployment is likely to account for only a small proportion of fatal crashes and few would advocate increased unemployment as a policy to reduce motor vehicle injuries.

The statistical technique (regression) used by NHTSA finds the line or curve that best describes the extent to which one factor predicts another. Regression coefficients indicate the increase (or decrease if minus) in a unit of the outcome variable per unit of the predictor variable. Correlation is how closely the data fit the line or curve, one if the fit is perfect and zero if the relationship between the variables is random scatter.

Correlation of aggregated data, such as injury rates and the economy, gives falsely high correlations. Year-to-year fluctuations in aggregated rates vary narrowly compared to the magnitude of the total rate above zero. The correlation is based not on the range of possible rates given combinations of driver, vehicle, and environmental factors, but on the marginal fluctuation of rates that fluctuate with the economy not accounting for the base rate maintained by the presence of the other factors. A regression equation with greater disaggregation of these factors is discussed in Chapter 7.

Ecological studies can be used to estimate the effects of changes in factors that affect a set of ecological units as a whole, such as changes in laws among states or other legal jurisdictions. For the results of such studies to be valid, the researcher must be able to specify that the change in law or other factor applied to the particular units of analysis associated with the injuries. As will be noted in Chapter 6, cross-sectional studies using ecological data have been especially misleading in that regard. Ecological studies are more convincing when a change in injury rates over time is shown to occur coincident with a change in law or other factor during a period in which other factors did not change appreciably.

Mixed designs

Many studies do not fit into a neat classification of study designs. The efficacy of a study design is not whether it can be easily classified, but whether it reveals usable information without substantial bias. It is better to describe the study procedure and the efforts made to account for bias rather than state that the study followed some design classification that may not be totally accurate in its implication for the procedures followed (Cummings et al., 1990).

DATA ANALYSIS

The analysis of data from a research project is substantially determined by the types of variables involved and the study design. Familiarity with the use and interpretation of various statistics appropriate to particular types of data and study designs is essential for data analysis and report preparation. Students and researchers in epidemiology should be familiar with statistical procedures (e.g., Armitage, 1971; Fleiss, 1981; Hellevik, 1984; Riegelman, 1981; Selvin, 1991), and those who are not should consult a statistician in the design stage of a research project. The best statistician in the world cannot produce some magical statistical trick to rescue what the study design has ignored or biased. Here a few basic principles and comparisons of analytical methods are reviewed as a basis for consideration of issues that commonly arise.

One consideration that is often ignored is the requirements of a given journal. Some journals require confidence intervals on estimates of percentages, rates, regression coefficients, rate ratios, odds ratios, and so on, rather than probabilities (p values) that an estimate could be the result of chance fluctuation in samples. Time and trouble can be saved by deciding, before analyzing data and writing the report, where the report will be submitted and checking out the requirements and style of the target publication.

Another consideration is the potential use of the results. Table 4.4 presents several measures used in summarizing the correlation of categorical data with two categories of each variable (partly from Abramson, 1985). There are obviously more potential measures of association of numbers in the table than there are numbers in the table. The statistic(s) to be used depends on the potential uses of the data.

If the results have potential for use in screening persons, vehicles, or environments for some intervention to reduce injury, the issue of statistical significance is much less relevant than the sensitivity and specificity of the factor as a basis for screening. Sensitivity is the proportion of persons injured that had the screening factor present prior to injury. Specificity is the proportion of persons not injured for whom the screening factor was absent. Assuming that the sample is not biased, if sensitivity is near 1.00, the factor will identify most of the people who would be injured. If specificity is near 1.00, the factor will not misidentify many people who would not be injured. From the public health standpoint, it is desirable that sensitivity be high. From the economic standpoint, if the intervention costs money, it is desirable that specificity be high. Too many missed cases (false negatives) greatly dilutes the potential effect of the countermeasure and too many cases included that would not be injured (false positives) makes the application of the countermeasure more expensive.

Notice in Table 4.4 that, if the factor is a necessary condition for injury, c would be zero and the odds ratio and rate ratio would each be infinite. The rate difference would be 1.00 only if the factor were a necessary and sufficient condition and could be small if the proportion injured of the population where the factor was present were small. The population excess risk would be even smaller if the latter were true. The attributable risk and attributable fraction in the population, however, would each be 1.00, indicating that all of the injuries could be eliminated by eliminating the risk factor. Yet the latter two statistics are seldom reported in analyses of injury data. If the researcher presents the data and the data are population-based, however, they can be calculated.

The advantage of the odds ratio is that studies with different designs can be compared. Rate ratio, rate difference, population excess risk, attributable risk, and attributable fraction in the population are not comparable among studies unless the data are population-based or are adjusted for the sampling fraction if based on a sample.

The use of the statistics measuring effects of a protective factor (Table 4.4)

TABLE 4.4. Common Measures of Association of Categorical Data

	INJURED	NOT INJURED	TOTAL
Factor present	a	b	$a+b$
Factor absent	c	d	$c+d$
Total	$a+c$	$b+d$	$N=a+b+c+d$

$$\text{Sensitivity} = \frac{a}{a+c}$$

$$\text{Specificity} = \frac{d}{b+d}$$

$$\text{Odds ratio} = \frac{ad}{bc}$$

$$\text{Rate ratio} = \frac{a/(a+b)}{c/(c+d)}$$

Assuming a risk factor:

$$\text{Rate difference} = \frac{a}{a+b} - \frac{c}{c+d}$$

$$\text{Population excess risk} = \frac{a+c}{N} - \frac{c}{c+d}$$

$$\text{Attributable risk} = \frac{a/(a+b) - c/(c+d)}{a/(a+b)}$$

$$\text{Attributable fraction in population} = \frac{(a+c)/N - c/(c+d)}{(a+c)/N}$$

Assuming a protective factor:

$$\text{Excess risk if unprotected} = \frac{c}{c+d - a(a+b)}$$

$$\text{Population excess risk} = \frac{a+c}{N - a(a+b)}$$

$$\text{Preventable fraction of the unprotected} = \frac{c/(c+d) - a(a+b)}{c/(c+d)}$$

$$\text{Prevented fraction in the population} = \frac{c/(c+d) - (a+c)/N}{c(c+d)}$$

$$\text{Preventable fraction in the population} = \frac{(a+c)/N - a/(a+b)}{(a+c)/N}$$

assumes that the protection examined is randomly distributed in the population at risk. If those at higher or lower risk are more or less likley to use the protection, the statistics will vary depending on the proportion of the population using the protection. In Chapters 6 and 7, the effects of differential use of seat belts by those at higher and lower risk of severe crashes and the estimates of seat belt effectiveness with and without belt use laws are discussed in that regard.

In this and the previous chapters, mention was made of regression and percentage of variation explained by regression. Unfortunately, these statistical techniques are often left out of the introductory biostatistics course. The calculations are complicated but the concept is straightforward. Figure 4.3 shows a regression line fitted to the plot of fatal, rollover rates of popular utility vehicles in the 1980s as a function of $T/2H$ (track width divided by twice the center of gravity height) where rollover did the first damage to vehicle or occupants (first harm). The computer program that fits the line minimizes the deviations of each observation from the line and gives the result in the form of the equation

$$\text{Rollover rate} = 106 - 86(T/2H)$$

If you know the $T/2H$ for a vehicle, you can put it in the equation and get the expected rollover rate. The scatter around the line occurs because of other factors. The number in parenthesis by each vehicle is the wheelbase, the distance from front to rear axle. Notice that the two vehicles substantially below the regression line (Bronco and SBlazer) have longer wheelbases than those near

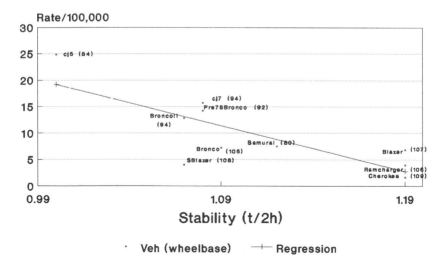

FARS 1982-1987

FIGURE 4.3. First harmful event rollovers per 100,000 vehicles in use per year.

the line at that *T/2H*. In Chapter 10, an equation that includes *T/2H,* wheelbase, and nonrollover for a larger sample of vehicles is discussed.

Wheelbase "explains" some of the variation not predicted by *T/2H.* Percent variation explained, called R^2, is one minus the ratio of squared deviations from the line to the total squared deviations from the average of the predicted variable, in this case rollover rates. If all the data points were on the line, the variation explained would be $1 - 0 = 1$, or 100 percent. If the scatter is totally random, the line would have no slope and the variation explained would be $1 - 1 = 0$, or 0 percent.

Notice also in Figure 4.3 that the line will cross zero at $0 = 105 - 86(T/2H)$, or, solving for *T/2H, T/2H* = 1.22. Since passenger cars have *T/2H* up to 1.62, it is obvious a straight-line regression will not fit the data if cars are included. In that case, a regression model that estimates two lines, one less than 1.2 and one at 1.2 or greater, can be used (Robertson & Maloney, 1997). There are also regression programs that fit curves rather than straight lines.

A variation on the concept of regression is logistic regression. The predicted outcome in a logistic regression is the logarithm of the odds of an outcome such as rollover. The equation that predicts back to the rate is not a straight line and is a little more complicated (Chapter 10), but the basic idea is to predict a particular outcome by knowing one or more risk factors, other things being equal. If those "other things" have been adequately controlled, it is then possible to say how much difference changing the risk factor will make in the outcome.

SUMMARY

Specification of causal paths in complex causal sequences, often a goal of "basic" science, can be misleading in injury control. Usually all of the potential risk factors can be ignored if a controllable necessary condition for harm is known. Since energy is the necessary and specific agent of injury, control of the energy or the way it is conveyed to the host will control the injury. A complex causal model may be useful for understanding sometimes out-of-control systems that affect injury, such as alcohol use. Generally, however, the more removed the hypothesized "cause" is from the energy that injures, the less likely that its control would reduce injury.

Commonly used epidemiologic study designs—case–control, cohort—can be used to investigate factors in injury incidence or severity. Controlled experiments are the most valid methods for evaluating injury control efforts, but they are seldom used. Study designs that rule out false inferences and the use of statistical techniques that quantify parameters that can be changed for injury control must be learned and applied.

REFERENCES

Abramson JH (1985) Cross-sectional studies. In Holland WW, Detels R, and Knox G (eds), *Oxford Textbook of Public Health. Volume 3. Investigative Methods in Public Health.* Oxford: Oxford University Press.

Armitage P (1971) *Statistical Methods in Medical Research.* New York: John Wiley and Sons.

Baker SP, Robertson LS, and Spitz WU (1971) Tattoos, alcohol, and violent death. *J Forensic Sci* 16:219–225.

Blalock HM Jr (1964) *Causal Inferences in Nonexperimental Research.* Chapel Hill: University of North Carolina Press.

Brown ST, Foege WH, Bender TR, and Axnick N (1990) Injury prevention and control: prospects for the 1990s. In Breslow L, Fielding JE, and Lave LB (eds) *Annu Rev Public Health* 11:251–266.

Cummings SR, Nevitt MC, and Kidd S (1988) Forgetting falls. The limited accuracy of recall in the elderly. *J Am Geriatr Soc* 36:613–616.

Cummings SR, Kelsey JL, and Nevitt MC (1990) Methodologic issues in the study of frequent and recurrent health problems. *Ann Epidemiol* 1:49–56.

Dean AD, Dean JA, Coulombier D, Burton JH, et al. (1994) *Epi Info Version 6: A Word Processing, Database, and Statistics Program for Epidemiology on Micro-computers.* Atlanta: Centers for Disease Control.

Donelson AC, Menich RP, Ray RM, and McCarthy RL (1994) Statistical analysis of vehicle rollover: causal modeling. *38th Annual Proceedings, Association for the Advancement of Automotive Medicine.*

Evans AS (1993) *Causation and Disease: A Chronological Journey.* New York: Plenum Publishing Co.

Fleiss JL (1981) *Statistical Methods for Rates and Proportions.* 2nd ed. New York: John Wiley and Sons.

Fulgham R (1989) A case-control study of road features in multiple-vehicle fatal crashes. Gallup, NM: Indian Health Service Hospital (mimeo).

Goodman RA, Mercy JA, Layde PM, and Thacker SB (1988) Case-control studies: design issues for criminological applications. *J Quant Criminol* 4:71–84.

Haddon W Jr, Valien P, McCarroll JR, and Umberger CJ (1961) A controlled investigation of adult pedestrians fatally injured by motor vehicles in Manhattan. *J Chronic Dis* 14:655–678.

Haddon W Jr, Kelley AB, and Waller JA (anonymously) (1968) *1968 Alcohol and Highway Safety Report.* Washington, DC: U.S. Government Printing Office.

Hedlund JH (1984) Recent U.S. traffic fatality trends. In Evans L and Schwing RC (eds), *Human Behavior and Traffic Safety.* New York: Plenum Publishing Co.

Hellevik O (1984) *Introduction to Causal Analysis.* London: George Allen and Unwin.

Insurance Institute for Highway Safety (1980) Serious rollover problems found in Jeep CJ-5 utility vehicles. *Status Report* 15 (December 22):1–4.

Joksch H (1983) Comments on the paper "Rollovers and serious driver injury differences among various utility vehicles, pickup trucks, and passenger car groups." *Q J Am Assoc Auto Med* 5:35–43.

Kellerman AL, Rivara FP, Rushforth NB, Banton JG, Reay DT, Francisco JT, Locci AB, Prodzinski J, Hackman BB, and Somes G (1993) Gun ownership as a risk factor for homicide in the home. *New Engl J Med* 329:1084–1119.

Kelsey JL, Thompson WD, and Evans AS (1986) *Methods in Observational Epidemiology.* New York: Oxford University Press.

King G (1997) *A Solution to the Ecological Inference Problem.* Princeton: Princeton University Press.

Krieger N (1994) Epidemiology and the web of causation: has anyone seen the spider? *Soc Sci Med* 39:887–903.

Leigh JP, and Waldon HM (1991) Unemployment and highway fatalities. *J Health Polit Policy Law* 16:135–156.

Loomis DP (1991) Occupation, industry, and fatal motor vehicle crashes in 20 states, 1986–1987. *Am J Public Health* 81:733–735.

Loomis TA, and West TC (1958) The influence of alcohol on automobile driving ability. *Q J Stud Alcohol* 19:30–46.

Lum H and Reagan JA (1995) Interactive Highway Safety Design Model: Accident Predictive Module. *Public Roads* 58:14–17.

McCarroll JR, and Haddon W Jr (1962) A controlled study of fatal automobile accidents in New York City. *J Chronic Dis* 15:811–826.

McClelland DC (1984) Drinking as a response to power needs in men. In *Motives, Personality, and Society.* New York: Praeger.

McMahon B, Pugh TF, and Ipsen J (1960) *Epidemiologic methods.* Boston: Little, Brown.

Michon JA (1985) A critical view of driver behavior models: what do we know: what should we do? In Evans L and Schwing RC (eds), *Human Behavior and Traffic Safety.* New York: Plenum Publishing Co.

National Center for Health Statistics (1972) *Optimum Recall Period for Reporting Persons Injured in Motor Vehicle Accidents.* Rockville, MD: U.S. Department of Health, Education and Welfare.

Needleman HL, Gunnoe C, Leviton A, Reed R, Peresie H, Maher C, and Barrett P (1979) Deficits in psychologic and classroom performance of children with elevated dentine lead levels. *New Engl J Med* 300:689–732.

Oster G, Huse DM, Adams SF, Imbimbo J, and Russell MW (1990) Benzodiazepine tranquilizers and the risk of accidental injury. *Am J Public Health* 80:1467–1470.

Powell EC, Sheehan KM, and Christoffel KK (1996) Firearm violence among youth: public health strategies for prevention. *Ann Emergency Med* 28:204–212.

Reagan JA (1994) The Interactive Highway Safety Design Model: Designing for safety by analyzing road geometrics. *Public Roads* 58:37–43.

Redelmeier DA, and Tibslirani RJ (1997) Association between cellular-telephone calls and motor vehicle collisions. *New Engl J Med* 336:453–458.

Renwick JH (1973) Analysis of cause—long cut to prevention. *Nature* 246:114–115.

Riegelman RK (1981) *Studying a Study and Testing a Test.* Boston: Little, Brown.

Robertson LS (1983) *Injuries: Causes, Control Strategies and Public Policy.* Lexington, MA: D.C. Heath.

Robertson LS (1989) Risk of fatal rollover in utility vehicles relative to static stability. *Am J Public Health* 79:300–303.

Robertson LS (1991) How to save fuel and reduce injuries in automobiles. *J Trauma* 31:107–109.

Robertson LS (1993) Fatal fires from rear-end crashes: the effects of fuel tank placement before and after regulation. *Am J Public Health* 83:1168–1170.

Robertson LS, and Kelley AB (1989) Static stability as a predictor of overturn in fatal motor vehicle crashes. *J Trauma* 29:313–319.

Robertson LS, and Maloney A (1997) Motor vehicle rollover and static stability: an exposure study. *Am J Public Health,* 87:839–841.

Robinson WS (1950) Ecological correlation and the behavior of individuals. *Am Sociol Rev* 15:351–357.

Selvin S (1991) *Statistical Analysis of Epidemiologic Data.* New York: Oxford University Press.

Snyder RG, McDole TL, Ladd WM, and Minahan DJ (1980) On-road crash experience of utility vehicles. Ann Arbor, University of Michigan Highway Safety Research Institute.

Stein HS, and Jones IS (1988) Crash involvement of large trucks by configuration: a case-control study. *Am J Public Health* 78:491–498.

Susser M, and Susser E (1996) Choosing a future for epidemiology: I. Eras and paradigms. *Am J Public Health* 86:668–673.

Tessmer J (1994) An analysis of fires in passenger cars, light trucks and vans. Washington, DC: National Highway Traffic Safety Administration.

Violenti JM, and Marshall JR (1996) Cellular phones and traffic accidents: an epidemiological approach. *Accident Anal Prev* 28:265–270.

Wechsler H, Kasey EH, Thum D, and Demone HW Jr (1969) Alcohol level and home accidents. *Public Health Rep* 84:1043–1050.

Wintemute GJ, Kraus JF, Teret SP, and Wright M (1990) Death resulting from motor vehicle immersions: the nature of the injuries, personal and environmental contributing factors, and potential interventions. *Am J Public Health* 80:1068–1070.

Wright PH, and Robertson LS (1976) Priorities for roadside hazard modification: a study of 300 fatal roadside object crashes. *Traffic Eng* 46:24–30.

Wright PH, and Zador PF (1980) A study of fatal rollover crashes in Georgia. Washington, DC: Insurance Institute for Highway Safety.

Zador PL, Jones IS, and Ginsburg M (1984) Fatal front-to-front car collisions and the results of 35 mph frontal barrier impacts. *28th Annual Proceedings, American Association for the Advancement of Automotive Medicine.*

5

HUMAN FACTORS AND ATTEMPTS TO CHANGE THEM

Most people who are injured are doing something at the time—driving, riding in a vehicle, walking, working, playing. So are people who are infected by microorganisms, but those who study injury place more emphasis on behavior than do those who study most infectious diseases. Notable exceptions are infectious diseases transmitted by sex.

Historically, manufacturers of injurious products emphasized behavior of the injured to divert attention from the products (Eastman, 1984). Despite the evidence that changes in vehicle crashworthiness accounted for most of the major reductions in car occupant fatalities per mile during the last third of the twentieth century (Chapter 7), employees of General Motors (GM) continued to argue that the major emphasis in injury control should be on behavior (Evans, 1996; Evans & Schwing, 1985). In the mid-1990s the head of the National Highway Traffic Safety Administration, who has legal responsibility for vehicle safety, joined the industry chorus (Frame, 1996).

The argument for behavioral causation is convenient for the industry and its apologists, particularly when industry negligence is alleged. For example, in its 1973–87 C/K pickup trucks, General Motors chose to place fuel tanks on the sides outside the frame of the vehicle next to external sheet metal to increase fuel capacity relative to competitive trucks. Other manufacturers placed the tank within the frame. The issue of risk of fire in GM pickups was publicized in 1992 when a family whose son died in a GM truck fire sued GM and demanded a trial rather than accept a private settlement from the company (Applebome, 1993).

The Center for Auto Safety petitioned the National Highway Traffic Safety Administration (NHTSA) to recall the vehicles based in part on data indicating higher fatal fire rates in GM compared to similar-sized Ford pickups during 1981–86. GM hired a consulting firm that claimed the GM trucks posed no unreasonable risk because some small cars and trucks had a higher fire risk, although its data clearly indicated a higher fatal fire rate in GM compared to similar-sized pickups (Lange et al., 1992). GM later retracted the claim that its pickups had a lower overall fatality rate than Ford's pickups—admitting that the total occupant fatality rate in GM C/K pickups was actually higher than Ford's of similar size (Meier, 1992). Then GM turned that argument on its head. In a submission to NHTSA, GM argued that its trucks have higher fatal fire rates because they were driven by "more aggressive" drivers (General Motors Corporation, 1993).

In 1988, GM introduced a redesigned pickup truck with the gasoline tank inside the frame. Comparison of GM and Ford full-sized pickups indicate that, when all fatal crashes, not just those fatal to occupants, are considered, pre-1988 GM trucks were no more involved than Ford trucks, contrary to the "aggressive driver" hypothesis. The fire rates in the pre-1988 GM trucks were substantially higher than in the Ford trucks, but the difference disappeared in the 1988 and subsequent models which had tanks inside the frames (Table 5.1). The differences in the pre-1988 vehicles are more remarkable when the data are limited to side impacts—clock positions 8–10 and 2–4 (Table 5.2).

GM also constructed an "Aggressive Driver Demographic Factors Index" by adding the percentage of 21 factors available in the Fatal Accident Reporting System to support its claim that drivers of its pickups were more aggressive. Some of these factors were driver characteristics and some, such as number of vehicles in the crash, ran off the road, and posted speed 55 miles per hour (mph) or greater, were not. Several of the factors are known to be highly correlated (age 29 years or younger, police indicates "driving too fast," one or more speeding convictions, vehicle speed 55 mph or greater). Posted speed is obviously not indicative of aggressive driving and the speed-related factors are obviously not additive. The summation of several indicators of the same phenomenon is methodologically indefensible. Also, data on actual vehicle speeds in the crashes are missing on more than half the cases in the Fatal Accident Reporting System.

Despite the claims of industry spin doctors and their echoes in government, injury control has never been a simple choice of changing agents and vehicles of injury versus changing behavior. The issue is: What factors can be changed

TABLE 5.1. Fatal Crash Rates per Million per Year of 1981–91 GM and Ford Pickup Trucks in Calendar Years 1981–92

	MODEL YEARS						
	1981–87				1988–91		
	GM		FORD		GM		FORD	
	N	RATE	N	RATE	N	RATE	N	RATE
Fire most harm								
Vehicles	139	5.1	85	3.4	23	3.2	26	4.2
Occupant deaths	164	6.0	104	4.2	29	4.1	32	5.2
All fires								
Vehicles	389	14.2	265	10.6	66	9.3	66	10.8
Occupant deaths	400	14.6	245	9.8	71	10.0	76	12.4
Nonfire								
Vehicles	9209	336.1	8376	336.0	2831	398.7	2241	365.8
Occupant deaths	4699	171.5	3595	144.2	1468	206.8	892	145.6

Cases in which fire is classified as "most harm" are also included in "all fires." The estimated years of use are, for 1981–87 models, GM, 27.41 million, Ford, 24.93 million, and for 1988–91 models, GM, 7.10 million, Ford, 6.13 million.

Source: Fatal Accident Reporting System (fatal crashes) and *Ward's Automotive Yearbook* (vehicle sales).

to reduce harm and how much difference can be achieved by deliberate attempts at changing the factors?

BEHAVIORAL THEORIES

The construction of behavior change strategies would be easier if behavioral and social scientists could agree on human behaviors that are changeable. For example, historical arguments regarding the best approaches to crime prevention turned on the issue of the extent to which behavior is modifiable at given stages of development (Tremblay & Craig, 1995).

The operant conditioning model prevalent among experimental psychologists portrays human beings as trainable by reward and punishment to do virtually anything; it often ignores biological limitations, as well as cognitions that intervene between the input of rewards and punishments and the output in behavior. The neoclassic economic model, and that of some cognitive psychologists, views human beings as rational "utility" (goal) optimizers, which allows little room for human physical or psychological limitations. In this model, rather

TABLE 5.2. Fatal Fire Rates in Side Impacts per Million per Year of 1981–91 GM and Ford Pickup Trucks in Calendar Years 1981–92

	MODEL YEARS							
	1981–87				1988–91			
	GM		FORD		GM		FORD	
	N	RATE	N	RATE	N	RATE	N	RATE
Fire most harm								
Vehicles	36	1.3	11	0.4	2	0.3	2	0.3
Occupant deaths	41	1.5	11	0.4	3	0.4	2	0.3
All fires								
Vehicles	72	2.6	30	1.1	7	1.0	6	1.0
Occupant deaths	84	3.1	31	1.1	9	1.3	8	1.3

than being mainly responsive to external stimuli as in the operant conditioning model, each person weighs the probability of each possible behavior for accomplishing or experiencing a utility and discounts the cost in terms of the time between the immediate situation and the ultimate goal. The origin of the "utilities" is often obscure in such theories.

Many sociologists view behavior as largely determined by the internalized cultural and social environment, including learned social customs and mores, socioeconomic status, and peer pressure. Socio- and psychobiologists emphasize the effects of genetics on the biological factors that contribute to motivations such as rivalry, emotions such as rage, cognitive limitations, and neuromotor function. Certain psychologists and psychiatrists look for the major motivations for behavior in the unconscious mind, largely determined by relationships with parents or guardians in infancy and early childhood.

Devotees to any one of these approaches may object to the oversimplification in a one-sentence description of what are often very complex and detailed theories. Also, the list is by no means exhaustive. There are numerous eclectic mixtures.

Each theory may have some merit for subsets of a population engaged in a given activity at a given time. Human beings are very complicated and, at any one time in the course of a lifetime, several of the factors emphasized by the various schools of thought may influence the behavior of the moment. Therefore, it is not surprising that behavioral or social scientists who have attempted to apply their disparate theories to behaviors that increase or decrease probability of injury have found one or more of their hypotheses supported to some degree by data. In many such instances, the hypothesis has some predictive value, but in others the research "results" are artifacts of research design or invalid assumptions about the data or their interpretation. The usefulness of the valid biological, psychological, economic, and social predictors of injury depends on the strength of the correlations and the extent to which the factors are subject to change by intervention.

DEVELOPMENTAL STAGES IN CHILDHOOD

Not only do the causal models of different schools of thought look quite different; the relative strength of a given causal path in any causal model of injury must differ dramatically depending on the stage of development of the individual (Kane, 1985). As noted in Chapter 4, age is a proxy for a mix of the factors emphasized in behavioral theories as well as differential vulnerability of tissue to energy insults, and the probability of being in situations where energy exchanges are more or less likely.

In 1976–77, the motor vehicle–occupant death rate per population of infants less than 1 year of age was twice that of those 1, but less than 2 years old. The rate declined as children grew older until age 6, where it leveled, and the rate among 6–12 year olds was about a third that of infants (Baker, 1979). Does this mean that parents were conditioned to love their children more and take better care of them as they grew? Do children increase in utility as they develop? Are the social and economic pressures on new parents so severe that their driving ability deteriorates enormously? Do some new parents have a subconscious hate for their newborn that is manifested in driving behavior, endangering themselves as well as the infant?

Perhaps a few of the behavioral and social scientists extremely dedicated to their respective theories would view such hypotheses as worthy of research, but scientists aware of anatomy and physics considered other hypotheses. The tissues of infants are less tolerant of energy insults, and certain positions in the vehicles increase the mechanical forces on them in crashes. By using the formula describing mechanical energy in Chapter 1, it can be shown that an unrestrained 10 pound baby becomes a 300 pound flying object in a 30 mile per hour crash. Furthermore, when placed in the lap of an adult, an infant in a frontal crash will be crushed between the interior-front structure of the vehicle and the similarly multiplied weight of an unrestrained adult attempting to hold the infant.

Social and behavioral factors undoubtedly affect the transportation of children in particular types of vehicles, their seating arrangement in the vehicles, and whether or not they are restrained. Children may also distract drivers, but probably no more at one year of age than at six years of age. The relative influence of these factors on the injury rates have not been studied in sufficient detail to weight them as contributors to injury.

During 1980–84, vehicle occupant death rates of children less than 1 year old declined 37 percent and those of 1–4 year olds declined 25 percent as child restraint use laws were adopted (Robertson, 1989). These reductions were associated with increases in observed child restraint use in urban environments that increased from less than 10 percent (Williams, 1976) to 49 percent (National Highway Traffic Safety Administration, 1989).

Child development may be modified by brain damage associated with low birth weight, in utero alcohol and drug exposure, serotonin deficiency, or head trauma in childhood. Such factors have been associated with later violent behavior, which led a National Research Council panel on violence to recommend longitudinal studies to better delineate their potential effects (Reiss & Roth, 1993).

As children develop motor skills, they become more active. For a time, the motor skills develop more rapidly than perceptual and cognitive skills. Children's injuries reflect the hazards in the environments in which they are placed or find themselves, and the behaviors that expose them to energy exchanges, as well as changing tissue vulnerabilities (Rivara, 1982b). They roll, and later crawl, off beds and from other elevated surfaces. Their heads are larger than their bodies, and those that work their bodies between crib slats are sometimes asphyxiated by hanging. They attempt to swallow foods and other objects that are large enough to block respiration when lodged in the trachea. Toxic chemicals and plants are also swallowed. They wander into swimming pools, hot tubs, and spas. They touch hot surfaces, pull over containers of hot liquids, and are placed in, or turn on, overheated water.

At given points in development, children apparently learn to largely avoid certain hazards to which they remain exposed in their environments. Head injuries associated with stairs and window or door glass decline by half from age 2 to age 3, and those associated with furniture and other household fixtures decline rapidly after age 6–7 (Rivara, 1982a). At age 4–9, children playing with matches and lighters start fires, disproportionate to their numbers in the population at that age (Cole et al., 1986). As they develop the ability to run, climb, and operate vehicles such as tricycles, bicycles, guns, skateboards, and motorized vehicles, children's involvement in injuries associated with these activities increases.

A variety of research questions have been raised by these distributions (Rivara, 1982b). To what extent does differential understanding of developmental stages by parents account for their children's exposure to hazards? If there are differences in knowledge, does giving information to the less informed result in reduced exposures and injuries? What are the capabilities of children relative to proposed countermeasures? For example, if fencing is the option chosen to reduce children's access to swimming pools, what types of fences can children breach (Rabinovich et al., 1994)? To know how to modify firearms to prevent child use, what is the limit of children's ability to pull the trigger of extant firearms (Naureckas et al., 1995)?

The age differences in injuries vary by sex in some cases and not in others. Are the differences in males and females learned, biological, or some combination of the two? What other characteristics of children, if any, are predictive of injury given similar exposure to hazards? Are such characteristics short-lived, or do they persist through several developmental stages? How does one distinguish cases of unintentional injury and child abuse (Kemp et al., 1994)? Are any of the predictive characteristics modifiable, and do attempts at modification result in reduced injury? One review of attempts to reduce antisocial behavior in children indicates that early interventions with prospective and new parents are more effective than later school-based approaches (Tremblay & Craig, 1995).

Less frequently considered are questions regarding stimuli generated outside the home. What influence does advertising have on decisions to purchase hazardous products? How much of such influence is exerted through programs and commercials directed at children? How many hazardous products are received as gifts and from whom? How often do the injuries associated with hazardous products occur from products that belong to neighbors, friends, relatives, and others outside the home?

The noted references indicate that epidemiologists and others interested in children's injuries have attempted to answer a few of the questions using a variety of methodological approaches. This is not the place for an exhaustive literature review, which should be undertaken before attempting new research. A biannually updated survey of research on interventions to reduce children's injuries is on the internet: http://weber.u.washington.edu/~hipre/childinjury.

ADOLESCENTS AND YOUNG ADULTS

The most severe injuries to teenagers and young adults occur in motor vehicles and assaults, particularly assaults on self or others with guns in the United States (Baker et al., 1992). Males are substantially more involved than females as drivers and assailants, and whites are more often killed in motor vehicles and suicides, while blacks are more often killed in assaults.

Again, behavioral theories contain all sorts of hypotheses as potential explanations, but the research in support of many of them is inadequate or nonexistent. Adolescence and young adulthood is a period of accelerated separation from parental influence, sexual maturity and establishment of sexual relationships, struggle for economic independence, and adaptation to changing expectations from peers and adults (Gilula & Daniels, 1969). Inexperience, risk-taking, sensation-seeking, impulsiveness, and alcohol and drug abuse are some of the terms used to describe the behaviors of adolescents and young adults that may contribute to injury.

One study in Canada found that motor vehicle crash rates of newly licensed drivers at age 17, 18, and 19 were similar to drivers of the same age who had been licensed one, two or three years (Pierce, 1977). Therefore, driving experience does not seem to be a major factor in the substantial decline in crash rates from age 16 to 19.

The term "risk-taker" implies that the person knows the risk and deliberately behaves in such a way as to increase risk to self. Certainly some suicide attempts and assaults are the result of deliberate choices, but the extent to which perception of risk is actually associated with various types of risky behavior is unknown. The involvement of alcohol, other drugs, and mental illness in many cases of presumed deliberate assaults on self and others raises doubt about the preinjury state of mind of the persons affected by these factors. The hypothesis that risk-denial or belief in personal invulnerability is a factor has at least equal plausability to the risk-taker hypothesis. Studies of perceived risk in motor vehicles indicate that younger drivers more often think their peers at higher risk than themselves, compared to such perceptions among older drivers (Bragg & Finn, 1982; Matthews & Moran, 1986), yet the authors of those studies persisted in calling the young drivers "risk-takers."

As noted in Chapter 4, motor vehicle injuries are common enough in the adolescent years such that prospective cohort studies could be undertaken to measure the extent to which knowledge of risk, beliefs about personal vulnerability, impulsiveness, mental illness, conflicts with parents, lovers, or peers, challenges from peers, and economic difficulties are predictive of becoming a driver in a crash-causing injury. Becoming the assailant or the injured in an assault may be subject to study by similar methods, although identification of cases not reported to police would be difficult given the potential for reluctance to report involvement.

Unwarranted conclusions have been drawn from the examination of patients after injury and inference of preinjury psychopathology. For example, one study of patients in a trauma center, excluding two-thirds (those with a Glasgow Coma Score less than 15 as well as children less than 18 and those receiving narcotics for pain), claimed that the patients had higher than normal "preinjury psychopathology." The measure of "psychopathology" consisted of a questionnaire with items such as "I feel isolated," "I have low/very low spirits" (Whetsell et al., 1989). Administered to people in a hospital after trauma, these items obviously are not necessarily measures of prehospital states of mind. No attempt was made to correlate the responses to the behavior of the respondents at the time of injury, that is, did the respondents' behavior contribute to the injury or not? Prospective studies of questionnaire measures of psychological traits and car crashes do not indicate a correlation (e.g., Schuster & Guilford,

1964), but temporary psychological states are not captured by such methods (Robertson, 1983).

The literature on assaults and homicides is mainly limited to descriptive studies. Some correlations among relationship of assailant and victim, weapon if any, and biological, psychological, social, and demographic characteristics have been reported, but there is substantial disagreement regarding causation, partly resulting from numerous methodological issues (Rosenberg et al., 1986). Characteristics of assailants and interactions among couples in domestic assaults have been described (Shupe et al., 1987), but no data were collected on couples not involved to be able to say that the alleged causal factors were less prevalent in those who do not have such problems.

Race is emphasized in many studies of homicide because of the very high rates among young black males. Studies of domestic homicide indicate, however, that the correlation with race disappears when household crowding is controlled statistically (Centerwell, 1995). It is the socioeconomic consequences of the way races have been treated historically that explains the differences in homicide, not the genetics of race.

Aggression has been studied extensively in controlled laboratory experiments under a wide variety of experimental conditions. The relevance of these studies to assaultive behavior in homes, streets and bars, or to aggressive driving, is open to debate. One well-designed study of alcohol and aggression in college students, for example, randomly divided the students into four groups: *(1)* alcohol and threatened, *(2)* alcohol and not threatened, *(3)* placebo and threatened, *(4)* placebo and not threatened. The alcohol and placebo were masked by strong flavoring. The subjects were placed in a situation where they were supposedly competing with a person in another room on a reaction-time task in which each subject could deliver an electric shock to the other. The situation was presumed as threatening, but those in the "nonthreatened" condition heard their "opponent" object to hurting someone. There was no difference in intensity of shock delivered to "opponents" between those with and without alcohol in the nonthreatened groups. Those in the threatened group delivered more intense shocks to their "opponents" and, if they had also consumed alcohol, they delivered very strong shocks to their "opponents" (Taylor et al., 1976).

Given knowledge of such results, an injury epidemiologist wants to know how much of the variation in assaultive injury can be explained by alcohol and threatening situations. How does one obtain unbiased samples of assailants and potential assailants in which alcohol can be measured? What constitutes a threat? Is there a relatively small set of threats that can be identified in large numbers of assault cases? Is the assault directed toward someone perceived as threatening or a scapegoat (e.g., child, spouse, lover)?

If the set of factors that are threatening to persons who are assaultive were limited to a few, such as unemployment or fear of unemployment, harassment by peers, and degradation of self-esteem by spouses or lovers, then it may be possible to find ways to help people cope with such threats. If the threats are so diverse that none accounts for a substantial part of the problem, then the probable success of changing threats to reduce assault is diminished.

Among the most publicized claims about causation of spouse and child battering is that the batterer was abused as a child. While being abused as a child may increase the risk of becoming an abusing adult, the majority of abusers were not abused as children (Rosenberg et al., 1986). Therefore, as desirable as reduction in child abuse would be, it would not reduce battering in the next generation as much as the publicized claims would have us believe.

One way of studying these issues in a population would be to identify from police records a sample of households that had one or more domestic disputes reported within the past year. Controls for comparison could be selected by identifying residents of other households in the same block and randomly choosing one or more that had no domestic disputes reported to police in the past year. Interviews with family members, preferably augmented by validity checks (e.g., employment history) where possible, might reveal a set of threats or other factors that, separately or in combination with alcohol, are amenable to change.

The advantage of police-reported cases is the potential for obtaining objective data on alcohol. A small pilot study could be undertaken to see whether cases and controls would cooperate with a request for breath alcohol, the controls at the same time of day and day of week as the dispute was reported in the cases.

The study design would be subject to criticism because it would not identify the set of battered women and children that do not come to the attention of police. Protocols for identifying such cases have been developed (Stark et al., 1981), and researchers with clinical affiliations should be able to identify many such cases in that setting, but objective measurement of alcohol in the batterer in those circumstances probably would not be feasible. Great care must be exercised in such research to avoid placing the battered person at greater jeopardy for having revealed the batterer, however inadvertently.

Descriptive studies of suicides of teenagers and young adults indicate clusters of types of problems (legal, interpersonal, history of mental illness), method used (firearm, hanging, drugs, gas), and age group (Gerberich et al., 1985). Case–control studies are needed to determine which from among the identified factors are substantial and changeable risk factors. Another design would select cases from each cluster and controls with similar problems to reveal the extent to which suicides within a given cluster are correlated to the misfit of personality and social environment, availablity of method used, and other variables in theories of suicide.

Little research has been conducted on attempts to change exposure to potential injury hazards by offering programs to youth that keep them from hazardous environments. In the United States, a proposed program to open schools and other facilities for "midnight basketball" for low-income youth was treated as a joke by political opponents of any government involvement, rather than taken seriously as a program to be studied. In Brazil, some 370 programs to engage so-called street children in productive activities were initiated, but the effect on injuries and other problems of these children has apparently not been evaluated (Berger & Mohan, 1996).

Immigrants to the United States apparently adapt to the gun culture quickly. Homicide rates are higher among many immigrant groups than among their counterparts of similar ethnic origin (Sorenson & Shen, 1996). A neglected area of research in adolescent and young adult injuries is the extent of recruitment to danger. To what extent is the use of cars and guns in hazardous ways a function of nightly doses of television portrayals of such behavior? To what extent do organized clubs for hazardous activities recruit new participants? What is the involvement of the industries that sell equipment for hazardous activities (e.g., hang gliding, scuba diving, sky diving, motorcycling, gun use, fast cars) in promoting the activity through clubs, magazines, and the like, and how many of the injured were led to the activity by such promotion?

ADULTHOOD

In the middle years of life, injury rates are lower for most types of injuries. Injuries to workers in certain occupations are major exceptions (Baker et al., 1992). The generally lower injuries in the midyears of life could be partly from greater knowledge of risks and partly from changes in exposure, such as reduced driving at night and reduced "partying" on weekends.

The effect of knowledge seems limited. Denial of risks is not confined to teenagers and young adults. After being presented the risks of gassing, hand burns, and child poisonings from household cleansers, a sample of consumers were asked how much more or less likely than average such injuries were in their homes. Only 2–3 percent said more likely and 40–65 percent said less likely (Viscusi & Magat, 1987). These results are similar to those obtained when a random sample of new-car buyers were asked whether their chances of being injured or killed in a car crash were greater than, the same as, or less than "people like yourself." Six percent said greater and 40 percent said less (Robertson, 1977). Whether the less extreme deniers are at more or less actual risk than the more extreme deniers has apparently not been studied.

Race and sex differences that persist in particular types of injury rates during middle age are often cited, but race and sex are no more modifiable than age. They are of interest only as identifiers of groups in which causal factors differ in kind or magnitude, or as identifiers for targeting programs to modify risk factors.

Too often conclusions about race and sex are based on stereotypes. When the author told colleagues he was reviewing the literature on injuries to Native Americans in the 1980s, virtually every one stated with conviction that alcohol accounted for the higher injury rates in that population.

The literature indicated that although alcohol is a problem among several Native American groups, it probably does not account for nearly the variation in injury rates that stereotypical thinking suggests. The only study found in which blood alcohol was measured among injured Native Americans indicated that more Native Americans were tested in the same jurisdiction relative to whites, 63 percent versus 45 percent (Westermeyer & Brantner, 1972). Therefore, the involvement of alcohol measured objectively was not available in a sample without potential selection bias. A recent study of Native Americans and others in fatal motor vehicle crashes in Arizona relied on invalid police reports for the majority of assessments of alcohol in Native Americans (Campos-Outcalt et al., 1997). Although the article claimed that there was no difference in the proportion chemically tested for alcohol concentration, recalculation of the numbers in the article indicates that 33 percent of Native Americans were tested and 56 percent of others were tested. If the police are more oriented to expecting alcohol in Native Americans, the estimate of alcohol involvement would be biased.

There was a 29-fold difference in deaths attributed to alcoholism, cirrhosis, or alcohol poisioning among different groups of Native Americans in Oklahoma (Stratton et al., 1978). Self-reported total abstinence from alcohol is twice as high among Native Americans as among whites. In groups where intoxication is frowned upon, drinking is done alone and in secret. In groups with a tradition of the seeking of visions and endurance dancing, heavy alcohol consumption in public is more acceptable, particularly among young males (Kunitz, 1976; Levy & Kunitz, 1974; May, 1982). The stereotype apparently evolved from historical accounts of "Indians and firewater" and the very noticeable public drinking in certain groups, particularly in towns near reservations.

The social factors that influence if, when, and where drinking occurs undoubtedly influence the risk of particular types of injuries, such as the high rate of deaths from cold and exposure among Native Americans in New Mexico (Sewell et al., 1989). Prior to declines associated with injury control programs for Native Americans (Smith & Robertson, in press), Native Americans had more than twice the injury death rates of the U.S. population as a whole. If one compares total injury death rates of Native Americans with those of rural isolated populations generally, however, the differences are small (Robertson, 1985).

Among U.S. Navy personnel, Native Americans were hospitalized for "alcoholism" three time more often per capita than whites or blacks, yet their hospitalizations for injury per capita were 13 percent less than those for whites and blacks (Hoiberg et al., 1981). Therefore, among races whose living and working conditions are similar, injury rates are similar. The major explanations for racial differences in injury rates are more likely to be found in the vehicles and environments to which they are exposed rather than in biological and personality theories or in racial stereotypes.

The extent to which differences in injury rates between sexes can be attributed to biological factors, social factors, or interaction among biological and social factors probably differs by type of injury. Women are usually at less risk of most types of injuries as teenagers and adults, but there are exceptions. In domestic violence that does not involve weapons, women often strike men as well as vice versa, but the severe injuries from violence in homes are most often to women and children (Rosenberg et al., 1986), probably because men are physically stronger, on average, than women and children. Most of the studies of dominance behavior, hormones, alcohol, and other potential factors in aggressive behavior have not included women (Mazur & Robertson, 1972).

GROWING OLD

Severe injury rates tend to increase among the elderly for several types of injury (Rice & MacKenzie, 1989). Although some exposures are decreased among the elderly (e.g., miles driven, driving at night), and injury incidence is lower, the consequences when injury occurs in length of hospital stays and mortality are more severe. Decreases in visual acuity, hearing, mental alertness, and so on, probably increase risk of incidence, but reduced exposure to factors such as driving, industrial machines, and farm equipment probably results in lower incidence. Certain exposures, such as use of stairs or walking on other surfaces that are conducive to falls, are not changed or may even increase after retirement. The elderly have particularly high injury rates from falls. In social environments where the young prey on or abuse the elderly, they are the victims of assault, and some resort to suicide to escape social circumstances or physical debilitation that they are no longer willing to tolerate.

Elderly people suffer various types of losses including friends, spouse, occasionally a child, job, status, income, power, self-esteem, self-confidence, hearing, sight, other aspects of personal control or competence, and health—losses that are thought to contribute to suicide (Osgood, 1985). Better research is needed to specify the extent to which suicide risk is associated with these and other factors for purposes of identifying those for whom support groups or other approaches might be helpful.

The exact contributions of exposure to energy exchanges by degree of energy generated versus tissue vulnerability to particular types of injury among the elderly have not been specified. Certainly the elderly person injured with the same degree of severity as a younger person is more likely to die than the younger person (Baker et al., 1974).

Attention to risk of falls in the elderly has increased. Among the factors related to falls potentially amenable to change are leg extension strength and gait (Graafmans et al., 1996; Tinetti et al., 1995b) and modifiable environmental factors, such as characteristics of stairs (Tinetti et al., 1995a), that have been found markedly different between the homes of fallers and controls (Locklear, 1991).

POSTTRAUMA BEHAVIOR

A very neglected area of research is the effect of trauma on subsequent behavior. Obviously, the lives of persons with noncorrected disabilities are changed— drastically in the case of severe spinal cord and brain injury. Documentation of the extent of these effects is important to understand the total, often nonquantifiable, costs of injury.

Other effects of injury may be more subtle or not appear immediately. How many people change their behavior as a result of injury? What is the effect on subsequent fear and anxiety of trauma to oneself or to relatives and friends? To what extent does neighborhood violence change the behavior patterns of people in the neighborhood? Does fear of falling result in less mobility among the elderly (Tinetti et al., 1994), further contributing to the risk? Does subtle brain injury contribute to intellectual or emotional deficits or increase risk of brain diseases such as Alzheimer's disease and epilepsy?

Some of these questions raise thorny methodological issues. To the extent that the hypothesized effect of trauma could also contribute to the incidence, posttrauma measurement may overstate the effect of trauma. For example, one research project measured intelligence quotients of persons who had been injured and correlated them to the injured persons scores on the Glasgow Coma Scale and the Injury Severity Score. Persons who were more severely injured had lower IQs (Gensemer et al., 1989). However, if lower IQ contributes to the probability of severe injury, the inference of a causal effect of trauma on IQ would be overstated.

A correlation of lower precrash IQs (measured at army induction) and fatal motor vehicle injury has been found (O'Toole, 1990).

Where preinjury measures are available, such as IQ scores from school, military, or other records, researchers interested in posttrauma effects should attempt to obtain the records. Where such measures are not available, the IQ of a sample of siblings or childhood friends of the injured could be used for comparison. To the extent that IQ is predictive, the issue of limits to modifiability of IQ is relevant to prevention.

Case–control studies of Alzheimer's disease consistently find a history of head trauma more frequent in persons with the disease—24 percent of cases and 8 percent of genetically unrelated relatives and friends matched by sex and approximate age in one study (Graves et al., 1990). The odds ratios were higher for those whose head injury did not result in loss of consciousness and among those with more recent head trauma. Although there are reasonable biological explanations for head trauma contributing to the disease and the average period between the head trauma and onset of symptoms was long—21.3 years for cases—it is not possible to exclude the disease or some correlate of the disease as a precursor to trauma rather than exclusively a posttrauma effect. It would be useful to compare cases in which the behavior of the person did or did not contribute to the injury, but recall of spouses or others regarding long-past incidents is a major methodological problem.

ATTEMPTS TO CHANGE HUMAN FACTORS

Programs aimed at changing human factors without resort to law are of three types: (1) attempts to change abilities such as driving skills, strength, and gait of the elderly; (2) attempts to change behaviors that are presumed to contribute to risk such as storage of materials hazardous to children, violent responses to peer challenges, speeding, and alcohol use; and (3) attempts to increase use of protection such as child restraints, seat belts, motorcycle and bicycle helmets, and certain sports equipment. Various techniques are used—information and motivation by education in schools and media campaigns, outreach programs for children and the elderly, behavior modification using incentives or punishments, and enhancement of perception.

Among the issues to be considered in attempting to modify behavior relative to childrens' injuries are the seriousness of the injuries, whether to focus on the parents' or guardians' behavior, the childrens' behavior, or the behavior of others, and the variety of injuries on which to focus in any one attempt to modify behavior.

One project that had an exemplary research design is questionable because of its focus. In a prepaid medical plan serving an upper-middle-class clientele, parents who brought children in for medical visits (excluding those with very acute illnesses or chronic conditions) were randomly assigned to experimental and control groups. Parents in the experimental group were counseled regarding a variety of hazards to children in the home and were given a booklet emphasizing ten such hazards and a packet of electrical outlet covers. In a follow-up telephone call, the parents in the experimental group were asked whether they had changed given hazards, and those who said no were encouraged to do so. In an unannounced home visit, the numbers of hazards observed were recorded in both experimental and control groups (Dershewitz & Williamson, 1977).

Two aspects of the research design are excellent: *(1)* The random assignment of experimental and control groups should equalize the potential effects of factors other than the counseling between the two groups. *(2)* Actual observation of certain targeted hazards rules out the potential biases of self-reporting. Such biases were indeed noted by comparing the results of the telephone interview and the observed hazards. While differences in the experimental and control groups were obtained in the telephone interviews, there were no differences between the two groups in hazards actually observed in the homes.

The problem with the approach is the lack of focus on one or a few hazards likely to result in severe injury. The types of hazards included were cleaning agents, prescription drugs, waxes and polishes, nonprescription drugs, coins, jewelry, watches, keys, appliances on countertops, matches, pins, needles, kitchen knives, and hazards on the floor. These differ substantially in associated injuries and severity. In light of other research, the lack of focus on one or a few of the most important may have defeated the purpose of the counseling.

Projects with a similar research design, but focused exclusively on a single problem, have found favorable effects of counseling parents. A 40 percent reduction in injuries from falls among infants was found relative to a control group after counseling in the experimental group (Kravitz, 1973). Counseling and demonstration of use of child restraints in two studies, and counseling regarding smoke detectors in another, found increased use in the counseled group when actually observed (Berger et al., 1984; Miller et al., 1982; Reisinger et al., 1981). A review of randomized trials of the effects of home visiting programs on injuries indicates some effectiveness (Roberts et al., 1996). Nevertheless, the use of this approach is apparently not extensive. For example, only 4.1 percent of pediatricians report counseling regarding drowning hazards and only 17 percent of those with training in such hazards offered counseling (O'Flaherty & Pirie, 1997).

These results raise other research questions. How many behaviors can be influenced at any one time by counseling? Given the demonstration of the effectiveness of counseling regarding certain behaviors, how many physicians actually use the information? If many do not, how can the behavior of physicians be changed?

Attempts at influencing childrens' behavior directly have also had some success. For example, based on research that indicated "dart-out" as the most important type of child pedestrian injuries up to age 9, a program directed at that specific behavior in that age group was developed. A cartoon character called Willy Whistle as well as older children, portrayed as role models, were shown in films, television spots, and posters in midblock and intersection situations. The characters in these media demonstrated to children that they should always stop at the edge of curbs and the road side of parked cars.

The materials were used by television stations and in the schools in three communities. Data were collected on childrens' knowledge, and observers at selected sites recorded child behaviors before and after the campaign. Also, police reports of pedestrian injuries were compared for the two periods. Knowledge increases were substantial, and correct behaviors observed among children on the streets increased somewhat. Midblock dart and dash injuries declined among three to seven year olds, but those at other locations did not change appreciably (Blomberg et al., 1983).

There are two problems with this approach, one methodological and one implementational. Without a comparison to control cities, it is not possible to estimate precisely how much of the observed injury reduction can be attributed to the campaign. Without continued implementation in these and other cities, the campaign is useful only to demonstrate a principle. An attempt to find out where the campaign was used some six years subsequent to the study found only one city in which it had been systematically implemented afterward.

Many of the educational and other behavioral change programs have not been subjected to careful study before being adopted. Seldom considered is the possibility that a program could be ineffective at best or potentially harmful. Driver education was introduced in the public schools without research on its effects, based on the premise that driving skills were a primary factor in the probability of a crash, and that those skills could be improved by training.

Decades later, the first controlled experiment indicated that high school driver training did not reduce individual drivers' crashes per mile driven, but increased the number of drivers licensed at an earlier age such that the risk per population was increased (Shaoul, 1975). The adverse effect was found to be widespread in an ecological study of teenaged licensure and involvement in fatal crashes in 27 U.S. states during a period when driver education was increased by federal funding supplements (Robertson & Zador, 1978). A case-control study of driver licensure and crash records of teenagers in schools that dropped the courses, compared to those in schools that retained the courses, found large reductions in months licensed before age 18 and parallel reductions in crashes among those in schools that dropped the courses (Robertson, 1980). Nevertheless, in many communities, teenagers continue to receive driver training in high schools.

Several principles are illustrated by this experience. The value of a program intended to reduce injuries is not necessarily a function of the good intentions of the program's proponents. Skill or behavior change programs can have unintended harmful effects and those effects are often found only by well-designed research. This is particularly true of programs that have the potential to increase exposure to hazards. Once a program becomes institutionalized, it is difficult to remove it no matter how ineffective or harmful its consequences.

A major barrier to the scientific evaluation of programs is the reluctance of those who develop, advocate, or profit from programs to have them evaluated objectively. In some cases, their investment in the programs is only psychological, but in others it is economic. Authors of textbooks used in driver education courses and an insurance company that sold driving simulators to schools were among the most adamant critics of the high school driver education studies. They pointed to old studies of differences in driving records of students who had the course and those who did not as indicative of efficacy. However, those studies did not account for selection of the courses by students, or their parents, who were different in other ways that accounted for the differences in driving records (McGuire & Kersh, 1969).

Although experimental–control studies of ensconced programs may be difficult to initiate, clever researchers can sometimes find ways to design studies that reveal biases in other types of evaluations. For example, the "defensive driving" course that is sold widely by the National Safety Council has apparently never been subjected to an experimental–control study. The effect of self-selection in the course was controlled in one evaluation—however, in a situation where everyone who selected the course could not be enrolled. Comparison of the driving records of those who took the course at one point and those who took it later found no difference in crashes in the interim period (Mulhern, 1977). Therefore, when self-selection was constant, the course had no apparent effect.

The number of programs attempting to reduce driving while intoxicated among young drivers is large. One survey identified 248. These are most commonly single sessions or short segments in the curricula of senior high schools. The programs vary in focus and some are multifocused. About 83 percent of surveyed programs emphasize personal knowledge and skills regarding decisions to drink and drive, and 48 percent include emphasis on resistance to peer pressure. Virtually none of these programs had been evaluated as to effectiveness in actually reducing injuries by strict scientific standards, although some data are available on pre- and postprogram knowledge, attitudes, and self-reported behavior (Vegega & Klitzner, 1988). Such data are known to be misleading (Chapter 3).

Virtually all attempts to reduce alcohol-related injuries are directed at driving while intoxicated. There seems to have been little notice that drunk walking, drunk arguing, or even drunk sleeping, given fire/smoke hazards, are also dangerous. If the preventive programs were successful in reducing driving while intoxicated without reducing intoxication, there would still be no certainty that the overall severe injury rate would be reduced, given the possibility that the intoxicated would engage in other activities in which risk is increased by intoxication. Not only does the lack of program evaluation suggest the need for research; the research should examine the effects on the total severe injury rate, not just that in motor vehicles.

Much of injury control in industry is oriented to worker education, but research on the effects of corporate programs is seldom published. Claims have been made that so-called back schools have reduced incidence, lost days, and workers' compensation costs from back pain and strain, but details on how the research was conducted were not indicated (Isernhagen, 1988). Since diagnosis of pain and strain is largely subjective, and willingness to work with back strain or pain has been shown to decrease substantially as a function of amount of workers compensation increases, adjusted for inflation (Robertson & Keeve, 1983), attention to measurement issues and what is actually affecting the changes observed is needed.

In the case of low back pain, the emphasis prevalent in this book on the physics of energy exchanges may not be as applicable. Low back pain is only slightly correlated to heavy lifting. While 47 percent of workers doing heavy lifting in a division of one company during a ten-year period reported such pain, 35 percent of those doing light or sedentary work also reported low back pain (Rowe, 1983). Therefore, carefully controlled experiments should be conducted to find to what extent any changes in claimed pain or strain related to "back schools" or other programs are a result of workers' gratitude for increased attention to their problems by management versus actual changes in lifting behavior related to the educational content of a given program (Snook & White, 1984). In this case, two control groups would be advisable—one in which increased concern is shown by management without specific ameliorative instruction, and one in which there is neither a program nor management attention to workers' back injuries.

Some successes of educational programs in industry have been reported. For example, participation in an 18–24 hour intensive course on emergency preparedness is associated with fewer drowning and hypothermia deaths among commercial fishermen in Alaska (Perkins, 1995). Miners were successfully trained in proficient use of gas masks but performance deteriorated rapidly after three months without repeated practice (Vaught et al., 1993).

Since television is viewed by the vast majority of the population, it is a potential medium for promoting behavior change. Two attempted uses of television to change behavior are public service advertising (e.g., "buckle up for safety") and integration of messages in dramatic programs (e.g., showing the consequences of drunk driving in dramatic series). Documentary presentations (on *Dateline NBC, 60 Minutes, 20/20*, etc.) and self-administered knowledge tests (e.g., "The National Driving Test") may also change behavior, but they are not primarily intended for that purpose.

While the ad-type messages are short and can be inserted relatively frequently in breaks in programming if the time is donated or a sponsor is found, the integrated messages in dramatic programs and documentaries are likely to be seen infrequently. The effects of ads and other programs could be studied experimentally in communities with split-cable television systems that advertisers use to study product advertising. When the outcome behavior is frequent and easily observable, such as seat belt use, the effects of the program can be measured unobtrusively (e.g., Robertson et al., 1974). The effects on behaviors such as alcohol use would require stopping a sample of drivers and obtaining breath tests, which could be done with police department cooperation, but the author is unaware of any such study related to television ad campaigns.

A rather large body of research has been conducted on attempts to persuade people to use seat belts, but very little on other important behaviors—type of vehicle purchased, purchase of smoke detectors, and the like. In contrast to the failure to increase belt use appreciably by advertising, various lotterylike incentive systems and direct warnings—for example, a sticker on the dash saying "Belt use required in this vehicle"—have been found to increase belt use, in some cases substantially (Geller, 1988). Despite the demonstrated success of the latter approaches, they have not been adopted for widespread use. The adoption of this approach to reduce health care and absentee costs in corporations should be attractive to their executives, but the number of industries with belt use or other incentive systems for injury-related behaviors is unknown. At the community level, governments have not undertaken such programs and apparently private organizations have not used such programs on a large scale.

There is a substantial literature indicating that if the behavior to reduce risk is needed frequently, it is more difficult to persuade people to do it than in cases where the behavior is required only once (Robertson, 1975). Therefore, one would expect that persuading people to use seat belts consistently would be more difficult than persuading them to purchase a relatively safer vehicle. Yet much research and programatic effort have been directed at belt use and virtually none at vehicle purchase behavior.

The effects of various therapies and exercise on agility and tissue vulnerability of the elderly are under active investigation. The emphasis in studies of falls among the elderly is often on perceptual and motor abilities, changes in blood pressure, and so-called drop attack, in which the person collapses for no apparent reason. Several experimental trials of various types of exercise and balance programs, modifications of polydrug prescriptions, and so on, indicate fewer falls among those in the programs (Buchner et al., 1993; Ory et al., 1993; Tinetti et al., 1993). Other approaches, such as use of energy-absorbing protective garments, are also under study (Wallace et al., 1993). Despite a multicenter set of trials, the studies suffer from insufficient sample sizes to generate high confidence in the conclusions (Province et al., 1995). It seems that some such studies have almost as many coauthors as elderly participants.

SCREENING ON HUMAN FACTORS

To the extent that measurable human factors are predictive of injury, these factors could be used to refuse employment or select people for some sort of injury reduction program. For example, among the 10 percent of applicants for positions in the postal service who had urine tests positive for marijuana (7.8 percent) or cocaine (2.2 percent), injury rates on the job were 85 percent higher than those negative for the drugs, controlling for several other factors (Zwerling et al., 1990). If persons who tested positive for the drugs had not been hired, the postal service would have experienced fewer injuries. However, the net benefit for society is more questionable. If those persons refused employment became employed in a more hazardous environment or were engaged in more hazardous activities if they remained unemployed, the net effect could be worse. Research on the subsequent injuries of persons refused employment on the basis of drug screens or other factors would be interesting and perhaps useful.

If, on the basis of screening, those at higher risk were placed in behavior change programs that reduce injuries, the screening could have a net benefit. If the screening is not sensitive or if the program is ineffective, the usefulness of such programs can be very limited or even harmful. Children with burn scars in Ghana were found to have repeated burns at a rate less, not more, than expected from the prevalent rate (Forjuoh, 1996). Therefore, prior burns are not sensitive in identifying new cases. The author examined the FARS data in counties in which more than 90 percent of fatally injured drivers were tested for alcohol and noted that about 80 percent of fatally injured drivers with illegal blood alcohol had no prior convictions for driving while intoxicated. Therefore, screening those with such convictions for treatment programs would have a maximum 20 percent effect even if the programs were perfectly effective. Persons assigned to an education–rehabilitation program rather than the usual court procedure in one county had a higher subsequent crash record, probably because license suspension is more effective than education–rehabilitation (Preusser et al., 1976). Evaluation of attempts to improve screening for commercial drivers' licenses found no effect (Hagge & Romanowicz, 1996).

MULTIPLE COMMUNITY CHANGES

Some experiments have adopted a more community-wide approach directed either toward one goal, such as reduction of injuries from fireworks or increased bicycle helmet use, or multiple goals, such as reductions in several high-priority injury rates simultaneously.

Study of fireworks injuries associated with New Years' celebrations in Naples, Italy, indicated 60 percent of injuries occurred from illegal fireworks and children's injuries were often from attempting to relight unexploded fireworks or from powder assembled from partially exploded fireworks. A community program to reduce the injuries in the holiday season at the end of 1993 included police seizure of 12.5 million illegal fireworks, street sweeping to remove partially exploded and unexploded fireworks, and an increased public information program relative to previous years. There were 48 percent fewer injuries from fireworks treated in 18 surveyed emergency rooms during that holiday season than in the previous year (D'Argenio et al., 1996).

A case–control study of head injuries to helmeted and unhelmeted bicyclists—showing 85 percent effectiveness of helmets (Thompson et al., 1989)—encouraged researchers to launch a study of a campaign to promote helmet use. A control community was included to measure the trend in bicycle helmet use where there was no campaign. The campaign, directed at both parents and children, had several features in addition to television spots and a program in elementary schools. Hang tags urging helmet purchase were placed on bicycles for sale. Coupons for free french fries at fast-food outlets and free tickets for baseball games were distributed to helmet users, and coupons for discounts of $25 toward helmet purchases were distributed at various organizations and events. Helmet use by bicyclists, observed at a sample of sites in the community, increased from 5.5 percent to 15.7 percent compared to an increase of only 2.6 percentage points in the control community that had no special effort to promote bicycle helmet use (DiGuiseppi et al., 1989). A study of such a program in Quebec found a similar effect overall but a much greater effect in middle-class and wealthy communities than in those less wealthy (Farley et al., 1996).

That is not to say that underprivileged communities cannot benefit from injury control programs if the programs are tailored to the needs of the children and their families. Based on surveillance of injuries in Central Harlem, a neighborhood including some 28,000 children in 1990, a program aimed at the most severe injuries to children 5–16 years old was initiated (Davidson et al., 1994). The targeted injuries included those from motor vehicles, falls, assaults, and firearms (intentional or not). Such injuries to same-aged children in a comparison neighborhood that had no program, Washington Heights, were examined to rule out trends not related to the program. The program included renovation of playgrounds, increased child supervision including involvement in skill training (dance, art, sports, horticulture, and carpentry), education in prevention of injury and violence, and lowered costs of bicycle helmets. An appealing aspect of the program is that many of the activities have intrinsic value even if they have no discernible impact on injuries.

Although the results were not entirely unambiguous, there was apparently a reduction in some of the targeted injuries. Since injuries also declined in the comparison community, other factors may have accounted for some of the observed reductions. The major evidence for efficacy of the program was that targeted injuries except falls declined in Harlem, but nontargeted injuries did not, whereas all injuries declined in Washington Heights. It also makes sense that children diverted from street activities would have decreases in motor vehicle and assault injuries without changes in fall injuries that occur in sports.

Particularly encouraging was the decline in assault and gun injuries, which decreased in Harlem while increasing in the comparison neighborhood during the intervention period (Durkin et al., 1996). This is likely due to diversion of children from the street culture rather than training in conflict resolution. Students in seventh-grade classes who had such training were compared to those from other classes without training. Contrary to the intended effect, the students with training reported an increase in aggression and delinquency relative to the comparison group (Colyer et al., 1996). Because of the questionable validity of self-reports, more definitive data on injuries related to training in conflict resolution is needed.

Various communities have developed coalitions, ad campaigns, school programs, clinical interventions, and the like, aimed at reducing violence, but there is precious little effort to evaluate their effects. One recent volume in which such efforts are described (Hampton et al., 1996) contains no reference to a study of ten communities where peer mediation in potentially violent situations was studied and found ineffective (Spiro & DeJong, 1991) or to the aforementioned success of alternative activities in Harlem.

GROUP BEHAVIOR

This chapter has noted several instances in which programs such as increasing supervision and alternative activities for children and adolescents, behavior-change counseling, and incentive systems resulted in reduced injuries, or behavior that would reduce risk. Some behavioral scientists have been defensive about the emphasis by epidemiologists on the agents, vehicles, and physical environmental factors that cause or contribute to injury, pointing to the noted studies as evidence that behavioral factors can also be changed. No one denies the latter, but as noted for some of the known effective behavior-change approaches, they are not being used. Perhaps behavioral scientists who emphasize the efficacy of a behavioral approach could design research that demonstrates how to remove barriers to the use of effective programs, whether oriented to behavior, agents, vehicles, or environments.

People behave in groups differently than they would as individuals. One interesting group phenomenon is "pluralistic ignorance" (Thibault & Kelley, 1965). In groups (corporations, governments, injury control coalitions), people will agree to action or inaction to which they would not personally commit in the absence of the group because they falsely believe the others in the group or its constituency support the action. One fascinating area for research is the extent to which revelation of pluralistic ignorance changes action.

An example occurred in White River, Arizona, where horses in the road were frequently struck by motor vehicles. The White Mountain Apache Tribal Council had years earlier adopted a law prohibiting horses in the road but there were no provisions for enforcement. When a health educator became concerned about the issue, he found that the injury surveillance system had identified the problem as a priority (Rothfus & Akin, 1988).

He talked with members of the council, but they were not convinced that other council members or the population would favor having to pay fines for their stray animals. He then conducted a community survey to see if there was support for removing horses from the road. The survey revealed overwhelming community desire for action. When the council was shown the survey, a wrangler was appointed to search for and round up stray animals daily and the owners were fined. The incidence of vehicle collisions with domestic livestock was greatly reduced (Anderson, 1995).

SUMMARY

Injury control efforts are inordinately oriented to behavior change. Theories of behavior contain conflicting hypotheses regarding behavioral motivations and limits on individual abilities, particularly in emergency situations. Injury rates at various stages in human development are a result of changing abilities, activities contibuting to differential exposures to energy, and changing susceptibility to energy.

Behavior change efforts are most successful when they decrease exposures and can be harmful if exposures are increased. Response to persuasion declines in relation to frequency of behavior necessary to reduce risk. Diffusion of effort toward many behaviors dilutes the effect. Personal counseling and community-based programs, particularly if incentives are included, are more effective than impersonal approaches such as advertising.

REFERENCES

Anderson HS (1995) An evaluation of the livestock control project on the Fort Apache Indian Reservation. White River, AZ: White Mountain Apache Health Education Department.

Applebome P (1993) GM is held liable over fuel tanks in pickup trucks. *New York Times,* April 5, p. 1.

Baker SP (1979) Motor vehicle occupant deaths in young children. *Pediatrics* 64:860–861.

Baker SP, O'Neill B, Haddon W Jr, and Long WB (1974) The injury severity score: a method of describing patients with multiple injuries and evaluating emergency care. *J Trauma* 14:187.

Baker SP, O'Neill B, Ginsburg M, and Li G (1992) *The Injury Fact Book* 2nd ed. New York: Oxford University Press.

Berger LR, and Mohan D (1996) *Injury Control: A Global View.* Delhi: Oxford University Press.

Berger LR, Saunders S, Armitage K, and Schauer L (1984) Promoting the use of car safety devices for infants: an intensive health education approach. *Pediatrics* 74:16–19.

Blomberg RD, Preusser DF, Hale A, and Leaf WA (1983) *Experimental Field Test of Proposed Pedestrian Safety Messages.* Washington, DC: National Highway Traffic Safety Administration.

Bragg WE, and Finn P (1982) Young driver risk-taking research: technical report of experimental study. Washington, DC: National Highway Traffic Safety Administration.

Buchner DM, Cress ME, Wagner EH, de Lateur BJ, Price R, and Abrass IB (1993) The Seattle FICSIT/MoveIt study: the effect of exercise on gait and balance in older adults. *J Am Geriatr Soc* 41:321–325.

Campos-Outcalt D, Prybylski D, Watkins AJ, Rothfus D, and Dellapena A (1997) Motor-vehicle crash fatalities among American Indians and non-Indians in Arizona, 1970 through 1988. *Am J Public Health* 87:282–285.

Centerwell BS (1995) Race, socioeconomic status and domestic homicide. *JAMA* 273:1755–1758.

Cole RE, Grolnick WS, Laurenitis LR, McAndrews MM, and Matkoski KM (1986) *Children and Fire.* Albany: New York Department of State.

Colyer E, Thompkins T, Durkin M, and Barlow B (1996) Can conflict resolution training increase aggressive behavior in young adolescents? *Am J Public Health* 86:1028.

D'Argenio P, Cafaro L, Santonastasi F, Taggi F, and Binkin N (1996) *Capodanno Senza Danno:* the effects of an intervention program on fireworks injuries in Naples. *Am J Public Health* 86:84–86.

Davidson LL, Durkin MS, Kuhn L, O'Connor P, Barlow B, and Heagarty MC (1994) The impact of the Safe Kids/Healthy Neighborhoods Injury Prevention Program in Harlem, 1988 through 1991. *Am J Public Health* 84:580–586.

Dershewitz RA, and Williamson JW (1977) Prevention of childhood household injuries: a controlled clinical trial. *Am J Public Health* 67:1148–1153.

DiGuiseppi CG, Rivara FP, Koepsell TD, and Polissar L (1989) Bicycle helmet use by children: evaluation of a community-wide helmet campaign. *JAMA* 262:2256–2261.

Durkin MS, Kuhn L, Davidson LL, Laraque D, and Barlow B (1996) Epidemiology and prevention of severe assault and gun injuries to children in an urban community. *J Trauma* 41:667–673.

Eastman JW (1984) *Styling vs. Safety: The American Automobile Industry and the Development of Automotive Safety, 1900–1966.* New York, NY: University Press of America.

Evans L (1996) Comment: the dominant role of driver behavior in traffic safety. *Am J Public Health* 86:784–786.

Evans L, and Schwing RC (eds) (1985) *Human Behavior and Traffic Safety.* New York: Plenum Publishing Co.

Farley C, Haddad S, and Brown B (1996) The effects of a 4-year program promoting bicycle helmet use among children in Quebec. *Am J Public Health* 86:46–51.

Forjuoh SN (1996) Burn repetitions in Ghanaian children: prevalence, epidemiological characteristics and socioenvironmental factors. *Burns* 22:539–542.

Frame P (1996) Has Martinez dropped the ball at NHTSA? *Automotive News,* June 24, p. 1.

Geller ES (1988) A behavioral approach to transportation safety. *Bull New York Acad Med* 64:632–661.

General Motors Corporation (1993) Evaluation of GM 1973–87 C/K Pickup Trucks, Part III: Analysis of FARS Fire Rates in Side Collisions for Fullsize Pickups and Supplemental Statistical Presentations. Submission to the National Highway Traffic Safety Administration, August 10.

Gensemer IB, Walker JC, McMurry FG, and Brotman SJ (1989) IQ levels following trauma. *J Trauma* 29:1616–1619.

Gerberich SG, Hays M, Mandel JS, Gibson RW, and Van der Heide CJ (1985) Analysis of suicides in adolescents and young adults. In Laaser U, Senault R, and Viefhues, H (eds), *Primary Health Care in the Making.* Berlin: Springer-Verlag.

Gilula MF, and Daniels DN (1969) Violence and man's struggle to adapt. *Science* 164:396–405.

Graafmans WC, Ooms ME, Hofstee HM, Bezemer PD, Bouter LM, and Lips, P (1996) Falls in the elderly: prospective study of risk factors and risk profiles. *Am J Epidemiol* 143:1129–1136.

Graves AB, White E, Koepsell TD, Reifler BV, van Belle G, Larson GB, and Raskind M (1990) The association between head trauma and Alzheimer's Disease. *Am J Epidemiol* 131:491–501.

Hagge RA, and Romanowicz PA (1996) Evaluation of California's commercial driver license program. *Acc Anal Prevention* 28:547–559.

Hampton RL, Jenkins P, and Gullotta TP (1996) *Preventing Violence in America.* Thousand Oaks, CA: Sage Publications.

Hoiberg A, Bernard SP, and Ernst J (1981) Racial differences in hospitalization rates among navy enlisted men. *Public Health Rep* 96:121–127.

Isernhagen SJ (1988) *Work Injury: Management and Prevention.* Rockville, MD: Aspen Publishers.

Kane DN (1985) *Environmental Hazards to Young Children.* Phoenix: Oryx Press.

Kemp AM, Mott AM, and Sibert JR (1994) Accidents and child abuse in bathtub submersions. *Arch Dis Child* 70:435–438.

Kravitz H (1973) Prevention of falls in infancy by counseling mothers. *Illinois Med J* 144:570–573.

Kunitz SJ (1976) Fertility, mortality, and social organization. *Hum Biol* 48:361–377.

Lange RC, Ray RM, and McCarthy RM (1992) Analysis of light-duty motor vehicle collision-fire rates. Menlo Park, CA: Failure Analysis Associates.

Levy JE, and Kunitz SJ (1974) *Indian Drinking: Navajo Practices and Anglo-American Thoeries.* New York: John Wiley and Sons.

Locklear G (1991) A retrospective case–control study of porch step falls occurring on the Fort Apache Indian Reservation, 1987 to 1989. Phoenix: Environmental Health Services Branch, Indian Health Service (mimeo).

Matthews ML, and Moran AR (1986) Age differences in male drivers' perception of accident risk: the role of perceived driving ability. *Accident Anal Prev* 18:299–313.

May P (1982) Substance abuse and American Indians: prevalence and susceptibility. *Int J Addict* 17:1185–1209.

Mazur A, and Robertson LS (1972) *Biology and Social Behavior.* New York: Free Press.

McGuire FL, and Kersh RC (1969) *An Evaluation of Driver Education.* Berkeley: University of California Press.

Meier B (1992) GM retreats on claims about fatal truck fires. *New York Times,* December 2, p. A20.

Miller RE, Reisinger KS, Blatter MM, and Wucher F (1982) Pediatric counseling and the subsequent use of smoke detectors. *Am J Public Health* 72:392–393.

Mulhern T (1977) The National Safety Council's Defensive Driving Course as an accident and violation countermeasure. Unpublished doctoral dissertation. College Station: Texas A and M University.

National Highway Traffic Safety Administration (1989) *Restraint System Use in the Traffic Population: 1988 Annual Report.* Washington, DC: U.S. Department of Transportation.

Naureckas SM, Galanter C, Naureckas ET, and Christoffel, KK (1995) Children's and women's ability to fire handguns. *Arch Pediatr Adolescent Med* 149:1318–1322.

O'Flaherty JE, and Pirie PL (1997) Prevention of pediatric drowning and near drowning: a survey of members of the American Academy of Pediatrics. *Pediatrics* 99:169–174.

Ory MG, Schechtman KB, Miller JP, Hadley EC, Fiatarone MA, Province MA, Arfken CL, Morgan D, Weiss S, and Kaplan, M (1993) Frailty and injuries in later life: the FICSIT trails. *J Am Geriatr Soc* 41:283–296.

Osgood NJ (1985) *Suicide in the Elderly.* Rockville, MD: Aspen.

O'Toole BI (1990) Intelligence and behavior and motor vehicle accident mortality. *Acc Anal Prevention* 22:211–221.

Perkins R (1995) Evaluation of an Alaskan marine safety training program. *Public Health Rep* 110:701–702.

Pierce JA (1977) *Drivers First Licensed in Ontario, October 1969 to October 1975.* Toronto: Ontario Ministry of Transportation and Communication.

Preusser DF, Ulmer RG, and Adams JR (1976) Driver record evaluation of a drinking driver rehabilitation program. *J Safety Res* 8:98–105.

Province MA, Hadley EC, Hornbrook MC, Lipsitz LA, Miller JP, Mulrow CD, Ory MG, Sattin RW, Tinnetti ME, and Wolf SL (1995) The effects of exercise on falls in elderly patients. A preplanned meta-analysis of the FICSIT trials. Frailty and injuries. Cooperative studies of intervention techniques. *JAMA* 273:1341–1347.

Rabinovich BA, Lerner ND, and Huey RW (1994) Young children's ability to climb fences. *Hum Factors* 36:733–744.

Reisinger KS, Williams AL, Wells JAK, John CE, Roberts TR, and Pogainy HJ (1981) The effect of pediatricians' counselling on infant restraint use. *Pediatrics* 67:201–206.

Reiss AJ, and Roth JA (1993) *Understanding and Preventing Violence.* Washington, DC: National Academy Press.

Rice DP, Mackenzie EJ (1989) *Cost of Injury in the United States.* San Francisco, CA:

University of California at San Francisco, and Baltimore, MD: Johns Hopkins University.

Rivara FP (1982a) Epidemiology of childhood injuries. In Bergman AB (ed), *Preventing Childhood Injuries.* Columbus, OH: Ross Laboratories.

Rivara FP (1982b) Epidemiology of childhood injuries: review of current research and presentation of conceptual framework. *Am J Dis Children* 136:399–405.

Roberts I, Kramer MS, and Suissa S (1996) Does home visiting prevent childhood injury? A systematic review of randomised controlled trials. *Br Med J* 312:29–33.

Robertson LS (1975) Behavioral research and strategies in public health: a demur. *Soc Sci Med* 9:165–170.

Robertson LS (1977) Car crashes: perceived vulnerability and willingness to pay for crash protection. *J Community Health* 3:136–141.

Robertson LS (1980) Crash involvement of teenaged drivers when driver education is eliminated from high school. *Am J Public Health* 70:599–603.

Robertson LS (1983) *Injuries: Causes, Control Strategies and Public Policy.* Lexington, MA: D.C. Heath.

Robertson LS (1985) *Epidemiological Assessment of the Contributing Factors of Injury Mortality and Morbidity among Native Americans.* Springfield, VA: National Technical Information Service.

Robertson LS (1989) Childhood injury prevention: some lessons learned. In Haller JA (ed), *Emergency Medical Services for Children.* Columbus, OH: Ross Laboratories.

Robertson LS, and Keeve JP (1983) Worker injuries: the effects of workers' compensation and OSHA inspections. *J Health Polit Policy Law* 8:581–597.

Robertson LS, Kelley AB, O'Neill B, Wixon CW, Eiswirth RS, and Haddon W Jr (1974) A controlled study of the effect of television messages on safety belt use. *Am J Public Health* 64:1071–1080.

Robertson LS, and Zador PL (1978) Driver education and crash involvement of teenaged drivers. *Am J Public Health* 68:959–965.

Rosenberg ML, Stark E, and Zahn MA (1986) Interpersonal violence: homicide and spouse abuse. In Last JM (ed), *Public Health and Preventive Medicine.* New York: Appleton-Century-Croft.

Rothfus GL, and Akin DP (1988) A study of motor vehicle crashes: White Apache Reservation, 1985–86. Phoenix: Indian Health Service.

Rowe ML (1983) *Backache at Work.* Fairport, NY: Perinton Press.

Schuster DH, and Guilford JP (1964) The psychometric prediction of problem drivers. *Hum Factors* 6:393–421.

Sewell CM, Becker TM, Wiggins CL, Key CR, Hull HF, and Samet JM (1989) Injury mortality in New Mexico's American Indians, Hispanics, and non-Hispanic whites, 1958 to 1982. *West J Med* 150:708–713.

Shaoul J (1975) *The Use of Accidents and Traffic Offenses as Criteria for Evaluating Courses in Driver Education.* Salford, England: University of Salford.

Shupe A, Stacey WA, and Hazelwood LR (1987) *Violent Men, Violent Couples.* Lexington, MA: D.C. Heath.

Smith RS, and Robertson LS (in press) Unintentional injuries and trauma. In Rhoades ER (ed), *The Health of American Indians and Alaska Natives.* Baltimore, MD: Johns Hopkins University Press.

Snook SH, and White AH (1984) Education and training. In Pope MH, Frymoyer JW, and Andersson G (eds), *Occupational Low Back Pain.* New York: Praeger.

Sorenson SB, and Shen H (1996) Homicide risk among immigrants in California, 1970 through 1992. *Am J Public Health* 86:97–100.

Spiro A, and DeJong W (1991) *Preventing Interpersonal Violence among Teens.* Final Report on National Institute of Justice Grant 87–IJ-CX, 009.

Stark E, Flitcraft A, and Zuckerman D (1981) *Wife Abuse in the Medical Setting: An Introduction for Health Personnel.* Washington, DC: Office of Domestic Violence, Monograph no. 7.

Stratton R, Zeiner A, and Paredes A (1978) Tribal affiliation and prevalence of alcohol problems. *J Stud Alcohol* 39:1166–1177.

Taylor SP, Gammon CB, and Capasso DR (1976) Aggression as a function of the interaction of alcohol and threat. *J Pers Soc Psychol* 34:938–941.

Thibaut JW, and Kelley HH (1965) *The Social Psychology of Groups.* New York: John Wiley and Sons.

Thompson RS, Rivara FP, and Thompson DC (1989) Prevention of head injury by bicycle helmets: a field study of efficacy. *New Engl J Med* 320:1361–1367.

Tinetti ME, Baker DI, Garrett PA, Gottschalk M, Koch ML, and Horwitz RI (1993) Yale FICSIT: risk factor abatement strategy for fall prevention. *J Am Geriatr Soc* 41:315–320.

Tinetti ME, Mendes de Leon CF, Doucette JT, and Baker DI (1994) Fear of falling and fall-related efficacy in relationship to functioning among community-living elders. *J Gerontol* 49:140–170.

Tinetti ME, Doucette JT, and Claus EB (1995a) The contribution of predisposing and situational risk factors to serious fall injuries. *J Am Geriatr Soc* 43:1207–1213.

Tinetti ME, Doucette J, Claus E, and Marttoli R (1995b) Risk factors for serious injury during falls by older persons in the community. *J Am Geriatr Soc* 43:1214–1221.

Tremblay RE, and Craig WM (1995) Developmental crime prevention. In Tonry M, and Farrington DP (eds), *Building a Safer Society: Strategic Approaches to Crime Prevention.* Chicago: University of Chicago Press.

Vaught C, Brnich MJ, Wiehagen WJ, Cole HP, and Kellner HJ (1993) An overview of research on self-contained self-rescuer training. Pittsburgh: U.S. Department of the Interior Bureau of Mines Bulletin 695.

Vegega ME, and Klitzner MD (1988) What have we learned about youth anti-drinking-driving programs? *Eval Program Plann* 11:203–217.

Viscusi WK, and Magat WA (1987) *Learning about Risk: Consumer and Worker Responses to Hazard Information.* Cambridge, MA: Harvard University Press.

Wallace RB, Ross JE, Huston JC, Kundel C, and Woodworth G (1993) Iowa FICSIT trial: the feasibility of elderly wearing a hip joint protective garment to reduce hip fractures. *J Am Geriatr Soc* 41:338–340.

Westermeyer J, and Brantner J (1972) Violent death and alcohol use among the Chippewa in Minnesota. *Minnesota Med* 55:749–752.

Whetsell LA, Patterson CM, Young DH, and Schiller WR (1989) Preinjury psychopathology in trauma patients. *J Trauma* 29:1158–1162.

Williams AF (1976) Observed child restraint use in automobiles. *Am J Dis Child* 130:1311–1317.

Zwerling C, Ryan J, and Orav EJ (1990) The efficacy of preemployment drug screening for marijuana and cocaine in predicting employment outcome. *JAMA* 264:2639–2643.

6

LAWS AND FORMAL RULES DIRECTED AT INDIVIDUAL BEHAVIOR

Governments sometimes impose laws applicable to the public or segments of the public in an attempt to change behavior to reduce injuries. Also, in organizations such as corporations, sports leagues, and summer camps, there are often formal rules that proscribe or require particular behaviors thought to be related to injury risk. For example, changing certain rules for sports events can reduce injury rates substantially (Roberts et al., 1996). This chapter is focused on the use of epidemiologic data to evaluate the effects of laws and their enforcement on injury incidence or severity.

Epidemiologic data may provide lawmakers and administrators with information to justify, change, or repeal laws or rules (Bergman, 1992). For example, the high infant and toddler mortality rates in motor vehicles during the 1970s, mentioned in Chapter 5, were used to persuade legislators to enact laws requiring restraint use among younger children. Postenactment analysis has identified gaps in coverage of child-restraint laws, indicating that 39 percent of children 0–5 years old killed as occupants were exempted from the laws and thus demonstrating a need for legislators to consider filling the gaps (Teret et al., 1986).

To simplify discussion, the word "law" is used here to refer to laws and adminstrative rules directed at individual behavior. Two types of laws have been adopted in attempts to reduce injuries: those that proscribe behavior thought to increase risk and those that require behavior thought to increase protection. Examples of proscribed behaviors are drunk driving and exceeding posted speed limits in motor vehicles. Protective laws include measures such as required use of hardhats at worksites, required use of helmets by motorcyclists, use of seat belts or child restraints by vehicle occupants.

The theoretical models regarding the effect of law on proscribed behaviors are called *deterrence theories* (e.g., Ross, 1982). These theories focus on several factors that may affect the behavior in question: probability of detection of the proscribed behavior by the enforcement authority, probability of conviction for the offense, time from detection to conviction, and severity of punishment if convicted.

Two types of deterrence are possible: *specific* deterrence of repetition of the proscribed behavior (recidivism) by those detected and *general* deterrence, which includes reduction in the proscribed behavior of those not detected. Research on detected recidivism is relatively easy using police, court, or medical records, but the inferences of the effects of law on general deterrence are more difficult to support with scientific evidence.

The "public health" and "criminal justice" approaches have been falsely characterized as a difference between prevention of first offenses and reduction of recidivism (Moore, 1995). Most theoretical criminologists have long recognized the possible general deterrent effects of laws and their enforcement. The public health approach may help lawmakers and law enforcers recognize that the effects of laws are influenced by factors in addition to incapacitation and punishment.

Required protective behaviors not only include use of protective equipment, such as seat belts in motor vehicles, but may also include procedures to be followed, such as the checklists of airline pilots. Although there is less theory regarding the effects of these laws than of those regarding deterrence, a body of research does suggest some generalizations whereby the probable success of the laws can be estimated. It can be argued that deterrence theory applies to protective laws as well, but coercing someone into doing something that would not ordinarily be done is not necessarily the same thing as deterring someone from doing something that he or she is wont to do.

The premises of deterrence theory are at least partly dependent on the question of the extent of intent in human behavior related to injury. If all homicides or assaults were well planned by people weighing the costs and benefits, as economic theories of "crime" would have us believe (Becker, 1968), then enough increase in the cost to the offenders should deter potential offenders from the acts. To the extent that assault is momentarily impulsive or reactive behavior without rational deliberation, or the result of mental illness, weighing of the potential consequences by the assailant may be inconsequential (Smith & Warren, 1978). Similarly, to the extent that alcohol use, seat belt use, or whatever behavior, is the result of psychological, social, or cultural factors that preclude or override concerns about detection or punishment, the effect of protective laws and their enforcement will be diminished. In some instances, the effects of laws may be diminished because people are exempted for reasons of religion or custom. For example, Sikhs in India and Great Britain are exempted from laws requiring helmet use on motorcycles because the turbans required by their religion do not accommodate commercially available helmets (Berger & Mohan, 1996). Turbans provide some protection but are not as effective as helmets (Sood, 1988).

Most drivers deliberately or inadvertently violate traffic laws daily and the discretion of the police in enforcement often looks arbitrary and sometimes looks capricious (Ross, 1960). How much this leads to disrespect for law and police beyond the road environment is unknown, but it is likely that frequent observation of law violations increases the probability of such behavior. Police may discriminate by race, sex, and socioeconomic status with impunity (Cressey, 1975) unless the incident escalates into violence, as several publicized cases have in recent years in the United States, further increasing the disrespect among those who feel singled out.

RESEARCH QUESTIONS AND STUDY DESIGNS

Most of the research on laws focuses on the effects of enforcement or punishment. Little attention has been paid to how laws aimed at injury reduction are enacted. No one familiar with the strong antigovernment strain in Tennessee politics would have expected that state to be the first to enact a law requiring children to be restrained in cars. Nevertheless, persistent lobbying by pediatricians and other groups of citizens was successful (Sanders, 1982). All U.S. states subsequently followed Tennessee's lead, albeit with significant gaps in the coverage.

Other laws have not been uniformly adopted, such as laws requiring seat belt use and gun control laws, and others have been difficult to retain once enacted, such as motorcycle helmet use laws. Although hypotheses regarding the social and political processes that lead to enactment or resistance to laws by legislators may not be viewed by epidemiologists as within their purview, those with backgrounds in sociology and political science may find the subject of interest.

One question that has been little explored is: What are the origin and sustenance of the lobbying in opposition to laws to reduce injury? No doubt many of the opponents are sincerely concerned that their rights or economic interests are at stake, but there may be a more cynical element. Some of the lobbyists, or magazine and newsletter publishers, may care less about the substance of an issue than about its potential to enrich them. By continuously stirring up opposition with claims that the rights of whatever group (gun owners, motorcyclists, etc.) are being violated, they promote collection of dues, subscriptions to magazines, newsletters sales, and other very profitable endeavors. Of course, proponents of laws can be exploited in a similar manner.

Once a law is enacted, the simplest question regarding a law is: Does it reduce injuries? The simplest research design to answer the question is to compare injury rates before and after the law. This can be misleading, however, for if other factors are changing that would have increased or reduced injuries during the same period of time, the change in injuries can be falsely attributed to the law.

For example, when a supervising judge in Chicago required seven day jail sentences for drunk driving during a period in 1970–71, the death rate declined and the rule was declared a success. Aware of the threats to validity in before–after comparisons (Campbell, 1969), researchers designed a quasi-experimental study to examine the effect of Chicago's judicial policy. Comparison of the death rates in Chicago and the nearby city of Milwaukee during the same period indicated that a similar decline occurred at the same time in Milwaukee, which did not have a policy of mandatory jail sentences (Robertson et al., 1973). The reduced fatality rates were likely the result of recession in the economy or changes in weather patterns that happened to occur concurrent with the judge's sentencing policy.

Most laws applied to individual behavior in the United States are enacted in state and local jurisdictions. Although this is disadvantageous in obtaining the uniform application of laws of known efficacy, it gives the researcher the opportunity to study the effect of laws of unknown or questionable efficacy in jurisdictions that introduce them relative to those that do not. Evaluation of the effect of enactment of laws that were in effect before data systems on relevant injuries were initiated is not possible, although the waxing and waning of enforcement may provide opportunities for study.

One of the threats to valid conclusions in before–after research designs without comparison jurisdictions, particularly in smaller jurisdictions where numbers fluctuate substantially in short periods of time, is so-called regression to the mean (Campbell, 1969). That is, if a new law or increased enforcement is initiated in areas based on a high injury rate in a short period, the rate would be expected to trend toward the average in a subsequent period irrespective of the change in policy. For example, the National Highway Traffic Safety Administration allocated $10 million in grants to states in 1973 for intensified law enforcement based on research indicating a reduction in fatalities after such enforcement in six counties. The counties were selected primarily on the basis of unusually high fatality rates. Using data from counties chosen on the basis of similar criteria in the same and another state, subsequent research showed that similar reductions in fatalities occurred in counties comparably chosen, but without special enforcement (Williams & Robertson, 1975).

Therefore, the reduction in the counties with special enforcement probably occurred because of return to normal from an unusual increase prior to the program, not because of special enforcement. While it makes sense to target efforts at areas where injuries are the most acute, claims of the effectiveness of a law or other injury control effort based on application in areas with unusually high rates prior to implementation is suspect. Effectiveness should be studied in areas that have no inordinate rates. If effectiveness is established, then efficient application dictates that the countermeasure with known effectiveness be targeted at areas with the highest rates.

When the law applies to a country as a whole, there may not be another country for comparison nearby that has comparable weather or other factors that could affect changes in injury rates. A research methodology that has been employed to evaluate the effect of laws in that circumstance is the interrupted time series (Campbell, 1969; Hoff, 1983). If one can obtain data on injury rates for an extended period of time before and after a law change, an abrupt and substantial change in the rates coincident with the change in law, enforcement, or punishment is usually indicative of the effect of the change in policy, particularly if such abrupt changes have not occurred in the rates in the past.

Sometimes gradual change in injury trends from before to after a change in law or enforcement is attributed to the law, but such inferences are highly questionable without replication in other jurisdictions and times. A trend may change for all sorts of reasons, and a continuation of a previous trend may occur for a reason different from the trend to that point. Lack of a change in trend may mask the effect of an efficacious policy if other factors are changing to offset it. For example, if the rural-to-urban migration of populations (that is usually accompanied by a downward trend in motor vehicle death rates, due to congestion and lower speeds in urban areas) slows about the time that an effective alcohol countermeasure is introduced, the effect of the alcohol countermeasure could be underestimated.

Both from the scientific and practical points of view, the extent of replication of research results is very important. *Replication* refers to finding a similar result when a study is repeated in a different study population. Particularly when there is no reasonable comparison or control group, replication is needed to assure that change in injuries at a time of change in law, enforcement, or punishment was not for reasons other than the legal effect. In the case of the effect of "crackdowns" on alcohol and driving, interrupted time series in several jurisdictions indicate that a publicized increase in police activity results in a temporary reduction in vehicle-related injuries, the time of the effect varying from a few months to a few years (Ross, 1982).

Most police crackdowns are locally determined and there is little research on why some communities undertake such efforts and others do not. Stimulation of community efforts by grant programs can have an effect, but many communities do not even apply for the funds. In Massachusetts, for example, communities were offered $70,000 per year for five years to initiate police enforcement and community activities to reduce drunk driving and alcohol use. Thirty responded and six were funded, resulting in reductions in motor vehicle injuries in those six compared to others that applied but were not funded (Hingson et al., 1996). Dozens of communities did not apply. It would be worthwhile to know why.

Perception of increased probability of arrest often has a deterrent effect, but changes in severity of punishment have little if any effect (Ross, 1982, 1992; Ross & Klette, 1995). The practical implication of the replicated findings is that crackdowns that increase the probability of arrest, or at least the perception of increased probability of arrest, will reduce the injury rate for a time, even in countries with somewhat differing cultures and legal traditions. The results leave open questions of how long such crackdowns can be maintained in terms of publicity and actual police activity, how often they can be repeated in the same population with the same effect, and whether a long-term change in behavior can be achieved with repetition (Hingson et al., 1988).

A decline in the proportion of fatally injured drivers with illegal blood alcohol was observed during the late 1980s and early 1990s in the United States (National Highway Traffic Safety Administration, 1995), partly due to the reenactment of 21-year-old drinking-age laws in several states (Robertson, 1989) and partly due to other laws and enforcement (Zador et al., 1988). Increased public attention to dieting and the marketing of beverages with less alcohol per volume may have also contributed to the reduction, but evaluation of the effect of such factors is difficult because of the lack of disaggregated data regarding these factors in drivers in crashes relative to those exposed to the same road and other conditions.

A more complex variation of time-series analysis is the multivariate analysis of the fluctuation of injury rates during a period of time in one or more ecological units (country, provinces, states, cities) relative to fluctuations in factors thought to affect those rates, including laws or aspects of law enforcement. In addition to the fact that ecological-level data do not necessarily reflect the characteristics of the individuals injured (or assailants, drivers in crashes, etc.), noted in Chapter 4 (the ecological fallacy), the specification of the statistical models and the intercorrelation of factors at the ecological level renders the estimates of effects from such analyses highly problematic. These problems have long been recognized in the analysis of economic data (Leamer, 1983; Orcutt et al., 1968), but economists particularly persist in performing such questionable analyses.

The effects of police staffing and police expenditures per capita have been studied with such models and the results vary remarkably depending on the ecological units used, the assumed causal variables controlled, and the types of outcomes measured. The unit of analysis and the type of crime analyzed may be more or less sensitive to the ecological fallacy or the direction and degree of effect. Use of smaller jurisdictions, such as cities, narrows the variation in factors such as poverty, concentration of minority populations, and other socioeconomic factors. If the increased enforcement merely moved the criminal activity to the suburbs, however, the estimate of effect would be overstated. The latter would not be true if the analysis were confined to domestic violence or crimes of passion, but in the noted studies, these are usually lumped together with all murders and police-reported assaults, or felonies generally. Use of larger ecological units, such as metropolitan areas or states, might give better estimates of the overall effect, but these estimates might be confounded in different ways by the variation of other factors as well as large differences in concentration of enforcement within smaller segments of such ecological units.

On the assumption that allocations of budgets for police and equipment are in response to crime as well as possibly having an effect on crime, the regression equations on the time series are sometimes estimated in two or more stages. One review of 11 such studies noted effects on several crimes varying from estimates of substantial effect of police staffing or expenditures, to no effect, to adverse effects (O'Connor & Gilman, 1978). The latter could occur, for example, if the police and certain criminals, or minorities who fear police as much or more than criminals, engaged in an arms race.

One of the more controversial issues that has been subjected to a variety of analyses is gun control legislation. Gun-related deaths and injuries are rare in most countries where the ownership of guns is tightly controlled or prohibited for most people. The population rate of all assaults in a region of Denmark in a year was about 75 percent of that in the Northeastern Ohio Trauma Study, but the Danish homicide rate was only 20 percent that in the Ohio study. The difference in homicide rates is mainly the result of greater use of guns in assaults in Ohio. Private ownership of guns is allowed in Denmark only for hunting (Baker, 1985).

Even countries that have substantial social and political unrest have lower gun deaths per capita than many cities in the United States. Detroit, Michigan, had more gun-related deaths in 1973 than Northern Ireland, with a similar-sized population, had during 5.5 years of renewed "troubles" in 1969–1974 (Zimring & Hawkins, 1987). Long-term comparisons of trends in violent crime as various countries imposed strict gun control indicates substantial effectiveness of such laws, but the weaker gun control laws typical in the United States had no discernible effects (Podell & Archer, 1994).

Opponents of gun control laws point to low gun death rates in Israel and Switzerland, where substantial numbers of citizens keep guns as part of the reserve defense forces. Important questions for research are: What criteria do these countries use to screen applicants to the defense reserves? How is the screening implemented? How many people are not allowed to have guns on the basis of the screening? Do the citizen–soldiers have loaded guns or are there conditions for the issuance of ammunition? Does the recipient of ammunition have to account for its wherabouts and use? The answers might provide guidance for more effective gun control in countries where guns are ubiquitous and where gun death rates are high.

The effects of new gun control laws in the United States are limited by the prelaw prevalence of gun ownership, and the effects of extant state and local laws are tempered by the movement of guns from jurisdictions with few restrictions to those with stricter laws. The results of studies of gun control laws in the United States are in substantial conflict, less so in the case of effects on suicide than in effects on homicide.

Using an index of strictness of combinations of various types of laws, comparisons of jurisdictions found gun-related deaths lower in jurisdictions with more strict gun control laws, and particularly where there is licensure of dealers, licensure of owners, and a waiting period between sale and delivery (Geisel et al., 1969). As indicated later in this chapter, when enforcement is augmented by persons in the community other than police—in this case dealers—laws tend to be more effective. The argument against studies showing a lower gun death rate related to gun control laws is: "You didn't control for X."

For example, other researchers found that when the region of the country is controlled statistically, the correlation of the gun strictness index and gun death rate is no longer statistically significant. This was interpreted as demonstration of a spurious correlation: gun death rates were said to be the result of the "frontier culture" of the South and Southwest rather than gun control laws, which are more prevalent in the North and East (Magaddino & Medoff, 1984). Since no one has attempted to measure "frontier culture," that is a dubious interpretation. For example, in Texas, a state that has been stereotyped as having a frontier culture, Dallas and Houston had the highest seat belt use in response to law, more than 15 percentage points higher than the highest use in 17 cities in other states (Goryl & Bowman, 1987). That hardly seems the manifestation of a frontier culture thumbing its nose at laws.

The effect of gun control on suicide rates is less controversial. Researchers who have questioned the effect on homicide rates found that suicide rates are substantially lower in areas with stricter gun control laws (Medoff & Magaddino, 1983).

Studies of severity of punishment of those who use guns have been limited. There is some evidence that mandatory sentencing for possession of a firearm during various crimes reduces homicides from firearms. Comparison of trends in percentage of homicides and suicides from firearms in New Jersey relative to the remainder of the United States before and after passage of a mandatory sentencing law in 1981 indicates a substantial reduction in gun involvement in homicides but not suicides (Fife & Abrams, 1989). Since New Jersey had relatively strict gun control laws prior to the mandatory sentencing law (Geisel et al., 1969), the results may not be generalizable to states without such combinations of laws.

Almost all studies of gun control are of aggregated data. It would be useful to compare individual-level data on homicides and suicides with guns in jurisdictions with different gun control laws regarding such factors as: How old was the gun? Was the gun legally or illegally possessed? How was the gun obtained? What was the history of the gun (e.g., a gun possessed illegally where the death occurred but purchased legally elsewhere)?

The augmentation of law enforcement by persons other than police in the community is probably a substantial factor in the effect of several laws known to reduce injuries. Examples are laws that prohibit driving by 16 year olds after a certain time in the evening. Since the police cannot easily see drivers at night, much less make a judgment regarding their ages, it is unlikely that arrest activity by police is effective in enforcement of such curfews. Yet comparisons of matched states with and without the laws indicates 25–62 percent reductions in crashes of 16-year-old drivers during the curfew hours (Preusser et al., 1984). A comparison of 47 cities with curfews for teenagers compared to 77 cities without curfews indicates a 23 percent reduction in motor vehicle deaths among 13–17 year olds (Preusser et al., 1993). It is likely that many parents enforce the law by requiring their youngsters to be home during the hours that the curfew is in effect. A comparison of other types of fatalities would be useful to assess what effect, if any, curfews have on deaths other than those related to motor vehicles.

With the exception of New Jersey, all states allow licensure to drive at age 16 and a few states permit licensure of even younger people. A comparison of the crash rates of 16 year olds in New Jersey, where the licensing age is 17 except for a special agricultural license, and Connecticut found 65–85 percent fewer 16 year olds as drivers in fatal crashes in New Jersey (Williams et al., 1983). Apparently most parents or guardians do not allow use of vehicles by unlicensed children. A complete analysis of the effects of curfews and licensing laws on injury would include injuries that could occur to teenagers when they are not driving. The issue here is whether activities substituted for driving are hazardous.

Several states have adopted "provisional licenses" for teenagers up to age 18. Some include curfews but others specify only conditions of obtaining and supervision while using a license or loss of license while in the probationary period. There is some evidence of reduced crash involvement of teenage drivers in states with such licenses (Jones, 1994), but the variations in the laws and studies make interpretation of effects of the particular aspects of the programs difficult.

Other jurisdictional comparisons have also suggested effectiveness of laws related to risks other than assaults and motor vehicles. Drownings of children in swimming pools were 65 percent less frequent in Honolulu, where pool fencing is required, than in Brisbane, Australia, with no requirement. The two cities had similar weather and pool-to-household ratios (Pearn et al., 1979). Comparison of adjacent affluent counties in Maryland and Virginia, with and without requirements for household smoke detectors, found 25 percent fewer deaths in housefires where smoke detectors were required (McLoughlin et al., 1985).

Since most legislative bodies are unlikely to enact a law for research purposes, the enactment of laws is not necessarily random, and research must be designed to account for prelaw differences among jurisdictions. The use of rules in corporate settings could be studied in randomized experimental–control studies, but if they are conducted, they usually are not reported in the literature. Attempts have been made to study the effects of differing sanctions by having judges randomly assign sentences but judges generally prefer to retain their discretion (Ross & Blumenthal, 1975).

Police departments have been somewhat more amenable to the use of randomized experimental designs in an attempt to find out if resources can be more effectively allocated or if certain procedures are more effective. For example, during more than a year, fifteen police districts in Kansas City were divided into three groups of five each: one set had the usual preventive patrol activity of a patrol car per district; a second had double to triple the usual patrol; and a third had no preventive patrol—the police responded only when called regarding a problem. Comparison of various crime rates and motor vehicle crashes among the areas, including victimization surveys as well as those reported to police, indicated no differences in assaults and motor vehicle crashes. The three comparisons that were statistically significant—sex crimes other than rape, home burglaries, and community vandalism—did not consistently support a case for more intensive patrols (Kelling et al., 1974).

Several subsequent experimental studies were undertaken in an attempt to define aspects of police procedure and response that might make a difference, but more recent efforts are focused on first defining the dimensions of the variety of problems that the police encounter and developing tailored prevention programs or responses (Goldstein, 1990). This is no less than the use of epidemiologic surveillance and analysis of relatively homogeneous subsets of the problem noted in Chapters 2 and 3. This approach requires a reorientation of policing from treating each incident as a case to be investigated and resolved to a search for patterns that can guide targeted efforts. The research evidence indicates that concentration of police activity in "hot spots" of crime, particularly in unpredictable patrol sequences for limited periods of time, reduces crime in those areas without displacing it elsewhere (Sherman, 1996). The severity of injuries related to guns has also been reduced using the hot-spot approach. In a controlled experiment in Kansas City, police concentrated in areas with high gun-related crime used traffic violations as probable cause to search for guns. Shots fired decreased 81 percent in the experimental area compared to 32 percent in the comparison area (Sherman, 1996).

Some of the literature on targeting countermeasures based on surveillance raises the question of whether the targets should be based on rates per exposure or total numbers. For example, one report from a police service in Canada compared police-reported motor vehicle crashes and convictions of drivers by age and sex relative to a survey of kilometers driven. Based on a narrowing of differences in crashes and convictions among age and sex groupings when considering rates per kilometer driven relative to proportionate involvement of those involved, the author of that study suggested that less attention should be paid to young and/or male drivers (Mercer, 1989). Yet, from a public health standpoint, one would target the groups with the largest numbers whether those numbers were generated by disproportionate exposure or not.

Particular aspects of the motor vehicle injury problem are known to be concentrated on certain roads at certain times of day. For example, Figure 6.1 presents illegal alcohol involvement in fatally injured drivers in the United States by type of road and time of day in counties where alcohol was actually measured in more than 90 percent of fatally injured drivers. While the amount of driving with illegal blood alcohol on these roads might be useful to indicate

FIGURE 6.1. Times and places of blood alcohol concentration (BAC) in fatally injured drivers, in percent.

how other conditions combine with alcohol to increase or decrease individual risk, the data are clear regarding enforcement of law. If the police are to maximize the apprehension of persons with illegal blood alcohol who will be in severe crashes, they will concentrate their alcohol squads on two-laned roads at night, where 61 percent of fatal crashes with illegally intoxicated drivers occur.

Can similar questions be raised about other types of injury that are known to involve alcohol? Do assaults in public occur repeatedly in certain bars, in other establishments, or on certain streets during certain hours? Do domestic assaults occur repeatedly in definable households at certain times of day and days of week?

Although assault among members of households resulting in injury requiring medical attention is more frequent than assault by strangers, arrest in domestic assault cases in the 1970s was about half as likely as in cases involving strangers (Berk & Loseke, 1980–81). A controlled experiment of the effect of arrest on specific deterrence of spouse battering was conducted in Minneapolis. In response to calls regarding domestic violence, police randomly applied one of three actions: they *(1)* arrested the assailant, *(2)* ordered the assailant away from the premises for eight hours, or *(3)* gave advice or attempted mediation. Follow-up study of police records and interviews with the persons assaulted indicated that arrest was the most effective policy to reduce recidivism (Sherman & Berk, 1984).

A retrospective study of 28 months of police records in a California county, controlling for factors that affected probability of arrest, found the same result (Berk & Newton, 1985). Since time in jail has implications for job or income loss, the authors of the latter study suggested another controlled experiment with treatments such as: *(1)* a citation (like a traffic ticket); *(2)* arrest, book, and immediate release; or *(3)* arrest and hold for a hearing. If the first or second was found as effective in deterring battering as arrest and hold, they would be preferable.

While many cities adopted an arrest policy as a result of the research, a substantial debate ensued regarding the methods of these studies, such as reliance on police records, and unmeasured effects, such as more severe injuries from escalation (Sherman, 1992). Replication of the Minneapolis experiment in other cities did not produce consistent results (Buzawa & Buzawa, 1996). This experience illustrates the difficulty both in policing private behavior and in learning whether police response has an effect because of questionable accuracy of reporting private behavior.

An example of an experimental study of detailed aspects of the effects on publicly observable behavior of a combined publicity and enforcement campaign is the research on elderly pedestrian behavior in Dade County, Florida. The experimental area was a street in Miami Beach with a high concentration of elderly residents and the control area was a comparable street with similar aged residents in Coral Gables. Observations of pedestrian behavior were obtained by cameras mounted high above the street and postcrossing interviews were also obtained, before, during, and after the increased enforcement of a law prohibiting jaywalking (crossing the street outside designated pedestrian crossing areas).

Prior to increased enforcement, news media coverage and speeches by police officers to 35 groups in the experimental area emphasized the law and the date enforcement would be increased. During a two-week special enforcement period, extra police foot patrols were deployed and about 300 tickets for jaywalking were issued, compared to about 40 per month ordinarily.

The results indicated that legal crossings increased during the enforcement period, especially when police were in sight, but declined to the preenforcement percentage when no police were present in the observation period after the special enforcement. Postcrossing interviews indicated that most people understood the law but prefered to rely on their own judgment regarding the movement of vehicles (Weiner, 1968). The effect on actual pedestrian collisions was not measured since too few would be expected in a two-week period for statistical power.

WHAT TO MEASURE

Most of the studies of effects of laws and rules measure the proscribed or required behavior or the incidence and severity of injuries thought to be affected by the behaviors. Preferably, both should be measured. For example, research on the effect of motorcycle helmet use included observations of helmet use by motorcyclists at selected sites in states with and without helmet use laws, as well as fatal injuries to motorcyclists in states with and without the laws before and after the laws were enforced. Since helmet use was almost universal in the states with laws requiring use, there was no question about differential use by those at differential risk after the law (Robertson, 1976).

Just because a law results in a change in the behavior required does not mean that the law is having proportional success in injury reduction. If compliance is not universal and those who comply with the law are more or less at risk, the ultimate effect of the law on injury will not be proportional to the technical effectiveness of the required behavior. That has apparently been the case with seat belt use laws.

The expected percentage change in injury rate as a result of a change in behavior (Robertson, 1983b) is

$$P_e = 100 \frac{E(U_2 - U_1)}{1 - U_1 E}$$

where

P_e = expected percentage change in injury rate
U_1 = proportion behaving in the prescribed way before the change
U_2 = proportion behaving in the prescribed way after the change
E = the technical effectiveness of the behavioral change

In Australia, where the first belt use law in a large jurisdiction (Victoria) was enacted, belt use increased from 20 to 70 percent from before to after the law. If the one-piece lap and shoulder belts used in Australia were 60 percent effective in reducing death as claimed, when used, $E=0.6$, $U_1=0.2$, and $U_2=0.7$. Therefore, the reduction in deaths should have been 35 percent. It was actually 10 percent in rural areas and 20 percent in urban areas, based on comparison of changes in death rates in Victoria relative to provinces without the law at the time (Foldvary & Lane, 1974). Even if belts, when worn, were 45 percent effective in reducing deaths (Chapter 7), that is, $E=0.45$, the reduction should have been 25 percent without selective use by those at less risk.

In the United States, enactment of belt use laws has been associated with death reductions of 5–15 percent, the lower reductions in states where citation for nonuse is allowed only when a driver is stopped for some other offense (Williams & Lund, 1988). That is less than in Australia, but the technical effectiveness in death reduction of belts in U.S. cars has been estimated at only 41 percent (Evans, 1986). This is at least partly because U.S. manufacturers of many models use "windowshade" devices, which allow substantial slack in the belts (Ciccone & Wells, 1988; Robertson, 1990).

When there are changes occurring simultaneously that could affect injury rates, then specification of changes in the behavior and specification of the injuries that should be affected by a law enacted at that time are essential for confidence in the research results. An example of multiple changing events occurred during the oil boycott that began near the end of 1972. The lack of gasoline and increased prices of fuel resulted in reduced driving; economic recession occurred; and the 55 mph speed limit was adopted on roads that had a higher limit, primarily to reduce fuel use—all in a matter of months. In the United States, there was a very notable reduction of about 8000 motor vehicle–related deaths per year in 1974–75 compared to the average in the five immediately prior years (interrupted time series), but the amount of the reduction that could be attributed to the reduced legal speed limit rather than the other factors was widely argued.

To estimate the effect of the speed limit, researchers noted that average speeds declined, particularly on rural interstates more than other roads. The percentage of drivers exceeding 65 mph decreased from 59 percent in 1973 to 10 percent in 1974, and those exceeding 55 mph declined from 93 percent in

1973 to 68 percent in 1974. The greatest reduction in deaths per miles traveled occurred on interstate and federal-aid primary roads—those where the speed limit was reduced. On the basis of reductions per miles traveled, about half of the total death reduction was attributed to the 55 mph limit (Kemper & Byington, 1977).

Eventually, due to an equivocal report from the Transportation Research Board (Altschuler et al., 1984) and an antiregulation Congress, the speed limits were raised. Deaths on rural interstate highways, where the limits were first raised, have increased.

Occasionally a situation arises that allows the researcher to obtain data regarding a hypothesis that is ordinarily difficult to test. For example, a police strike in Finland provided evidence of the effect on vehicle speeds of public knowledge that police would not be on the road (Summala et al., 1980). The average speed increased only slightly but the standard deviation increased about 20 percent. Apparently, those who took advantage of the police strike to drive faster were offset by those who drove more slowly, perhaps for fear of other drivers in a period of no enforcement. Unfortunately, crash data were not included, perhaps because the strike lasted only two weeks and the numbers would have been too small for statistical power.

Generally, the effects of laws on behavior and the evaluation of the effects are enhanced if the behavior is easily observable. If the researcher can observe the behavior, so can the police. It is not surprising, therefore, that laws requiring observable behavior, such as limits on vehicle speed, child restraint use, seat belt use, and motorcycle helmet use are usually more effective than laws directed at phenomena not observable without stopping persons—such as limits on blood alcohol of drivers or the carrying of concealed weapons (Robertson, 1983a).

UNINTENDED CONSEQUENCES

Generally laws that apply to publicly observable behaviors have proved more effective than nonlegal persuasive approaches (e.g., Mock et al., 1995). Few studies have paid attention to the possibility that laws requiring or proscribing a particular behavior could result in alternative behaviors that could place the individuals affected at more or less risk. For example, if children are required to be placed in child restraints while riding in cars, it is doubtful that families who could not afford child restraints would make fewer trips resulting in the child being in a more or less safe environment, given the availability of restraint loaner programs. But if child restraints were required on commercial airplanes, it has been argued, a large enough proportion of children that now fly free in adult arms would be driven rather than flown if the airline required payment for use of a seat. The relative risk in motor vehicles compared to cars would result in more injuries to children, or so the theory goes.

Since no data are available on what people would actually do, those who argue the issue one way or another are less than well-informed. One can conceive of a study in which child restraints would be required on a set of experimentally assigned air routes, and the numbers of child passengers in airplanes, motor vehicles (including busses), and trains would be counted by observers of the different modes of traffic among the experimental and randomly selected control routes before and after the restraint rule was put in effect. If there were apparent substitution of mode of travel, the net effect on risk to children could be estimated given known risk per mile by each mode of travel, and the observed use of child restraints in the two environments.

Laws that proscribe participation in certain activities also raise the issue of the extent to which the alternative activities are more or less dangerous. Numerous studies were done of the effects of the minimum legal drinking age on involvement of teenagers as drivers in fatal crashes without consideration of potential effects on other injuries. Although the estimates of effects on vehicle crashes were somewhat biased toward underestimate of the effect of the laws because proxy measures for alcohol involvement (night and single-vehicle crashes) were not as indicative of alcohol in the younger drivers (Robertson, 1990), the studies usually found reduced fatal motor vehicle crashes of the drivers in the age groups affected by the laws (General Accounting Office, 1987).

These studies left open the question of what teenagers who were drinking in bars or other settings, where drinking was legal, would have been doing had they not been there. Not only did no one consider that those drinking legally were placed at risk of other injuries related to alcohol (e.g., assaults in bars), no one considered that if they could not drink, they might be doing something even more dangerous.

Finally, one research project, based on one state that changed its legal drinking age compared to one that did not, found no statistically significant effect of changing the drinking age on mortality not related to motor vehicle injury (Hingson et al., 1985), but the statistical power was limited by the small sample. A larger study, based on all the states, estimated the effect of the legal minimum drinking age on all fatal injuries to persons 16–24 years of age and found a net beneficial effect on all injuries (Jones et al., 1992). Several potential effects were considered. Did the law affect injuries to persons younger than the drinking age, presumably because alcohol may be more easily obtained if adjacent aged peers can drink legally? Was there a spurt in injuries at the age that drinking became legal—the initiation effect? Did injuries decline as persons aged beyond the drinking age—the experience effect? The data indicated that, for most types of injuries, the higher the legal minimum drinking age, the lower the injury death rates in correlation with the number of years between the individuals' ages and the legal age. The hypothesized initiation effect was found only for homicides, and increased rather than decreased injury death rates occurred in correlation with presumed drinking experience (age at death minus legal drinking age).

Laws that prohibit alcohol sales in a limited geographic area have the potential to increase the risk of injury if the law results in driving or walking by intoxicated persons returning to the "dry" area from the "wet" area. During a brief period of legal alcohol use on an American Indian reservation, the arrests of reservation residents for intoxication in the neighboring county were reduced about one-third with no increase in such arrests on the reservation (May, 1975). Since arrests do not necessarily reflect alcohol use or the other behaviors associated with its use, the data are inadequate for a strong conclusion, but the issue is worthy of research. One study comparing retail availability of alcohol among states found no correlation between "single-vehicle" fatal crashes at night and alcohol retail outlets when other factors were taken into account (Greunewald & Ponicki, 1995).

Following the oil boycott in the mid-1970s, most states in the United States adopted a law allowing right turns on red at signalized intersections after drivers stopped to assure that the turn could be made safely, unless a particular intersection was specified otherwise. The purpose of the law was to conserve fuel that was being burned during the waits for lights to change. However, observations of driver behavior indicated that the number of drivers who turned right at signalized intersections without stopping increased from 47 percent to 70 percent in one state (Baumgartner, 1981). The unintended effect was an increase in total crashes and, particularly, injuries to pedestrians and bicyclists (Zador, 1984).

A theory of unintended consequences says that drivers whose crash protection is increased will drive more riskily and endanger other road users—so-called risk compensation, or risk homeostasis, theory. The origin of this theory has been claimed by modern neoclassical economists (Lave & Weber, 1970; Peltzman, 1975), but it was used to oppose the requirement of safety equipment on trains in the nineteenth century (Adams, 1879). The typical study claiming to support the theory employs an ecological design: cross-sectional or time-series data on fatality rates correlated to aggregated data on seat belt use or regulation of vehicle characteristics. The latter studies will be discussed in Chapter 7.

Among the problems in such studies is that the drivers who were more protected were not disaggregated from those less protected and motorcyclists were included as "pedestrians." For example, one study attempted to correlate occupant and other road user fatalities among states to belt use and factors such as vehicle miles driven, percent urban population, average speed on rural roads, alcohol sales per capita, percent youth in the population, and income per capita. States with higher belt use, according to the behavioral risk factor survey of the Centers for Disease Control, had higher nonoccupant fatalities, controlling statistically for the other factors (Garbacz, 1990).

In the study, "nonoccupants" included all motorcyclists, many of whom were killed in single-vehicle crashes involving no other drivers, belted or not. As noted in Chapter 3, the behavioral risk factor survey on belt use is not valid. Numerous differences among the states that could be confounded with belt use and fatal injuries—child restraint laws, motorcycle helmet use laws, mix of large and small cars, tractor-trailer trucks, and so on—were not considered.

The studies that have examined disaggregated data on the effects of belt use laws on behavior of drivers, or belt use in crashes, have not found evidence of risk compensation. Several important driving behaviors were observed on the road before and after the belt use law was enforced in Newfoundland, and in Nova Scotia during the same period without a law. Belt use increased from 16 percent to 77 percent in Newfoundland and remained virtually unchanged in Nova Scotia. Four driver behaviors—speed, stopping at intersections when the control light was amber, turning left in front of oncoming traffic, and gaps in following distance—were measured at various sites before and after the law. Changes in these behaviors in Newfoundland were similar to those in Nova Scotia, except that drivers in Newfoundland drove slower on expressways after the law, contrary to the theory (Lund & Zador, 1984). There is no study of appropriately disaggregated data that finds an effect on other road users of increased driver belt use.

Detailed data from Suffolk County, New York, on all motor vehicle–related injuries (including nonoccupants) seen in emergency rooms (or that were fatal), before and during the first two quarters of the seat belt use law in New York, indicate a substantial reduction in severe injuries. Total injury cases decreased slightly in the first quarter and increased slightly in the second quarter, compared to the same periods in the year before, but larger increases were expected based on trends in Rhode Island without a law (Barancik et al., 1988; Rockett et al., 1988). In Suffolk County, the fatalities per emergency room case declined 20 percent in the first six months of the belt use law compared to the same period a year earlier, whereas in Rhode Island, without a law, the fatalities per case increased 24 percent. These and the previously mentioned studies of the effects of belt use laws were not mentioned by the economist claiming that risk compensation behavior offsets the effects of belts.

Changes in laws can have unintended consequences if they affect substitution of a less effective countermeasure for one having some effect. In Nassau County, New York, drivers convicted of driving while intoxicated were assigned randomly to the usual sentence or an education–rehabilitation program. The drivers who had the latter program had worse subsequent driving records than those who received the usual sentences (Preusser et al., 1976). Contrary findings occurred in an experiment in two Canadian cities. When "accidental" and violent injuries were combined, convicted drunk drivers who received rehabilitation were less likely to die in the subsequent decade (Mann et al., 1994).

The effect of law on economic incentives or disincentives may also have unintended consequences. In Quebec, Canada, the government did not subsidize driver education, as was done in the United States, but required it for licensure before age 18 at a cost to the potential licensee of about $200. In 1983, the law was amended to require driver education of all newly licensed drivers. Since, thereafter, drivers could not avoid the cost of driver education whatever their age, the economic incentive to delay licensure to age 18 was removed. Licensure of 16–17 year olds increased 12 percent among males and 19 percent among females in the year after the law was changed (Potvin et al., 1988).

Laws and rules regarding work practices have unintended consequences that could be changed to reduce injuries. Comparison of fatalities in the periods around the one hour change from daylight saving and standard time indicate that some 900 fatal crashes could be avoided annually if daylight savings time were retained year round (Ferguson et al., 1995). The self-reported crash rate of hospital nurses working in rotating shifts is twice that of those working fixed shifts (Gold et al., 1992).

Unintended consequences of changes in law are not always adverse to injury control, for example, the death reductions when the 55 mph speed limit was enacted. Required deposits on cans and bottles for various drinks and other uses has been required in some jurisdictions to reduce cleanup costs and for conservation. In Maryland, the adoption of such legislation was associated with a 60 percent reduction of glass-related lacerations to children (Baker et al., 1986).

Replicated quasi-experiments of the relation of alcohol taxes to alcohol consumption indicate substantial effects. Increase in the cost of alcoholic beverages is associated with a reduction in motor vehicle fatalities as well as mortality due to cirrhosis (Cook, 1981). Replication of that research is needed on the effects of alcohol taxes on other injuries, including homicide and suicide.

SUMMARY

Compliance with laws or rules aimed at reducing injury is influenced by degree of consensus regarding the justification for the law and probability of detection of a violation. If violations are not publicly observable or the behavior can be changed easily when enforcers are approaching, the effect is diluted. Severity of punishment is less important than its prominence in political debate would indicate.

The clustering of violence, drunk driving, and similar behaviors, in space and time, if revealed by surveillance, has been used to increase the efficiency and effects of law enforcement. Persons at increased risk of injury less often use protection required by law, which reduces the real protection to less than would be expected technically. Evidence regarding offsetting behavior by those who do comply, however, does not support that theory.

REFERENCES

Adams CF (1879) *Notes on Railroad Accidents.* New York: G.B. Putnam's Sons.

Altschuler AA, (ed) (1984) *55: A Decade of Experience.* Washington, DC: Transportation Research Board Special Report 204.

Baker MD, Moore SE, and Wise PH (1986) The impact of "Bottle Bill" legislation on the incidence of lacerations in childhood. *Am J Public Health* 76:1243.

Baker SP (1985) Without guns, do people kill people? *Am J Public Health* 75:587–588.

Barancik JI, Kramer CF, Thode HC, and Harris D (1988). Efficacy of the New York State seat belt law: preliminary assessment of occurrence and severity. *Bull New York Acad Med* 64:742–749.

Baumgartner WE (1981) After stop, compliance with right turn on red after stop. *Inst Transp Eng J* 51:19–27.

Becker G (1968) Crime and punishment: an economic approach. *J Polit Econ* 76:169–217.

Berger LR, and Mohan D (1996) *Injury Control: A Global View.* Delhi: Oxford University Press.

Bergman AB (ed) (1992) *Political Approaches to Injury Control at the State Level.* Seattle: University of Washington Press.

Berk RA, and Newton PJ (1985) Does arrest really deter wife battery? An effort to replicate the findings of the Minneapolis spouse abuse experiment. *Am Sociol Rev* 50:253–262.

Berk SF, and Loseke DR (1980–81) "Handling" family violence: situational determinants of police arrests in domestic disturbances. *Law Soc Rev* 15: 317–333.

Buzawa ES, and Buzawa CG (eds) (1996) *Do Arrests and Restraining Orders Work?* Thousand Oaks, CA: Sage Publications.

Campbell DT (1969) Reforms as experiments. *Am Psychol* 24:409–429.

Ciccone MA, and Wells JAK (1988) Improper shoulder belt use by Maryland drivers. *Hum Factors* 30:359–366.

Cook PJ (1981) The effect of liquor taxes on drinking, cirrhosis and auto accidents. In Moore MH and Gerstein DR (eds), *Alcohol and Public Policy: Beyond the Shadow of Prohibition.* Washington, DC: National Academy Press.

Cressey DR (1975) Law, order and the motorist. In Hood R (ed), *Crime, Criminology and Public Policy.* New York: Free Press.

Evans L (1986) The effectiveness of safety belts in preventing fatalities. *Accident Anal Prev* 18:229–241.

Ferguson SA, Preusser DF, Lund AK, Zador PF, and Ulmer MA (1995) Daylight savings time and motor vehicle crashes: the reduction in pedestrian and vehicle occupant fatalities. *Am J Public Health* 85:92–95.

Fife D, and Abrams WR (1989) Firearms' decreased role in New Jersey homicides after a mandatory sentencing law. *J Trauma* 29:1548–1551.

Foldvary LA, and Lane JC (1974) The effectiveness of compulsory wearing of seatbelts in casualty reduction. *Accident Anal Prev* 6:59–81.

Garbacz C (1990) Estimating seat belt effectiveness with seat belt usage data from the Center for Disease Control. *Econ Lett* 34:83.

Geisel MS, Roll R, and Wettick RS Jr (1969) The effectiveness of state and local regulation of handguns: a statistical   analysis. *Duke Law J* 1969:647–676.

General Accounting Office (1987). *Drinking-Age Laws: An Evaluation Synthesis of Their Impact on Highway Safety.* Washington, DC: U.S. Congress.

Gold DR, Rogacz S, Bock N, Tosteson TD, Baum TM, Speizer FE, and Czeisler CA (1992) Rotating shift work, sleep, and accidents related to sleepiness in hospital nurses. *Am J Public Health* 82:1011–1014.

Goldstein H (1990) *Problem Oriented Policing.* Philadelphia: Temple University Press.

Goryl ME, and Bowman BL (1987) *Restraint System Usage in the Population.* Washington, DC: National Highway Traffic Safety Administration.

Greunewald PJ, and Ponicki WR (1995) The relationship of the retail availability of alcohol and alcohol sales to alcohol-related traffic crashes. *Accident Anal Prev* 27:249–259.

Hingson R, Merrigan D, and Heeren T (1985) Effects of Massachusetts raising its legal drinking age from 18 to 20 on deaths from teenage homicide, suicide, and nontraffic accidents. *Pediatr Clin North Am* 32:221–232.

Hingson R, Howland J, Heeren T, and Levenson S (1988) Effects of legal penalty changes and laws to increase drunken driving convictions on fatal traffic crashes. *Bull New York Acad Med* 64:662–677.

Hingson R, McGovern T, Howland J, Heeren T, Winter M, and Zakocs R (1996) Reducing alcohol-impaired driving in Massachusetts: the Saving Lives Program. *Am J Public Health* 86:791–797.

Hoff JC (1983) *A Practical Guide to BOX-JENKINS Forecasting.* Belmont, CA: Lifetime Learning Publications.

Jones B (1994) The effect of provisional licensing in Oregon: an analysis of traffic safety benefits. *Accident Anal Prev* 25:33–46.

Jones NE, Pieper CF, and Robertson LS (1992) The effect of the legal drinking age on fatal injuries of adolescents and young adults. *Am J Public Health* 82:112–115.

Kelling GL, Pate T, Dieckman D, and Brown CE (1974) *The Kansas City Police Patrol Experiment.* Washington, DC: Police Foundation.

Kemper WJ, and Byington SR (1977) Safety aspects of the 55 MPH speed limit. *Public Roads* 41:58–67.

Lave LB, and Weber WW (1970) A cost-benefit analysis of auto safety features. *Appl Econ* 4:265–275.

Leamer EE (1983) Let's take the con out of econometrics. *Am Econ Rev* 73:31–43.

Lund AK, and Zador P (1984) Mandatory belt use and driver risk taking. *Risk Anal* 4:41–53.

Magaddino JP, and Medoff MH (1984) An empirical analysis of federal and state firearm control laws. In Kates DB (ed), *Firearms and Violence: Issues of Public Policy.* Cambridge, MA: Ballinger.

Mann RE, Anglin L, Wilkins K, Vingilis ER, MacDonald S, and Sheu WJ (1994) Rehabilitation for convicted drinking drivers (second offenders): effects on mortality. *J Stud Alcohol* 55:372–374.

May PA (1975) Arrests, alcohol, and alcohol legalization among an American Indian tribe. *Plains Anthropol* 20:129–134.

McLoughlin E, Marchone M, Hanger SL, German PS, and Baker SP (1985) Smoke detector legislation: its effect on owner occupied homes. *Am J Public Health* 75:858–862.

Medoff MH, and Magaddino JP (1983) Suicides and firearm control laws. *Eval Rev* 7:357–372.

Mercer GW (1989) Traffic accidents and convictions: group totals versus rate per kilometer driven. *Risk Anal* 9:71–77.

Mock CN, Maier RV, Boyle E, Pilcher S, and Rivara FP (1995) Injury prevention strategies to promote helmet use decrease severe head injuries at a level I trauma center. *J Trauma* 39:29–33.

Moore MH (1995) Public health and criminal justice approaches to prevention. In Tonry M and Farrington DP (eds) (1995), *Building a Safer Society.* Chicago: University of Chicago Press.

National Highway Traffic Safety Administration (1995) *Traffic Safety Facts 1994.* Washington, DC: U.S. Department of Transportation.

O'Connor RJ, and Gilman B (1978) The police role in deterring crime. In Cramer JA (ed), *Preventing Crime.* Beverly Hills, CA: Sage Publications.

Orcutt GH, Watts HW, and Edwards JB (1968) Data aggregation and information loss. *Am Econ Rev* 58:773–787.

Pearn JH, Wong RK, Brown J, Ching Y, Bart R, and Hammar S (1979) Drowning and near-drowning involving children: a five-year total population study from the city and county of Honolulu. *Am J Public Health* 69:450–454.

Peltzman S (1975) The effects of automobile safety regulations. *J Polit Econ* 83:677–726.

Podell S, and Archer D (1994) Do legal changes matter? The case of gun control laws. In Costanzo M and Oskamp S (eds), *Violence and the Law.* Thousand Oaks, CA: Sage Publications.

Potvin L, Champagne F, and Laberge-Nadeau C (1988) Mandatory driver training and road safety. *Am J Public Health* 78:1206–1209.

Preusser DF, Ulmer RG, and Adams JR (1976) Driver record evaluation of a drinking-driver rehabilitation program. *J Safety Res* 8:98–105.

Preusser DF, Williams AF, Zador PL, and Blomberg RD (1984) The effect of curfew laws on motor vehicle crashes. *Law Policy* 6:115–128.

Preusser DF, Zador PL, and Williams AF (1993) The effect of city curfew ordinances on teenage motor vehicle fatalities. *Accident Anal Prev* 25:641–645.

Roberts WO, Brust JD, Leonard B, and Hebert BJ (1996) Fair-play rules and injury reduction in ice hockey. *Arch Pediatr Adolescent Med* 150:140–145.

Robertson LS (1976) An instance of effective legal regulation: motorcyclist helmet and daytime headlamp laws. *Law Soc Rev* 10:456–477.

Robertson LS (1978) Automobile seat belt use in selected countries, states and provinces with and without laws requiring belt use. *Accident Anal Prev* 10:5–10.

Robertson LS (1983a) *Injuries: Causes, Control Strategies and Public Policy.* Lexington, MA: D.C. Heath.

Robertson LS (1983b) Public perception and behavior in relation to vehicle passenger restraints. In Covello VT, Flamm WG, Rodricks JV, and Tardiff RG (eds), *The Analysis of Actual Versus Perceived Risks.* New York: Plenum Publishing Co.

Robertson LS (1989) Blood alcohol in fatally injured drivers and the minimum legal drinking age. *J Health Polit Policy Law* 14:817–825.

Robertson LS (1990) Shoulder belt use and belt effectiveness in cars with and without "windowshade" adjustable belts. *Hum Factors* 32:235–242.

Robertson LS, Rich R, and Ross HL (1973) Jail sentences for driving while intoxicated in Chicago: a judicial policy that failed. *Law Soc Rev* 8:55–67.

Rockett IRH, Hollingshead WH, and Lieberman ES (1988) A preliminary assessment of change in motor vehicle traffic trauma incidence and outcome in Rhode Island, 1984–1985. *Bull New York Acad Med* 64:750–756.

Ross HL (1960) Traffic law violations: a folk crime. *Soc Probl* 8:231–241.

Ross HL (1982) *Deterring the Drinking Driver: Legal Policy and Social Control.* Lexington, MA: D.C. Heath.

Ross HL (1992) *Confronting Drunk Driving: Social Policy for Saving Lives.* New Haven, CT: Yale University Press.

Ross HL, and Blumenthal M (1975) Some problems in experimentation in a legal setting. *Am Sociol* 10:150–155.

Ross HL, and Klette H (1995) Abandonment of mandatory jail for impaired drivers in Norway and Sweden. *Accident Anal Prev* 27:151–157.

Sanders RS (1982) Legislative approach to auto safety: the Tennessee experience. In Bergman, AB (ed), *Preventing Childhood Injuries.* Columbus, OH: Ross Laboratories.

Sherman LW (1992) *Policing Domestic Violence.* New York: Free Press.

Sherman LW (1996) The police. In Wilson JQ, and Petersilia J (eds), *Crime.* San Francisco: Institute for Contemporary Studies Press.

Sherman LW, and Berk RA (1984) The specific deterrent effect of arrest for domestic violence. *Am Sociol Rev* 49:261–272.

Smith DL, and Warren CW (1978) Use of victimization data to measure deterrence. In Cramer JA (ed), *Preventing Crime.* Beverly Hills, CA: Sage Publications.

Sood S (1988) Survey of factors influencing injury among riders involved in motorized two-wheeler accidents in India: a prospective study of 302 cases. *J. Trauma* 28:530–534.

Summala H, Naatanen R, and Roine M (1980) Exceptional condition of police enforcement: driving speeds during the police strike. *Accident Anal Prev* 12:179–184.

Teret S, Jones AS, Williams AF, and Wells JAK (1986) Child restraint laws: an analysis of gaps in coverage. *Am J Public Health* 76:31.

Weiner EL (1968) The elderly pedestrian: response to an enforcement campaign. *Traffic Safety Res Rev,* December.

Williams AF, Karpf RS, and Zador PL (1983) Variations in minimum licensing age and fatal motor vehicle crashes. *Am J Public Health* 73:1401–1403.

Williams AF, and Lund AK (1988) Mandatory seat belt use laws and occupant crash protection in the United States: present status and future prospects. In Graham JD (ed), *Preventing Automobile Injury: New Findings from Evaluation Research.* Dover, MA: Auburn House.

Williams AF, and Robertson LS (1975) The fatal crash reduction program: a reevaluation. *Accident Anal Prev* 7:37–44.

Zador PH (1984) Right-turn-on-red laws and motor vehicle crashes: a review of the literature. *Accident Anal Prev* 16:241–245.

Zador PH, Lund AK, Fields M, and Weinberg K (1988) Fatal crash involvement and laws against alcohol-impaired driving. Washington, DC: Insurance Institute for Highway Safety.

Zimring FE, and Hawkins G (1987) *The Citizen's Guide to Gun Control.* New York: Macmillan.

7

CONTROLLING AGENTS, VEHICLES, AND ENVIRONMENTS

Injuries have been reduced through control of energy, vehicles that convey the energy, and characteristics of environments that contribute to the concentration of energy and vehicles. Manufacturers of products and builders of roads, housing, and other structures, have the opportunity to modify their products to reduce the incidence and severity of injurious energy exchanges. The vast majority of serious injuries originate with use of the products of industry and builders in everyday or frequent use: among them, motor vehicles, road characteristics, guns, agricultural and industrial machines, stairs, cigarettes, matches, propane lighters, stoves and space heaters, clothing, bedding, swimming pools, and watercraft.

Many low-income countries are repeating the mistakes that occurred during the industrialization of Europe and the United States. As human and animal power is replaced by electrical and internal combustion engines, exposure of people to energy is vastly increased, often with no attention to features or alternatives that would minimize harm (Berger & Mohan, 1996; Krishnan et al., 1990).

Well-designed epidemiologic studies can reveal the injuries associated with the characteristics of products and environments. They can also aid in the evaluation of the effectiveness of modifications of products, protective equipment, and environments in injury control.

Decisions that influence the rate of injuries associated with a given product may include design characteristics, quantity per package and type of package, quality control in manufacture or building the product, and extent and target of marketing efforts. Most of the efforts by government to influence these decisions for injury reduction have been focused on standards affecting designs or on recalls of products that have design or manufacturing defects. The agreement between the U.S. Consumer Product Safety Commission and the manufacturers of all-terrain vehicles that the vehicles would not be marketed for use by children, the very occasional banning of a product by the Commission, and labeling requirements by various agencies are exceptions to the general lack of attention to marketing and its targets.

PRODUCT DESIGN

Research that relates product or environmental designs to injury rates and patterns can inform manufacturers, builders, and governmental regulatory agencies, although there is often resistance to the inference that injury is "caused" by the design. Such research is frequently attacked on the grounds that every conceivable behavioral factor was not controlled or was inadequately controlled. In contrast, when a behavioral factor is correlated to rates of injury, questions regarding controls for characteristics of products involved are rarely raised by scientists, much less by manufacturers or the government.

Not only is analysis of causation sometimes a "long cut to prevention" (Chapter 4), so is the argument about causation with respect to injury from product characteristics. If children are being poisoned by aspirin, what are the causes: the children's natural tendency to put things in their mouths, the parents' or others' failure to store the aspirin inaccessible to children, the attractiveness of the aspirin package, the number of pills per package, or the color of the pills?

If the number of pills per package can be reduced or the cap on the bottle can be made child-resultant, why argue about primal causation or launch expensive studies to specify the affects of various risk factors, some of which are much less controllable than a product modification? In the case of child poisonings from aspirin, the aspirin manufacturers were informed by pediatricians and consumer groups that they could make a difference in child poisonings by modification of quantity per package and type of packaging and did so. The child poisonings from aspirin declined 80 percent (Done, 1978).

The hazardous characteristics of certain products are obvious but their consequences are often ignored. Examples are points and edges on interior and exterior surfaces of motor vehicles, sharp edges on the ends of roadside guardrails, the height of playground equipment relative to the hardness of the surface under it, the concealability of handguns, and exposed moving parts of industrial, agricultural, and recreational machines.

Clinical case studies can be a rich source of hypotheses regarding such characteristics of products, as they were historically in investigations of motor vehicles and aviation (e.g., Woodward, 1948; Gikas, 1972; Snyder, 1975; Champion et al., 1986; Clark et al., 1987). The epidemiologist can draw attention to a given problem and provide estimates of the effects of modification by correlating the incidence and severity of injuries to variations in relevant characteristics of the products or environments.

Even products that are sometimes used to injure intentionally may be changed to reduce severity. As noted in Chapter 1, the physics of bullets and shotgun pellets have been described in detail (Ortog et al., 1988; Sykes et al., 1988), but their relative contribution to severity of injuries in shootings has only recently been subjected to epidemiologic investigation.Trends toward higher caliber weapons that remain small enough to be concealed will probably increase the fatalities per shooting (Wintemute, 1996). The companies that aggressively promoted the cheap "Saturday-night specials" are increasing their marketing of more powerful, concealable handguns (Wintemute, 1994).

Suicide by cutting and piercing declined about 80 percent among males in England in parallel with the replacement of straight razors by safety razors (Farmer, 1992). Apparently no one studied the exact extent of razor involvement, but at least some of the reduction is likely from replacement of a potentially lethal instrument easily at hand. The removal of carbon monoxide from domestic gas was associated with a reduction of about one-third in the net suicide rate in England and Wales, but apparently not in Scotland or the Netherlands (Clarke & Mayhew, 1988; Kreitman, 1976). In the United States, suicide by motor vehicle exhaust increased among males as that by domestic gas decreased, but there was an apparent net decrease in suicides among females (Lester, 1990).

Characteristics of products and environments that may not be obvious, but that are likely contributors to injury incidence or severity, can be learned by review of elementary physics or chemistry (Chapter 1). Examples are stability of vehicles; energy-absorbing capability of vehicle components as well as trees, poles, guardrail, and other roadside objects; cigarette burn rates; flammability of clothing, furniture, and bedding; and toxicity of drugs, household chemicals, and chemicals used in farming and industry. Again, the epidemiologist can learn the variations among products and, by observing the patterns of such variations in relation to relevant injury rates, estimate the effect of potential modifications with well-designed studies.

Too often these factors are neglected. For example, early studies of injuries from all-terrain vehicles focused primarily on variations in user characteristics—age, sex, height, weight, alcohol use, use of helmets, gloves, goggles, or boots—and certain circumstances such as number of riders, setting, terrain, estimated speed, maneuver, and type of crash (hit object, overturned, etc.). Variations in potential effects of stability of the vehicles, maximum speed capability, exposed moving parts, and seating allowing passengers were not examined (Newman, 1985; Smith & Middaugh, 1986).

The U.S. Consumer Product Safety Commission subsequently concluded that children were incapable of operating larger vehicles safely. Apparently no study has questioned, much less specified, the proportion of adults who lack the abilities and coordination to simultaneously operate throttle, gear shift, and brakes (sometimes requiring both hands and one or both feet), as well as judge speed and anticipate variations in terrain that require shifts in weight to maneuver over various types of terrain or around objects, without the vehicle tipping over or plowing into obstacles such as trees, boulders, and fences. For a substantial proportion of adults, these vehicles might be more appropriately called "no-terrain" or "limited-terrain" rather than all terrain.

The specific pattern of injuries relative to the design of products is often apparent. For example, drivers of tractor-trailer trucks in crashes have disproportionately large percentages of abdominal injuries, mostly attributable to steering wheel design. The steering wheel in many such trucks is almost parallel to the ground, the edge aimed at the abdomen of the driver (Baker, 1983). To conduct such studies, the epidemiologist must gain access to clinical details of the injuries from morgues or hospital records and correlate them with specific vehicle characteristics that are likely to produce such injuries as predicted from physics and biomechanics.

If the design does not damage directly, a case–control study may indicate degree of contribution of designs to risk. For example, comparison of defective steering and brakes on tractor-trailer trucks in crashes and those stopped at the same time of day and day of week near the same locations found that those with steering defects had twice the risk of crashing and those with defective brakes had 1.5 times the risk of crashing (Jones & Stein, 1989).

It is often possible to infer the effects of design from correlational studies, as illustrated by the studies of height of center of gravity relative to track width contributing to rollover of certain vehicles (Chapter 4). The height of such vehicles has also been found related to pedestrian injuries. A study of children less than five years old struck by vehicles during five years in Washington state found that more than a third of these cases occurred off the road; mainly children were backed over in driveways and parking lots. In about 76 percent of such cases, the vehicle was a truck, utility vehicle, or van, but in on-road pedestrian fatalities to children, the vast majority of the vehicles were cars (Brison et al., 1988). While the exact risk is not calculable from such a comparison, it is doubtful that children's exposure to vehicles being operated in reverse in driveways is substantially different between cars and trucks, vans, or utility vehicles in use on the road. It makes sense that the increased height of these vehicles decreases the ability of the drivers to see the area behind the vehicle when backing it. A subsequent case–control study of children struck in driveways falsely claimed that no studies of driveway injury had been done and ignored vehicle factors (Roberts et al., 1995). The study did note that shared driveways among households increases the risk and removal of play areas from driveways reduces the risk.

Biomechanical studies in the laboratory also suggest hypotheses for epidemiologic investigation. Laboratory studies of simulated pedestrian collisions using bumpers of varying height indicated that bumpers 25 or more inches from the road surface produced more severe injuries (Weiss et al., 1977). Epidemiologic study of the injuries to people struck on the road showed more severe injury related to higher bumper height (Ashton, 1982).

Collaboration of biomechanical and epidemiologic researchers can contribute to understanding of injury tolerances of subsets of the population. For example, tolerances of children to head impacts have been studied by examinations of severity and circumstances of injuries to children in free falls and biomechanical simulations of the events (Mohan et al., 1979).

It is also important to know whether product modifications intended to reduce risk are functioning as intended. For example, of 20 families who had antiscald devices attached to bathroom faucets, 19 had removed them within 9 months because of sediment buildup in the devices (Fallat and Rengers, 1993).

Epidemiologists sometimes are afforded opportunities to study relatively rare phenomena at the site for other reasons. For example, when an area in Guatemala where nutrition studies were under way experienced an earthquake, epidemiologists were able to correlate injury with housing characteristics and other factors (Glass et al., 1977).

ENVIRONMENT AND BEHAVIOR

The extent to which physical and social environments can be modified to reduce violence is an important area for research. Apparently night lighting of high-crime areas reduces fear far more than incidence (Murray, 1996). Of the numerous approaches that have been proposed, those employed include various types of barriers (e.g., bulletproof windows in cash windows of service stations and other establishments), bus stop placement, and street closures (Clarke, 1992). Convenience store robberies are reduced by having two or more clerks in the store, signs indicating limited cash, access control, and location of stores in areas of high traffic (Hunter and Jeffery, 1992).

Although some researchers claim that the vast majority of motor vehicle crashes are the result of "driver error" (e.g., Treat, 1977), they do not specify the extent to which the error is enhanced by vehicle characteristics or environmental conditions. Perception of speed by vehicle occupants is related more closely to sound than to vision (Evans, 1970). Yet some vehicle manufacturers attempt to minimize sound and maximize speed capability. What, if any, is the difference in crash rates between vehicles that filter out varying degrees of noise, controlling for radio use and other factors?

Drivers underestimate their speeds when asked to reduce speed after driving at higher speeds for a time (Schmidt & Tiffin, 1969). They also underestimate their speeds taking curves, older drivers more than the young (Milosevic & Milic, 1990). The crashes of drivers turning left across the paths of motorcycles are ten times more frequent than crashes of motorcyclists turning left in front of cars (Griffin, 1974), perhaps because of misperception of speeds of smaller vehicles.

Several studies indicate that vehicle and environmental changes to enhance perception can be effective. Experiments in which vehicles in corporate and government fleets were equipped with a variety of rear brake-light configurations found that a high-mounted center light substantially reduced rear-end crashes while braking (e.g., Reilly et al., 1980). Similar research is needed on the effect of the so-called heads-up display of the speedometer—that is, display of the speed of the vehicle nearer the driver's line of sight.

Crash rates of vehicles at intersections are related to the length of the amber phase of traffic control lights (Zador et al., 1984b). Controlled experiments are needed to specify the extent to which incidence and severity of injury are affected by changes in light timing.

Evidence that road lighting greatly reduces crashes where they cluster at night was noted in Chapter 3. Lines painted across the road at exponentially decreased intervals reduces speed of drivers crossing them; studies at sites in England indicate this tactic substantially reduced crashes at certain sites (Denton, 1980). Various road markings at curves have a differential effect on speed, depending on type of vehicle (cars versus trucks), and the effect on crash incidence and severity deserves further study (Shinar et al., 1980). Crashes of aircraft on runways also raise the issue of the extent to which runway versus taxiway markings are clear.

EVALUATION OF REGULATIONS

Most governmental standards for products are performance standards that do not directly dictate design but set minimum limits for performance in injury reduction or, in the case of worker injuries, set standards and allow for inspections of workplaces. The U.S. Federal Motor Vehicle Safety Standards, for example, specify criteria for performance of components, such as the energy absorption of steering assemblies in frontal crashes, but do not indicate how the component is to be designed to meet the standard.

The effectiveness of a regulation depends on the technical effectiveness of the regulation relative to the performance of the regulated product, process, or environment prior to the regulation as well as the degree of compliance to the regulation by manufacturers (or other relevant organizations). There is also the argument, noted in Chapter 6, that persons whose risk is reduced will behave differently, offsetting the effect of laws or regulation. Conclusions of the research on the effect of regulation conflict, mainly based on differences in research methodology. These issues are instructive regarding the misleading results that are often obtained from insufficiently disaggregated data.

Motor vehicles were essentially unregulated in the United States until the 1960s except for a few consensus standards adopted by the states, such as for headlamps. Installation of lap belts in front outboard seats was required by several states in the early 1960s, and by 1964 the manufacturers installed them in passenger cars as standard equipment. The federal government required certain standards, such as energy-absorbing steering assemblies and windshields, in 1966 and later models sold to the government, and the manufacturers included these features in public sales of certain models that also were sold to the government in substantial numbers. In 1968 and subsequent model years, the federal government required numerous standards, including several to reduce energy exchanges between occupants and vehicles in crashes and several to reduce crash incidence, such as reduced glare in drivers' eyes, redundant brakes, and side running lights.

Since national data disaggregated by type, make, and model of vehicles in crashes were not available until the Fatal Accident Reporting System began in 1975, it was necessary to assemble state data to obtain such detailed information. The author undertook such a study using fatal crashes in Maryland to evaluate the overall impact of Federal Motor Vehicle Safety Standards. The data indicated that, during the calendar years 1972–75, occupant deaths averaged 44 fatalities per 100,000 cars in pre-1964 model cars, 35/100,000 for 1964–67 cars, and 27/100,000 for 1968–75 model cars, a decline of 39 percent from unregulated pre-1964 cars to the federally regulated cars (Fig. 7.1). Deaths to pedestrians struck by the cars by model year were not significantly different— 8/100,000 for pre-1964 cars, 10/100,000 for 1964–67 cars, and 9/100,000 for 1968–75 cars (Robertson, 1977a).

Factors such as driver age and vehicle age, which later came into contention regarding the effect of regulation, were not found in the author's Maryland study. Percentage of youthful drivers (in this case less than 26 years old) was slightly less in the older, unregulated cars—opposite to subsequent conjectures that older cars had higher rates because they were driven by younger drivers. The death rate of the preregulation cars during 1972–75 in Maryland was 44/

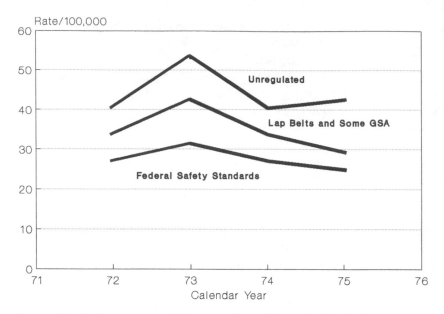

FIGURE 7.1. Fatal car occupant injury rates by model year in Maryland.

100,000, the same as the national death rate for passenger cars in the calendar years 1960–63. Therefore, age of vehicle did not explain the reductions in deaths to occupants of regulated vehicles.

After completion but before publication of the Maryland study, an economist published a study using aggregated trends in motor vehicle fatalities and other factors in an attempt to evaluate the effect of motor vehicle safety regulations on fatality rates. He argued that drivers with increased occupant protection would drive more "intensively"—the risk compensation, or risk homeostasis, hypothesis mentioned in Chapter 6—and kill more pedestrians.

His study design involved projections of expected death rates based on correlations of death rates and trends in other aggregated data over time. He included separate regressions of total occupant and supposed "pedestrian" death rates during 1947–65, using as predictors alcohol consumption per capita, average speeds on rural roads, linear trend, ratio of younger to older persons in the population, income, and "cost of crashes" in those years. The regression equations were then used to project the expected death rates in 1966–72 based on year-to-year indicators of the other variables during that time. The actual occupant rates were less than expected but the "pedestrian rates" were greater than expected, the latter offsetting the former. The results, he said, supported risk compensation theory and indicated no net benefit of regulation (Peltzman, 1975).

Having found no effect of regulation on pedestrian deaths in the Maryland study, this author obtained the data used in the econometric analysis in an attempt to account for the difference in results of the two studies. The econometric study was laced with methodological errors. Not only were regulated and nonregulated cars not separated, occupants of unregulated trucks and "pedestrians" struck by them were not disaggregated from regulated cars. Motorcyclists were included as pedestrians and single-vehicle motorcycle crashes were not disaggregated from those in collisions with other vehicles. Also, motorcycle registrations were doubling every five years, guaranteeing a substantial increase in their deaths.

There were also problems with the predictor variables. The alcohol-consumption variable excluded beer. The crash-cost index was based on the Consumer Price Index for auto repair services, which includes such things as oil changes and filters, but not the cost of auto parts damaged in crashes. The youth variable was ratio of 15–24 year olds to older persons in the population rather than their percentage as licensed drivers or drivers in crashes, which was known for all but three of the earliest years studied. A regression equation based on 1947–60 data did not predict the rates in 1961–65, a simple check on the validity of the model that would have ruled out its use to evaluate regulation. Some of the predictor variables were virtual substitutes for one another, a condition called multicolinearity, which distorts regression coefficients, and their correlations changed drastically in the pre- and postregulation periods, guaranteeing invalid projections (Table 7.1). Although just what was considered as "intensive" driv-

TABLE 7.1. Correlation Matrix of Data Used by Peltzman to Project Fatality Rates, 1947–65 (1966–72 in parentheses)

	1	2	3	4	5
Crash cost index					
Income/capita age 15+	−0.87				
	(0.88)				
Linear trend	−0.92	0.97			
	(0.80)	(0.95)			
Alcohol consumption	−0.85	0.90	0.91		
	(0.72)	(0.95)	(0.91)		
Average rural speed	−0.89	0.98	0.98	0.89	
	(0.68)	(0.88)	(0.85)	(0.96)	
15–24 year olds/older population	−0.34	0.29	0.37	0.57	0.32
	(0.78)	(0.95)	(0.99)	(0.91)	(0.99)

ing was not specified, the most likely candidate, speed, was used as a predictor variable rather than an outcome variable.

Despite the documentation of these errors, the editors of the *Journal of Political Economy (JPE)*, who published the econometric study, refused to publish a critique, and it was published elsewhere (Robertson, 1977b). Since the *JPE* publication of the original study, it has been cited frequently as gospel in the economic literature, usually without reference to the critique and other research contradicting it, including one study on similar regulations in Sweden published later in the same journal (Lindgren & Stuart, 1980).

When the Fatal Accident Reporting System (FARS) data became available for a number of years (1975–78), it was possible to examine separately data on regulated and unregulated vehicles nationally. Using a survey of mileage per vehicle by vehicle age, the effects of state and federal regulations on death rates per mile of occupants and of pedestrians, motorcyclists, and pedalcyclists in collisions with specific vehicles were estimated in a regression equation, controlling for age of vehicle and type of vehicle (cars versus trucks). The data indicated that significant reductions in car occupant death rates were associated with state regulations, and deaths both to car occupants and nonoccupants struck by cars were lower for vehicles subject to federal safety standards. These results were consistent with the fact that state lap belt requirements and standards for government cars in 1964–67 models were exclusively aimed at occupant protection in crashes while the 1968 and subsequent federal standards included crash avoidance. The occupant death reduction was similar to that found in the Maryland study, 40 percent (Robertson, 1981).

The study of the FARS data was attacked by an economist who claimed that it was inappropriate to compare cars to trucks, and because age of vehicle and model year was correlated, the critic said that the regulatory effect was greatly reduced mainly by his estimate of a vehicle-age effect (Orr, 1984). His estimate of lives preserved, however, was miscalculated by 38 percent using his own regression coefficients.

The most misleading characterization of the alleged vehicle-age effect was presented in a conference at General Motors. Model year differences were graphed by calendar year, removing rather than demonstrating the vehicle-age effect, and totally and mistakenly attributing all model year differences to vehicle age (Adams, 1985).

Since more data are accumulated each year in the Fatal Accident Reporting System, the opportunity to evaluate the effects of safety standards and other factors is available as conditions change. Adoption of safety standards virtually ceased from 1978 to 1987. The federal standard that required seat belts that automatically encircle front-outboard occupants or, in the alternative, air bags, was rescinded by the Reagan administration. It was restored in the late 1980s only after the courts ruled that the administration had acted illegally. The National Highway Traffic Safety Administration did continue frontal crash tests of a selection of cars annually and published the results. Manufacturers were embarrassed enough by the reported forces on occupant test dummies at 35 miles per hour that on occasion they requested a retest after modifying the vehicles.

The crash tests indicated incremental improvement in crashworthiness during the 1980s, as evidenced by reduced forces on crash-test dummies. Research on fatalities to occupants in frontal crashes indicated reduced deaths in frontal crashes of vehicles that performed well in the crash tests (Kahane, 1994; Zador et al., 1984a), but the research designs of these studies did not allow for the possibility of offsetting behavior, the alleged increased risky driving. Seat belt use laws, enacted by the states from 1985 to 1990, largely accounted for more than doubling of seat belt use (National Highway Traffic Safety Administration, 1975–91), and alcohol in fatally injured drivers declined about 20 percentage points during the 1980s (National Highway Traffic Safety Administration, 1995) due to a variety of factors.

FARS data can be combined with data from other sources on vehicle use and belt use to assess the effects of the various mentioned government policies. Death rates per 100 million miles use in which passenger cars were involved, by model year of the vehicles and whether the death was to one or more occupants of the cars, were tabulated for model years 1961–90 in each of the calendar years 1975–91. The miles per vehicles of a given age in a 1988 mileage survey (Energy Information Administration, 1990) were adjusted to other years by multiplying them by the ratio of average miles driven in other years to the 1988 average (Federal Highway Administration, 1975–92). The mileage survey included periodic calls to the same households to obtain odometer readings, which is probably more valid than asking people their annual mileage. Rates are available on 254 combinations of vehicle model year and calendar year.

Two sets of rates per 100 million miles were analyzed separately: *(1)* occupant fatalities and *(2)* crashes fatal to nonoccupants (occupants of the other vehicle in multiple-vehicle crashes, pedestrians, and bicyclists). The first allows an estimate of the effects of safety standards, improved crashworthiness, and the other factors on all occupant deaths. The second examines possible effects on other road users. If there is offsetting behavior, nonoccupant death rates should increase in relation to regulation, crash-test publicity, or belt use.

Since some safety standards were imposed by the General Services Administration in 1966 on cars sold to the government and the standards for all cars began to be imposed in 1968, the absence of standards is correlated with vehicle age. Data on the 1975–77 models were available for a full 15 years of vehicle use. The death rates (each of the two sets separately) per mile were calculated for these model years for each year of age and averaged among the three model years. The death rates were neither linear nor monotonic as the vehicles aged (Robertson, 1996). Ten- to fifteen-year-old 1975–77 models had substantially lower death rates than the ten- to fifteen-year-old preregulation vehicles. The 1975–77 rate for a given-aged vehicle was used as an expected rate for a vehicle of that age to control for variation attributable to vehicle age.

Other factors considered were the "downsizing" of vehicles and economic conditions during a given calendar year, both of which have been correlated to death rates; observed seat belt use in a given calendar year; and percentage of drivers with alcohol greater than 0.10 percent by weight in a given calendar year. Smaller vehicles have higher occupant death rates because of less interior space to decelerate, and deaths per mile are marginally higher in years of greater economic prosperity. Wheelbase, the distance from the front to rear axle, has been shown to be the best predictor of differences in fatality rates due to vehicle size (Robertson, 1991).

To control for vehicle size, the death rates per mile in calendar year 1988 were calculated for seven categories in five-inch increments of wheelbase (from <95.1 to 120.1 +), using the 1988 mileage survey and decoded vehicle identification numbers for make and model of vehicle in the fatal file and mileage survey file. Expected fatalities were calculated by multiplying the 1988 rate for each size times the numbers of vehicles of those sizes sold in a given model year, discounted for scrappage as they aged (Flammang, 1992; *Ward's Automotive Yearbook,* 1960–92). The expected number was then divided by the mileage previously estimated for each model and calendar year. The index of industrial production was used as an indicator of economic activity (Council of Economic Advisors, 1994). Belt use in a given model–calendar year was included from the annual survey of 19 cities and their environs, extrapolating for a few years in which the survey was not done (National Highway Traffic Safety Administration, 1975–91). Percentage of alcohol in fatally injured drivers for each model–calendar year was obtained from FARS in states that test 80 percent or more of such drivers.

Ordinary least-squares regression (Chapter 4) was used to estimate the effects of the various factors. The variable for minimum safety standards was zero for pre-1966 models, incremented from 1 to 12 in 1966–77 models and assigned 12 for 1978–91 models. As noted, the reduction in occupant death rates has been shown to be incremental in 1966–77 models, partly because of the imposition of new standards in various years of that period and partly because of delays in meeting the standards in some models. The publication of crash test data from the New Car Assessment Program (NCAP) results began in 1979, so the NCAP variable is zero for 1961–79 models and incremented by 1, from 1 to 11 consecutively, for 1980–90 models, based on the assumption that crashworthiness was improved incrementally as the crash test results for particular makes and models became known.

The regression coefficients for the predictor variables are presented in Table

7.2. Controlling for the expected effects of vehicle age and size differences, the incremental model years in which minimum standards were imposed and the model years during which NCAP tests were publicized are strong predictors of reduced occupant death rates and are somewhat related to *reduced* nonoccupant fatal crash rates.

In the 1966–77 model passenger cars, the occupant death reduction was an average 0.26 death per 100 million vehicle-miles (mvm) per model year across 12 model years for a total reduction of 3.12 deaths per 100 mvm (0.26×12). The reduction in 1980–90 models was 0.077 per model year, a total of 0.847 per 100 mvm in 11 model years (0.077×11). The effect of belt use increases and alcohol reductions were much less. A 40 percentage point increase in belt use reduced the rate 0.28 (i.e., 40×0.007) and a 20 percentage point reduction in alcohol reduced the rate 0.14 (20×0.007).

The rates increase marginally in more economically prosperous years, as indicated by the predictive coefficient on the index of industrial production. There is no significant linear trend in the rates independent of the other predictor variables, as indicated by the coefficient on calendar year.

The results support the conclusion that vehicle-related fatalities were reduced substantially by increased crashworthiness and somewhat by increased seat belt use and reduced alcohol use. Contrary to offsetting behavior theory, the evi-

TABLE 7.2. Regression Estimation of Passenger Car Rates per 100 Million Vehicle Miles, 1961–90 Cars in Calendar Years 1975–91

VARIABLE	OCCUPANT DEATHS		NONOCCUPANT CRASHES	
	EFFECT	95% CI +/−	EFFECT	95% CI +/−
Standards	−0.260	0.023	−0.055	0.010
NCAP publicity	−0.077	0.033	−0.029	0.020
Belt use, %	−0.007	0.006	−0.006	0.004
Alcohol > 0.10, %	0.007	0.006	0.007	0.005
Calendar year	−0.017	0.036	−0.016	0.022
Industrial production	0.029	0.014	0.019	0.009
Expected age of vehicle	0.444	0.212	0.289	0.096
Expected from wheelbase	1.066	0.454	1.252	0.299
Intercept	−0.793		−1.950	
R^2	0.92		0.86	

CI = confidence interval.

dence indicates that the reduction of fatalities per mile attributable to increased crashworthiness of passenger cars and increased seat belt use was not attenuated by increased risk to others from more protected drivers. Indeed, more regulated vehicles were in fewer crashes fatal to other road users.

There are reasonable explanations for the latter. The minimum safety standards included crash avoidance standards (redundant brakes, reduced glare in driver's eyes, side running lights, etc.) as well as crashworthiness standards. The period of NCAP tests and increased seat belt use was also the period of increased aerodynamic designs to save fuel, which may, coincidentally, reduce severity of pedestrian and cyclist impacts. The points and edges on older models were related to increased risk to pedestrians (Robertson, 1990). The "crumple zones" that absorb more energy may help reduce the velocity changes to occupants of other vehicles in crashes with the more crashworthy vehicles.

Although most of the reductions in occupant deaths are model-year–specific during the period of regulation or publicized crash tests, and therefore vehicle-rather than driver- or environment-based, the data do not allow the conclusion that all of the reduction is attributable to regulation or embarrassment. Some aspects of crashworthiness might have been adopted without government standards had there been no regulation, although the failure of most manufacturers to adopt available technology until required to do so in the 1960s, and the 18 year battle against the airbag in the 1970s and 1980s, suggests otherwise. And concern for sales lost to manufacturers of vehicles that had better crash indices in the NCAP tests may have motivated improvements, irrespective of embarrassment.

The most recent claims of offsetting behavior (Chirinko & Harper, 1993) apparently resulted from failure to separate passenger cars from pickup trucks and utility vehicles in a time-series analysis. This will give false results on the effects of regulation on passenger cars, not because the regulated cars are more often hitting trucks, as claimed by recent proponents of the risk compensation hypothesis, but because the government has failed to impose standards to reduce rollover of unstable pickup trucks and utility vehicles, whose use has grown substantially (Chapters 4 and 10).

Another test of the hypothesis that increased protection would be offset by behavior was provided by the introduction of airbags in cars. Those drivers protected by airbags could have reduced their belt use to partly offset the reduced risk provided by the airbags, but they did not. Belt use by drivers in airbag-equipped cars was not significantly different than in cars without airbags (Williams et al., 1990).

This seemingly academic quarrel over study designs had ominous results. The antiregulation administrators of federal agencies in the 1980s were often advised by neoclassic economists, and those who attempted some feeble extension of safety regulations were blocked by the neoclassic economists and others in the Office of Management and Budget in the White House. The long delay in the adoption of airbags was but one of many delays in regulations influenced by intragovernmental debates.

The evidence on the effectiveness of the initial motor vehicle safety standards does not mean that all regulation is effective or that regulation is always the most effective way to achieve injury reductions. The time necessary for unregulated products to be discarded is also a factor in accomplishing the full effects of regulation, or product changes undertaken voluntarily. In the case of passenger cars, the average life of the vehicles is ten years, so it took longer than that for the initial regulations to have full effect as the older vehicles were scrapped. Other products, such as mattresses, may be used longer, and some, such as children's cribs, may be used for generations. Research on trends in child suffocations and strangulations suggests that standards for refrigerator or freezer entrapment and warnings on plastic bags reduced fatalities from those sources, but regulations regarding crib design have had less, if any, effect (Kraus, 1985).

Regulation that provides for inspections, such as the workplace inspections of the Mine Safety and Health Administration and the Occupational Safety and Health Administration, could have effects analogous to those discussed for legal controls of individual behavior in Chapter 6—general deterrence and specific deterrence. If corporate executives in a position to make changes wish to avoid citations and fines, they could make the changes in the absence of actual inspections (general deterrence). Some may make changes only when they are cited by inspectors (specific deterrence) and others may not respond even under those conditions.

A substantial increase in regulation of coal mines followed the enactment of the Federal Coal Mine Health and Safety Act of 1969. Death rates of miners showed no trend in the prior ten years but declined rapidly in the 1970s (Weeks & Fox, 1983). Apparently no attempt has been made to study differential effects in mines inspected versus others to delineate specific versus general deterrence. The inspections of coal mines were intense relative to other occupational settings, about 34,641 inspections of 2131 active underground mines in 1977, for example.

The probability of inspection of workplaces regulated by the Occupational Safety and Health Administration (OSHA) was much lower than that of mines in the 1970s and declined substantially in the 1980s. A business could expect to be inspected once per 20 years in 1977 if the inspections were random (Mendeloff, 1979). OSHA targeted industries with higher injury rates for more frequent inspections and some plants were inspected every few years. Several econometric analyses of trends in worker injuries found no effect of OSHA

(Mendeloff, 1979; Smith, 1976; Viscusi, 1979). Further analysis of disaggregated data found an effect in one instance but not significantly so in another (Smith, 1979).

One of the economists who found no effect of OSHA inspections claimed that increased protection of workers would be offset by behavior changes (risk compensation again), and that fines for plants cited were too low to provide an incentive for workplace modification in any case (Viscusi, 1979). In a project originally intended to study the epidemiology of worker injuries in three metal-working plants during eight years, the author and a colleague serendipitously discovered new data on the issue of the effects on injury rates of workplace inspections (Robertson & Keeve, 1983).

Individual differences in injuries in the plants were mainly correlated with the type of work being done in specific departments with some correlations to worker age, formal education, and number of previous employers. Using regression estimates of the effects of these factors at the individual level, the expected injury rate in a given year in a given plant was calculated and compared to the actual rate. The actual rates were separated into injuries that could be observed objectively in the plants' clinics (lacerations, burns, amputations), which we called "objective injuries," and those that were discernible as to incidence or severity primarily by patient complaint (mainly back pain), which we called "subjective injuries." Figure 7.2 is a comparison of the actual and expected rates per year in one of the plants.

Noting that the actual rates varied from the expected rather sharply in certain years, we asked ourselves what other factors might have affected the rates in a given year. Two obvious external factors were OSHA inspections and workers' compensation available to workers who missed work because of injury. When the effects of these factors were examined, "objective" injuries declined relative to those expected in the year following OSHA inspections and "subjective" injuries increased more than expected when workers' compensation increased above inflation (Robertson & Keeve, 1983).

The lack of the effect of OSHA in the studies of aggregated data was apparently due to failure to control for workers' compensation effects. Changes in lost workdays from 1975 to 1976 among industries in 20 states were also examined, and the injuries decreased in correlation to an increase in OSHA inspections but increased in relation to increases in workers' compensation. If "risk compensation" occurred at all, it did not offset the effects of OSHA inspections, but actual compensation that allowed the workers to take time off apparently did affect their absence when they could afford to be away from work, particularly for pain and strain, when working and not working is more discretionary.

The economic theory that the fines for OSHA violations were too small for deterrence did not seem a factor in the plants studied. The researchers were given free access to correspondence regarding OSHA citations and it was obvi-

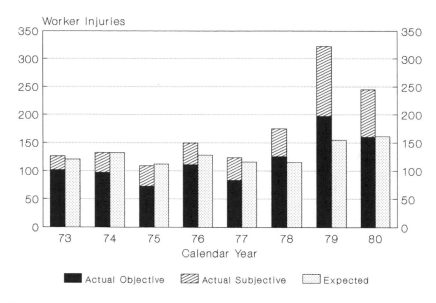

FIGURE 7.2. Expected versus actual worker injuries.

ous that management took the citations very seriously, in some cases spending more in time and travel to persuade OSHA to reduce a fine than the amount of the fine. The deterrent effect of OSHA inspections did appear to be specific and temporary. Lagged correlations indicated no effect of an OSHA inspection beyond the first year following an inspection.

EVALUATION OF PROTECTIVE EQUIPMENT AND ENVIRONMENTS

Irrespective of the means employed to increase use of protection (persuasion, laws directed at individuals, regulation or voluntary changes in products and processes), the effect of the protection in use is often worthy of epidemiologic study. Engineers who design and test protective equipment can indicate precisely the energy absorbed, reduction of access to moving parts, and so on, but other factors cannot always be anticipated—the range of uses and factors affecting lack of use, the amounts of energy involved in actual injuries, and the possibility of misuse. Epidemiologic data on the use and effectiveness of potentially injurious energy sources can be helpful in modifications of design or attempts to change how the equipment is used.

For example, estimates of the effectiveness of seat belts have varied substantially, partly because of variations in belts or their effectiveness in crashes of different severity, and partly because of variations in research methodology.

Nineteen studies of belt effectiveness in reducing severe and fatal injuries, available by the mid-1970s, indicated estimates ranging from 7.5 percent to 82.8 percent effectiveness. That variation was examined by two potential factors that might explain it—the seriousness of the injuries included and the potential bias in claimed belt use (Robertson, 1976).

Table 7.3 illustrates the potential biases that could occur by inclusion of injuries of different severity or if some people who were uninjured claimed to use belts when they actually did not. Such false claims were found to occur when use in traffic was observed and people were later questioned about their belt use (Waller & Barry, 1969). As Table 7.3 shows, if 5 percent (500 of the 10,000 hypothetical occupants) of the persons in crashes claimed to use belts but did not, the effectiveness of belts would be overestimated. If only injured

TABLE 7.3. Hypothetical Data Illustrating Potential Systematic Error in Estimating Belt Effectiveness

	BELT USE		
	BELTED	UNBELTED	TOTAL
All vehicle occupants in crashes	2,500	7,500	10,000
No injuries	2,040	5,700	7,740
Minor injuries	400	1,500	1,900
Severe injuries	60	300	360
Percent severe of all occupants	2.4	4.0	
Percent severe and minor of all occupants	18.4	24.0	

Estimated belt effectiveness in reducing all injuries $= \dfrac{24 - 18.4}{24} = 0.233$, or 23 percent

Estimated belt effectiveness in reducing severe injuries $= \dfrac{4.0 - 2.4}{4.0} = 0.40$, or 40 percent

If only injury cases are used to estimate effectiveness:
Estimated belt effectiveness $= \dfrac{16.7 - 13.0}{16.7} = 0.221$, or 22 percent

If 500 noninjured occupants claimed to use belts but did not:

	CLAIMED BELT USE	
	BELTED	UNBELTED
All vehicle occupants in crashes	3,000	7,000
Percent severe of all occupants	2.0	4.3

Estimated belt effectiveness $= \dfrac{4.3 - 2.0}{4.3} = 0.535$, or 54 percent persons were considered, belt effectiveness would be underestimated. In the 19 studies examined, belt effectiveness was primarily correlated to claimed use, suggesting that the higher estimates of belt effectiveness were influenced by false claims of belt use.

Controls for crash severity in estimating belt effectiveness have been attempted by estimates of vehicle damage. The method involves comparison of vehicles in crashes to photographs of vehicle damage and coding crash severity. Based on data thus controlling for crash severity, researchers in North Carolina estimated belt effectiveness in reducing injuries with an Abbreviated Injury Score of 2 or more at 62 percent in 1973–75 model cars (Reinfurt et al., 1975). Researchers who use hospitalized injuries to estimate the effects of belts and other equipment (e.g., Orsay et al., 1988) should be aware that without inclusion of the fatally injured and the uninjured, the estimates are substantially biased.

Another method that attempts to control for a variety of factors, a *double-pair comparison* (Evans, 1986a) is a variation of a case–control design applied to fatal crashes in which there is more than one occupant. The relative risk (R) of a fatality to a given set of occupants is calculated as a ratio of ratios. For example, the calculation of the relative risk of belt use for drivers and passengers is noted in Table 7.4, using the cross-tabulation of who was using belts and who died in the formula as indicated. Belt effectiveness in percent is then $100(1-R)$. Estimates of the effectiveness of belts by this method, using FARS data for 1975–84 car models in calendar years 1975–83, produced a weighted average of belt effectiveness in preventing death at 41 percent, averaged among age groups (Evans, 1986b). One of the virtues of the method is that it is not sensitive to misreported belt use unless the misreporting is different for the fatally injured and survivors.

The consistency among studies can be checked by the mathematical relationships among equipment use, equipment effectiveness, and total injury reductions. For example, the regression coefficient in Table 7.1 indicates a reduction of 0.007 in fatal crashes per 100 million vehicle-miles for each percentage point increase in belt use. Belt use was approximately 53 percent in 1991 (National Highway Traffic Safety Administration, 1975–92). If the remaining 47 percent of car occupants had been restrained, the occupant fatality rate of 1.6 per 100 million miles would have been reduced by about 21 percent. This result is obtained by multiplying the coefficient in Table 7.1 by the percentage of unused belts $(0.007 \times 47 = 0.329)$ and dividing the result by the death rate $(0.329/1.6 \times 0.21)$. The implied effectiveness of belts when used is 21/47, or 45 percent, near the 41 percent estimate using the double-paired comparison method.

There is a hypothesis that nonusers of belts are more likely to crash at higher speeds, resulting in an overestimate of the effects of belts. Tests of the hypothesis, however, rely on data that is inadequate to support or reject the hypothesis.

TABLE 7.4. Double-Pair Comparison of Drivers and Passengers in Fatal Crashes by belt Use and Who Was Killed

	PASSENGER			
	KILLED		ALIVE	
DRIVER	BELTED	UNBELTED	BELTED	UNBELTED
Killed				
Belted		c		a
Unbelted	f	1	d	j
Alive				
Belted		b		
Unbelted	e	k		

$$\text{Driver } R \;=\; \dfrac{\dfrac{a+c}{b+c}}{\dfrac{j+1}{k+1}} \quad \text{Passenger } R \;=\; \dfrac{\dfrac{d+f}{e+f}}{\dfrac{k+1}{j+1}}$$

For example, Evans (1996) compared "delta-v" in crashes, an estimate of velocity change in the crash, from the National Accident Sampling System (NASS) during 1982–91, between belted and unbelted drivers. Delta-v is missing in 60 percent or more of cases in each of those years and the percent missing is related to injury severity. Competent epidemiologists do not rely on data with such high potential for bias in selecting vehicles to measure delta-v based on the outcome in injury severity. Evans also used a data set from North Carolina that measured injury by the police codes, combining A + K, which is biased by the overwhelming number of A injuries that are relatively trivial.

One means of estimating potential bias in selection of cases or controls is the use of more than one control group in a case–control study. A good example of such a study involved estimation of the effect of bicycle helmets in reducing head injuries. Cases were persons who were seen at five hospitals for head injuries suffered while bicycling. One comparison group was bicyclists who came to the emergency rooms of the same hospitals for injuries other than to the head. Another comparison group of injured bicyclists was identified from the records of a group health plan. The claimed helmet use in the two comparison groups was nearly the same but was substantially lower in the head-injured group. Data obtained on several potential confounding factors in the three groups allowed adjustment for these factors in the estimate of helmet effectiveness given an injury while bicycling, which suggested a reduction in risk of head injury of bicyclists using helmets of about 85 percent (Thompson et al., 1989).

The researchers had no way of verifying that helmets were actually used in the groups studied. To check on claims of use versus actual use, observed users and nonusers would have to be identified unobtrusively and later questioned regarding use. To control for whether bicylists who are injured are more or less likely to be using helmets, a third control group would be needed—those bicycling at the same times and places as the injured.

Again, the best research design is the experimental–control design where feasible. For modifications of higher priced products, experimental–control designs are usually not feasible for sales to the general public, but if large volumes are bought for use by corporations or the government, random assignment to users in those organizations is possible. For example, the effect of the high-mounted brake light on crashes of cars while braking was studied experimentally in corporate and government fleets (e.g., Reilly et al., 1980).

If the government or other agencies distribute certain products, studies can be done experimentally. The New York Health Department undertook an experimental–control study of potential problems with a type of child-resistant cap for medicine containers (the "Palm-'N'-Turn" cap) by randomly distributing them in municipal hospitals and conducting follow-up home visits in experimental and control groups (Lane et al., 1971). The substantial effect of breakaway bases on reduced injuries to softball players was demonstrated by randomly rotating teams among fields with and without the breakaway bases (Janda et al., 1988).

Modifications of environments under the jurisdiction of corporations or governments can usually be studied experimentally, although they seldom are. Extensive reviews of the literature on road modifications are available (Federal Highway Administration, 1982). Much has been learned from cross-sectional studies of road features and before–after studies of modifications. Often the differences in crashes or severity in before–after studies of environmental modifications are so large that the reduction is unlikely due to biased study design, but the lack of control sites and the potential for regression to the mean (Chapter 6), where the modifications were targeted only at high incident sites, raise doubts about the exact magnitude of some effects.

For example, installation of flashing lights at rural stop signs was associated with an 80 percent reduction in fatal crashes at those sites (Hagenauer et al., 1982). Removal of trees from near roadsides or use of impact attenuators at fixed objects was estimated to reduce fatal crashes by 50–75 percent (McFarland et al., 1979).

An analysis of various studies that claimed large reductions in motor vehicle crashes at high incidence sites (so-called black spots) claims that those with controls for regression to the mean show fewer or no effects (Elvik, 1997). The study did not distinguish between reduced incidence and reduced severity. For example, a guardrail may reduce severity without reducing incidence. While modifications at sites that had temporarily high incidence rates would be expected to return to the average without the modifications, studies that are based on long experience of severe injuries at particular sites show remarkable reductions over similarly long follow-up periods when the modification would be expected to have a long-term effect, such as guardrail installations (Short & Robertson, 1997).

Case–control studies have indicated the high-risk sites for these and other severe crashes where vehicles left the road (Chapter 4). Epidemiologists who become familiar with the literature and gain agreement with highway authorities to aid in study designs could make an enormous contribution to increased precision of estimates of the effects of road modifications.

QUALITY CONTROL

The detection of defects that occur during production may also be important for reducing product-related injuries. In any manufacturing process, variances will occur in the products produced. Prudent manufacturers employ an inspection system to identify and correct safety defects from variances in manufacturing processes, as well as other aspects of quality of the product. Some manufacturers install internal checks on operability of safety and other systems even after the product is sold. For example, the airbags and some other systems in motor vehicles are checked electronically each time the vehicle is started.

An important issue in quality control of the manufacturing process, particularly for products or components that can increase injury and death, is how many to inspect and the criteria for rejection of a defective product or inspection of a total batch for defects when one or more is found in a sample. The cost of inspection is a small proportion of the cost of relatively expensive products, such as cars, but adds proportionately more to the price of inexpensive items, such as matches, propane lighters, or hand tools. In some cases, the inspection of every unit produced may not be feasible and a sample of the products in a batch are inspected.

The probability of finding a defect or percentage of defects in a batch is highly sensitive to the size of the sample inspected. The Poisson probability distribution can be used to provide a good estimate of the probability of a proportion of defects escaping detection in inspection of a sample from each batch (Burr, 1953). Assuming that a defect found in a sample prompts inspection of the entire batch and removal of all defective products found, the probability *(P)* of accepting a batch with a proportion *(p)* of the batch being defective in samples of size *n* is

$$P = e^{-pn}$$

If a sample of 100 is inspected and no defect is found in the sample, there is a 37 percent chance that 1 percent of the products in the batch are defective. That chance can be reduced to 14 percent if a sample of 200 is inspected, to 5 percent if 300 are inspected, to 2 percent if 400 are inspected, and to 0.7 percent if 500 are inspected (Fig. 7.3). The probability of injury from the product is the risk of injury per product times *P.* Obviously, manufacturers can greatly reduce the injuries from their products by using larger samples in their inspection systems.

The size of samples used in quality control is proprietary to the manufacturers. The author is aware of no federal or state standards for sample size to detect defects from manufacturing variances. Motor vehicle manufacturers are required to report known design defects or defects due to manufacturing variances to the National Highway Traffic Administration, but known defects have not always been reported.

A requirement that manufacturers reveal public sample sizes used for detecting defects as well as the numbers found, and the procedure for inspecting the batch given defects in the sample, would likely result in greater manufacturer attention to the problem. It would also give epidemiologists a tool to correlate the types of quality control and sample sizes to injury incidence and severity related to product variations.

FIGURE 7.3. Sample size and probability of 1 percent defects.

SUMMARY

Changes in agents, vehicles, and environments can be made voluntarily by designers, manufacturers, and marketers of products based on the research on hazardous characteristics. Regulations to impose standards for products and processes that injure have been associated with large reductions in death rates.

Environments may affect behavior in addition to exposing people to hazards. They can be modified to reduce violence as well as exposure to inanimate energy. The best studies of reduced risk from product or environmental modifications indicate no effect on offsetting behavior, but claims for compensation are influenced by increased availability of money, above inflation, for such claims.

REFERENCES

Adams J (1985) Smeed's law, seat belts, and the emperor's new clothes. In Evans L and Schwing RC (eds), *Human Behavior and Traffic Safety*. New York: Plenum Publishing Co.

Ashton SJ (1982) Vehicle design and pedestrian injuries. In Chapman AJ, et al. (eds), *Pedestrian Accidents*. London: John Wiley and Sons.

Baker SP (1983) Killer truck steering wheels: a challenge to designers. *Design News*, September, 5.

Berger LR, and Mohan D (1996) *Injury Control: A Global View*. Delhi: Oxford University Press.

Brison RJ, Wicklund K, and Mueller BA (1988) Fatal pedestrian injuries to young children: a different pattern of injury. *Am J Public Health* 78:793–795.

Burr IW (1953) *Engineering Statistics and Quality Control*. New York: McGraw-Hill.

Champion HR, Copes WS, Craig M, Morelli S, Keast S, and Bain L (1986) *A Preliminary Study of Head and Neck Trauma of Automobile Crashes, and Their Consequences*. Washington, DC: National Highway Traffic Safety Administration.

Chirinko RS, and Harper EP (1993) Buckle Up or Slow Down? New Estimates of Offsetting Behavior and Their Implications for Automobile Safety Regulation. *J Policy Anal Manage* 12:270–293.

Clark CC, Jettner E, Digges K, Morris J, Cohen D, and Griffin D (1987) Simulation of road crash facial lacerations by broken windshields. Warrendale, PA: Society of Automotive Engineers Paper No. 870320.

Clarke RV, and Mayhew P (1988) The British gas story and its criminological implications. *Crime Justice* 10:79–116.

Clarke RV (ed) (1992) *Situational Crime Prevention: Successful Case Studies*. New York: Harrow and Heston.

Council of Economic Advisors (1994) *Economic Indicators*. Washington, DC: U.S. Government Printing Office.

Datta TK, and Guzek P (1990) *Restraint System Use in 19 U.S. Cities: 1989 Annual Report*. Washington, DC: National Highway Traffic Safety Administration.

Denton GG (1980) The influence of visual pattern on perceived speed. *Perception* 9:393–402.

Done AK (1978) Aspirin overdosage: incidence, diagnosis, and management. *Pediatrics* (suppl) 59:890–897.

Elvik R (1997) Evaluations of road accident blackspot treatment: a case of the iron law of evaluation studies? *Accident Anal Prev* 29:191–199.

Energy Information Administration (1990) *Household Vehicles Energy Consumption, 1988.* Washington, DC: U.S. Department of Energy.

Evans L (1970) Speed estimation from a moving automobile. *Hum Factors* 13:23–27.

Evans L (1986a) Double pair comparison—a new method to determine how occupant characteristics affect fatality risk in traffic crashes. *Accident Anal Prev* 18:217–227.

Evans L (1986b) The effectiveness of safety belts in preventing fatalities. *Accident Anal Prev* 18:229–241.

Evans L (1996) Safety belt effectiveness: the influence of crash severity and selective recruitment. *Accident Anal Prev* 28:423–433.

Fallat ME, and Rengers SJ (1993) The effect of education and safety devices on scald burn prevention. *J Trauma* 34:560–563.

Farmer R (1992) Epidemiology of suicide. *Int Clin Psychopharm* 6 (suppl 6):1–11.

Federal Highway Administration (1982) *Synthesis of Safety Research Related to Traffic Control and Road Elements.* Washington, DC: U.S. Department of Transportation.

Federal Highway Administration (1975–92). *Highway Statistics.* Washington, DC: U.S. Department of Transportation.

Flammang JM (1992) *Standard Catalog of Imported Cars, 1946–1990.* Iola, WI: Kraus Publications.

Gikas PW (1972) Mechanisms of injury in automobile crashes. *Clin Neurosurg* 19:175–190.

Glass RI, Urrutia JJ, Sibony S, Smith H, Garcia B, and Rizzo L (1977) Earthquake injuries related to housing in a Guatemalan village. *Science* 197:638–643.

Griffin LI III (1974) *Motorcycle Accidents: Who When, Where, and Why.* Chapel Hill: North Carolina Highway Safety Research Center.

Hagenauer GF, Upchurch D, and Rosenbaum MJ (1982) Intersections. In Federal Highway Administration, *Synthesis of Safety Research Related to Traffic Control and Roadway Elements.* Washington, DC: U.S. Department of Transportation.

Hunter RD, and Jeffery CR (1992) Preventing convenience store robbery through environmental design. In Clarke RV (ed), *Situational Crime Prevention: Successful Case Studies.* New York: Harrow and Heston.

Janda DH, Wujtys EM, Hankin FM, and Benedict ME (1988) Softball sliding injuries: a prospective study comparing standard and modified bases. *JAMA* 259:164–166.

Jones IS, and Stein HS (1989) Defective equipment and tractor-trailer crash involvement. *Accident Anal Prev* 21:469–481.

Kahane CJ (1994) *Correlation of NCAP Performance with Fatality Risk in Actual Head-On Collisions.* Washington, DC: National Highway Traffic Safety Administration.

Kraus JF (1985) Effectiveness of measures to prevent unintentional deaths of infants and children from suffocation and strangulation. *Public Health Rep* 100:231–240.

Kreitman N (1976) The coal gas story. *Br J Prevent Soc Med* 30:86–93.

Krishnan R, Subramanian N, and Adnan A (eds) (1990) *Proceedings of the First Malaysian Workshop on Accident Prevention.* Kuala Lumpur: University of Malaya.

Lane MF, Barbarite RV, Bergner L, and Harris D (1971) Child-resistant medicine containers: experience in the home. *Am J Public Health* 61:1861–1868.

Lester D (1990) The effects of detoxification of domestic gas on suicide in the United States. *Am J Public Health* 80:80–81.

Lindgren B, and Stuart C (1980) The effects of traffic safety regulations in Sweden. *J Polit Econ* 88:412–417.

McFarland WF, Griffin LI, Rollins JB, Stockton WR, Phillips DT, and Dudek CL (1979) *Assessment of Techniques for Cost-Effectiveness of Highway Accident Countermeasures.* Washington, DC: U.S. Department of Transportation.

Mendeloff J (1979) *Regulating Safety: An Economic and Political Analysis of Occupational Safety and Health Policy.* Cambridge, MA: MIT Press.

Milosevic S, and Milic J (1990) Speed perception in road curves. *Accident Anal Prev* 21:19–23.

Mine Safety and Health Administration (1978) *Annual Report of Achievements: Fiscal Year 1978.* Washington, DC: U.S. Department of Labor.

Mohan D, Bowman BM, Snyder RG, and Foust DR (1979) A biomechanical analysis of head impact injuries to children. *J Biomechan Eng* 101:250–260.

Murray C (1996) The physical environment. In Wilson JQ, and Petersilia J (eds), *Crime.* San Francisco: Institute for Contemporary Studies.

National Highway Traffic Safety Administration (1975–91) *Restraint System Use in the Traffic Population.* Washington, DC: U.S. Department of Transportation.

National Highway Traffic Safety Administration (1995) *Traffic Safety Facts 1994.* Washington, DC: U.S. Department of Transportation.

Newman R (1985) Survey of all terrain vehicle related injuries (1985) (preliminary report). Washington, DC: U.S. Consumer Product Safety Commission.

Orr LD (1984) The effectiveness of automobile safety regulation: evidence from the FARS data. *Am J Public Health* 74:1384–1389.

Orsay EM, Turnbull TL, Dunne M, Barrett JA, Langenberg P, and Orsay CP (1988) Prospective study of the effect of safety belts on morbidity and health care costs in motor-vehicle accidents. *JAMA* 260:3598–3603.

Ortog GJ, Wasserberger J, and Balasubramaniam S (1988) Shotgun wound ballistics. *J Trauma* 28:624–631.

Peltzman S (1975) The effects of automobile safety regulation. *J Polit Econ* 83:677.

Reilly RE, Kurke DS, and Bukenmaier CC (1980) *Validation of the Reduction of Rear-End Collisions by a High-Mounted Auxiliary Stoplamp.* Washington, DC: National Highway Traffic Safety Administration.

Reinfurt DW, Silva CZ, and Hochberg Y (1975) A statistical analysis of seat belt effectiveness in 1973–1975 model cars involved in towaway crashes. Chapel Hill: University of North Carolina Highway Safety Research Center.

Roberts I, Norton R, and Jackson R (1995) Driveway-related child pedestrian injuries: a case-control study. *Pediatrics* 95:405–408.

Robertson LS (1976) Estimates of motor vehicle seat belt effectiveness and use: implications for occupant crash protection. *Am J Public Health* 66:859–864.

Robertson LS (1977a) State and federal new-car safety regulation: effects on fatality rates. *Accident Anal Prev* 9:151–156.

Robertson LS (1977b) A critical analysis of Peltzman's "The effect of automobile safety regulation." *J Econ Issues* 11:587.

Robertson LS (1981) Automobile safety regulations and death reductions in the United States. *Am J Public Health* 71:818–822.

Robertson LS (1984) Automobile safety regulation: rebuttal and new data. *Am J Public Health* 74:1390–1394.

Robertson LS (1990) Car design and risk of pedestrian injuries. *Am J Public Health* 80:609–610.

Robertson LS (1991) How to save fuel and reduce injuries in automobiles. *J Trauma* 31:107–109.

Robertson LS (1996) Reducing death on the road: the effects of minimum safety standards, publicized crash tests, seat belts and alcohol. *Am J Public Health* 86:31–34.

Robertson LS, and Keeve JP (1983) Worker injuries: the effects of workers' compensation and OSHA inspections. *J Health Polit Policy Law* 8:581–597.

Robertson LS, and Maloney A (1997) Motor vehicle rollover and static stability: an exposure study. *Am J Public Health* 87:839–841.

Rogers GB, Tinsworth DK, Polen C, Cassidy S, Trainor CM, Heh SR, and Donaldson MF (1994) *Bicycle Use and Hazard Patterns in the United States.* Washington, DC: U.S. Consumer Product Safety Commission.

Schmidt F, and Tiffin J (1969) Distortion of drivers' estimates of automobile speed as a function of speed adaptation. *J Appl Psychol* 53:536–539.

Shinar D, Rockwell TH, and Malecki JA (1980) The effects of changes in driver perception on rural curve negotiation. *Ergonomics* 23:263–275.

Short D, and Robertson LS (1997) Motor vehicle death reductions from guardrail installation (mimeo).

Smith RS (1976) *The Occupational Health and Safety Act: Its Goals and Its Achievements.* Washington, DC: American Enterprise Institute.

Smith RS (1979) The impact of OSHA inspections on manufacturing injury rates. *J Hum Resourc* 14:145.

Smith SM, and Middaugh JP (1986) Injuries associated with three-wheeled, all-terrain vehicles, Alaska, 1983 and 1984. *JAMA* 255:2454–2458.

Snyder RG (1975) Crashworthiness investigation of general aviation accidents. Warren, PA: Society of Automotive Engineers.

Summala H (1984) Modeling driver behavior: a pessimistic prediction? In Evans L, and Schwing RC (eds), *Human Behavior and Traffic Safety.* New York: Plenum Publishing Co.

Sykes LN, Champion HR, and Fouty WJ (1988) Dum-dums, hollow-points, and devastators: techniques designed to increase wounding potential of bullets. *J Trauma* 28:618–623.

Thompson RS, Rivara FP, and Thompson DC (1989) A case-control study of the effectiveness of bicycle safety helmets. *New Engl J Med* 320:1361–1367.

Treat JR (1977) Tri-level study of the causes of traffic accidents: an overview of final results. *21st Annual Proceedings, American Association for the Advancement of Automotive Medicine.*

Viscusi WK (1979) The impact of occupational safety and health regulation. *Bell J Econ* 10:117.

Waller PF, and Barry PZ (1969) Seat belts: a comparison of actual and reported use. Chapel Hill: University of North Carolina Highway Safety Research Center.

Ward's Automotive Yearbook (1960–92) Detroit: Ward's Communications.

Weeks JL, and Fox M (1983) Fatality rates and regulatory policies in bituminous coal mining, United States, 1959–1981. *Am J Public Health* 73:1278–1280.

Weiss EB, Pritz HB, and Hassler CR (1977) Experimental automobile-pedestrian injuries. *J Trauma* 17:823–828.

Whitfield RA, and Jones IS (1995) The effect of passenger load on unstable vehicles in fatal, untripped rollover crashes. *Am J Public Health* 85:1268–1271.

Williams AF, Wells JAK, and Lund AK (1990) Seat belt use in cars with air bags. *Am J Public Health* 80:1514–1516.

Wintemute GJ (1994) *Ring of Fire: The Handgun Makers of Southern California.* Sacramento, CA: Violence Prevention Research Program.

Wintemute GJ (1996) The relationship between firearm design and firearm violence. *JAMA* 275:1749–1753.

Woodward FD (1948) Medical criticism of modern automotive engineering. *JAMA* 138:627–631.

Zador PL, Jones IS, and Ginsburg M (1984a) Fatal front-to-front car collisions and the results of 35 mph frontal barrier impacts. *28th Annual Proceedings, American Association for the Advancement of Automotive Medicine.*

Zador PL, Stein H, Shapiro S, and Tarnoff P (1984b) Effect of signal timing on traffic flow and crashes at signalized intersections. Washington, DC: Insurance Institute for Highway Safety.

8

RESEARCH ON TREATMENT AND REHABILITATION

Research questions regarding the treatment of injuries and rehabilitation range from the profound issue of who survives trauma to the more mundane estimates of costs and who pays. Only a small minority of physicians and other professionals delivering care to traumatized patients conduct research, but because of their familiarity with the treatment and rehabilitation scene, these persons are usually in a better position to ask good research questions about treatment than academic epidemiologists (Findley, 1989).

Mortality from trauma has a trimodal distribution as a function of time after injury. Half or more of the deaths occur in the first hour, mainly from massive nervous system or heart and blood vessel damage. A second peak occurs within 1.5–2 hours, usually from internal injuries and blood loss. A third peak occurs at three to four weeks posttrauma, often due to infection or multiple organ failure. Many of the injuries to those who do not survive the first hour are not treatable, but there is substantial evidence that the timing and quality of emergency response and treatment can increase survival, particularly in the other groupings (Trunkey, 1983).

More and better research in the delivery of emergency services and on specific treatment and rehabilitation regimens would lead to increased survival and a better quality of life for those impaired by injury. Although research on the efficacy of modes of treatment and rehabilitation has accelerated, many practices are based on impressions from experience rather than quantitative evidence (Basmajian & Banerjee, 1996).

Issues include placement of emergency responders to minimize response time, amount and type of treatment at the scene, safety of transportation modes (ambulances, helicopters, fixed-wing aircraft), triage to designated trauma centers, designation of trauma centers, referral to rehabilitation, and efficacy of specific treatments in acute care and rehabilitation (Committee on Trauma Research, 1985). The injury epidemiologist who becomes knowledgeable in these issues can provide assistance in study design and statistical analysis to other health and organizational researchers involved in their investigation.

EMERGENCY RESPONSE

The effect on survival of delay in treatment of injuries has been inferred from the extent of delay and survival in war (Table 8.1). The bypassing of field treatment and transport to M.A.S.H. units in Korea and the transport directly to surgical units for definitive treatment in Vietnam are thought to be the major factors in reduced mortality (Trunkey, 1983), although controls for type and extent of wounds and improved surgical technique and technology might raise or lower the estimates somewhat.

Civilian emergency response systems have evolved from ambulance services, about half operated by morticians (who had an obvious conflict of interest), to a variety of systems based in hospitals, fire or police departments, volunteer services, and for-profit organizations (Boyd, 1983). The study of the effect of response times is complicated by the fact that response times are longer in remote rural areas where the injuries are also more severe and the quality of care upon arrival at a hospital is more often inferior. Controlling for types of motor vehicle crashes that would affect survival among rural counties in Texas,

TABLE 8.1. Delay between Injury and Surgery and Percent Mortality of the Injured in Wars

WAR	DELAY (HOURS)	MORTALITY (PERCENT)
World War I	12–18	8.5
World War II	6–12	5.8
Korea	2–4	2.4
Vietnam	1.1	1.7

Source: Trunkey, 1983.

the extent of access to emergency response systems apparently reduced the ratio of mortality to disabling injuries, but the cost-effectiveness of improving systems in remote areas was questioned (Brodsky & Hakkert, 1983). A major problem is that the rural areas with the lack of adequate emergency services are often those that can least afford them (Martin et al., 1990).

Some national data are available on emergency response times to fatal motor vehicle crashes in the Fatal Accident Reporting System, although nonreporting is a problem. For fatal crashes in urban areas during 1995, the emergency service arrived within 10 minutes of notification in about 88 percent of cases and within 20 minutes in 98 percent of cases. For fatal rural crashes, arrival occurred within 10 minutes in 55 percent of recorded cases and within 20 minutes in about 90 percent of recorded cases, but the response times were missing in about 38 percent of cases (National Highway Traffic Safety Administration, 1996). Time from first call to arrival at the hospital is problematic because data on hospital arrival time were missing in 49 percent of cases. Since these data are for fatal cases only, they do not allow correlation between response time and survival, but control data on survivors could be obtained from a sample of emergency response systems.

In an area with a regionalized trauma system in which patients with severe trauma are supposed to be taken to a special treatment center, probability of survival was not directly related to time at the scene or transport time. Time at the scene averaged 16.7 minutes for survivors and 15.2 minutes for nonsurvivors. Transport time was an average 13.0 minutes for survivors and 11.9 minutes for nonsurvivors (Shackford et al., 1989). While there does not appear to be a difference in an area with the range of response times studied, that does not mean that response time would not have an effect in areas where it is longer.

TREATMENT AT THE SCENE

Emergency responders and the public generally should learn how to clear breathing passages, stop obvious hemorrhage, stabilize the spine, and perform cardiopulmonary resuscitation in the absence of pulse or breathing (Jacobs & Bennett, 1983). Many questions remain about the advisability of delivering other kinds of treatment at the scene of injury versus delaying definitive treatment before transport. The main controversies revolve around various practices at the scene, such as intravenous infusion of fluids and the use of a pneumatic antishock garment, endotracheal intubation, and esophageal obturator airways (Lewis, 1983).

Many of these techniques were used by paramedics in the Vietnam War and were adopted in civilian emergency systems, particularly early on in those manned by veteran paramedics returned to civilian life. Some have become routine and in a few cases availability, at least, is mandated by law. For example, the pneumatic antishock garment was required equipment on ambulances in one-third of the states by the early 1980s despite lack of evidence of its efficacy (Lewis, 1983).

A study of the use or nonuse of the pneumatic antishock garment, assigned for use in the recommended circumstance on alternating days, indicated that an average of 4 minutes was added to time at the scene on the days that the garment was used. Survival was 69 percent on days when the garment was used and 75 percent on days it was not used. Although the assignment was not random, as claimed, it is doubtful that day-to-day differences biased the results. The authors concluded that the use of the garment had no net positive effect on survival and possibly a negative effect (Mattox et al., 1989).

That study does not quite lay the issue to rest because survival was higher when the garment was used (38 percent versus 29 percent when not used) among those with systolic blood pressures less than 50, although the difference was not statistically significant due to the small number of patients with those blood pressures. The remaining issue is whether more selective use of the garment on a sample and control group of sufficient size would indicate statistically significant benefit for selected patients.

Such controlled trials are unusual in the evaluation of prehospital emergency systems. The use of intravenous fluids before arrival at the hospital—studied retrospectively—indicates no advantage to trauma patients in several important subcategories of severity and clinical status. Patients taken to six hospitals in San Diego County during a 2.5 year period were studied (Kaweski et al., 1990). The use of fluids appeared to be random relative to severity of diagnosis and clinical status—some 56 percent received prehospital fluids. Time to the hospital was also similar in most severity groups, the exception being a 5 minute longer time among those who received fluids in the group with Injury Severity Scores 25–50 and systolic blood pressure greater than 90. Survival was similar in those treated with and without fluids in subgroups with various combinations of Injury Severity Score and Trauma Score.

Another type of study involves retrospective review of procedures and outcomes by a committee of emergency room physicians, trauma surgeons, and neurosurgeons. For example, one such study concluded that advanced life support (the care delivered by the best trained paramedics including intravenous fluids, endotracheal intubation, and pneumatic shock garments) "appears to be beneficial in the treatment of multisystem trauma in a rural state" (Reines et al., 1988). This despite the fact that advanced life support took an average 5 minutes more at the scene and a ten physician review committee judged the treatment not in compliance with recommended practice in 74 percent of cases for endotracheal intubation and 54 percent of cases for pneumatic garments. In the cases where the techniques were applied, the review committee judged advanced life support as "helpful or essential in 85 percent of cases" and harmful in less than 2 percent.

An ecological study also found a correlation between levels of training of emergency response personnel and fatality rates per population among counties in North Carolina. Counties with advanced or paramedic training had lower fatality rates after adjusting statistically for numerous other differences among the counties. Since all urban counties had advanced training, however, it was not possible to totally disaggregate the possible effects of other factors (Messick et al., 1992).

Clearly, there is conflict in the results of the clinical trial of the pneumatic garment and the results of the postinjury review study. Since the methodological power of randomized field trials is far superior to ecological studies and retrospective judgment, such trials must be employed to evaluate more definitively the efficacy of particular procedures. Of course, if the procedures are substantially unused even when there is a policy regarding their use, or policy guidelines are not followed, the issue is largely moot.

The efficacy of modes of transportation of injured patients is also a matter of controversy. Many hospitals have purchased helicopters ostensibly to reduce travel times, although the use in transplant programs, as well as publicity and pride of ownership, also no doubt contribute to the decision to purchase. While the use of helicopters to transport trauma patients from remote locations is seldom questioned, research has raised doubts of its net benefit in urban areas.

For example, based on comparison of patients suffering from blunt trauma with survivable Injury Severity Scores and Glasgow Coma Scores, no advantage of helicopter transport was indicated within a metropolitan area in patient outcomes (Schiller et al., 1988). Other studies suggest increased survival in helicopter transfers (Schwartz et al., 1989). A complete assessment of the efficacy of the available forms of transportation would require assessment of the costs of helicopter systems as well as injury to patients and emergency personnel in crashes during transport by whatever mode. Since helicopters cannot fly in certain weather conditions or where there is insufficient landing space, they are an incremental rather than a substitutable expense. Land-based ambulance systems cannot be eliminated when a helicopter is purchased.

Assessment of the effect of changing any one system component is complex because of the intercorrelation of various factors. Attempts to assess survival, length of hospital stay, and costs as a function of mode of transport and direct transport to a trauma center versus an interim stop at another hospital must control at least for age and injury severity. The numbers of cases in certain combinations of the factors become thin even when beginning with a large sample size. Given these limitations, the available data suggest that arrivals at a trauma center from interhospital transfers have longer length of stay and greater costs than those brought directly to the trauma center (Schwartz et al., 1989). Among spinal cord patients, the increased time in hospital is a result of increased need for acute care; time in rehabilitation is not significantly different (Oakes et al., 1990). This could be partly because only the more severe cases or cases with complications are transferred, but those who are not transferred are known to be at greater risk in many community hospitals.

TRAUMA CENTERS

Once the injured person is en route to a hospital, the hospital of choice is at issue. Although time to the hospital may be a factor in outcome in some cases, if the medical care received on arrival is inadequate or misdirected, the probability of survival can be reduced. There is little doubt that the treatment received in hospitals makes a difference in chance of survival (e.g., Baker et al., 1971; Smith et al., 1990).

Some patients are apparently dead on arrival (DOA) at the hospital but the question of what criteria to use for attempting resuscitation remain under investigation. Based on a literature review and discussion, one trauma team defined DOA as follows:

—All blunt trauma and penetrating trauma of the abdomen, head, neck or groin: prehospital CPR (cardiopulmonary resuscitation) >5 minutes, age >12 years, no pulse on arrival
—Penetrating trauma of the chest: prehospital CPR >15 minutes, age >12 years, no pulse on arrival
—Child with any of the above that has in-hospital CPR >15 minutes (open or closed) without pulse. (Pasquale et al., 1996)

Of 86 patients studied by this trauma team who met the DOA criteria, none survived despite continued resuscitative efforts on 70 at a cost of more than $4000 each. Of 20 patients who did not meet the criteria, 3 survived. Children were excluded from the analysis because of the small number.

The authors of the study noted that there are potential cost savings from the application of DOA criteria. They also noted that use of the criteria in their institution was "erratic." Two issues are raised by this research. First, the sample is relatively small and a multicenter study is needed to specify factors predictive of survival probability. Second, if criteria are established, will they be followed?

The movement to designate certain hospitals as trauma centers and to transport severely injured patients to such centers evolved from the understanding that the necessary experience and training to treat severe trauma, as well as efficient use of technology, could occur only in facilities that treat large numbers of cases. While this has been accomplished in many areas, the extent of compliance with designation in a given area varies. For example, Illinois was among the first states to have regionalized trauma centers. Yet Chicago, where the fire department managed the emergency medical system, did not join the state system and the old practice of transporting a patient to the nearest hospital continued. A study of the patients' destinations relative to their trauma scores indicated no correlation between serious injury and the probability of being taken to a trauma center (Cadigan, 1985).

One question for research in any given area is the extent to which the guidelines for transportation of patients to designated trauma centers are being followed. One surgeon has hypothesized that persons taken to community hospitals who have insurance (assessed by "wallet biopsy") are more likely to be retained there while the rest are sent to trauma centers (Gann, 1989).

The survival rate of seriously injured patients among hospitals is inversely correlated to the volume of patients seen. In one study, for example, the survival rate was 30 percent higher in hospitals that treated more than 110 such patients per year than in those that treated 75 or fewer (Smith et al., 1990). Detailed data on severity scores were not available for more refined adjustment of the estimate and more research incorporating such data is needed. When adjusted for injury severity within a hospital, patients treated by a trauma team were more likely to survive that those treated by others (Petrie, 1996).

Traditionally, two methods—the autopsy method and the clinical method—have been used in the assessment of adequacy of treatment (West & Cales, 1983). The *autopsy method* involves examination of autopsy records for certain types of cases—eliminating prehospital deaths, dead-on-arrivals, and central nervous system cases for which treatment is ineffective. Deaths to persons less than 50 years old, those that occurred less than six hours after arrival, those in which laparotomy or thoracotomy was not done, and deaths from hemorrhage are examined in particular detail and preventability is assessed.

The autopsy method has identified substantial proportions of preventable deaths among the defined subsets of all deaths, a process that helped justify the designation of trauma centers and helped substantially reduce deaths judged preventable in those subsets (West et al., 1983). The method is not adequate to assess the overall effect of trauma center designation, however. If the designation were to result in deaths due to longer transport times, and more deaths in emergency vehicle crashes en route due to longer travel distances, for example, those would have to be subtracted from the net lives preserved rather than eliminated from the analysis before counting.

The *clinical method* includes audit of the prehospital as well as hospital records, identification of fatalities thought to be survivable, and determination of the phase of response or treatment that failed. The use of the method is dependent on the quality of the records of paramedics, hospitals, and coroners as well as the lack of bias in those who audit the cases. Use of the method in Orange County, California, before and after the implementation of a comprehensive trauma system, indicated a reduction in preventable deaths from 34 percent to 15 percent despite the fact that the average age and Injury Severity Scores of the patients audited increased during the study period (West & Cales, 1983).

The use of committees to review records of deaths to judge the numbers that were preventable by treatment has been brought into serious question by reliability studies. When the same cases were reviewed by separate panels, the agreement was poor (MacKenzie et al., 1992; Wilson et al., 1992).

The designation of trauma centers can concentrate a cost burden on the designated hospitals which threatens their ability to continue the service. In an attempt to control rising medical care costs, average costs in diagnosis-related groups (DRGs) are used by insurance companies and governments to determine the amounts hospitals will receive for given diagnoses (Waller et al., 1989).

There is substantial evidence that DRGs are inadequate for determining costs of trauma treatment and certainly should not be used for quality assurance. Since only one DRG category is assigned per patient, multiple injuries are not adequately reflected, as they are in more detailed classification systems (Chapter 2). Comparison of DRG classifications of trauma patients and other classifications of criteria for injury management indicate that DRGs are relatively poor predictors of cost of treatment (Young et al., 1990).

The overall impact on hospital financial status of the costs of treatment of severely injured patients compared to the amounts specified for reimbursement in DRG systems have produced conflicting results depending on case mix examined. While some studies find that the less severe injuries are reimbursed at more than cost, offsetting insufficient reimbursement of the more severe injuries (Waller et al., 1989), other hospitals have substantial net shortfalls. In the trauma center for southern New Jersey, the average cost per case in 1985 was $7137 and the average reimbursement was $3574, resulting in the hospital losing a total of almost $1.9 million in revenues. The research indicates that the Injury Severity Score could be used to predict costs to some extent (Schwab, 1988).

More research from other trauma centers would perhaps lead to an adjustment of DRGs based on case-mix criteria. For example, a DRG category was added for certain burn injuries, but the categories in use apparently remain inadequate. The categories in use do not distinguish subtantial variations in costs of burn treatment (Chakerian et al., 1990). Four Multiple Significant Trauma DRGs were added in 1991 to account for trauma to more than one body site. Nevertheless, a study of 49 consecutive patients that met the criteria for the new DRGs during 5 months found that 38 percent of the cost of care was not covered by the DRGs, a shortfall of $492,057, or about $10,000 per patient (Jacobs and Jacobs, 1992).

The finances of 70 trauma centers in 12 metropolitan areas with populations exceeding 1 million indicate that public hospitals were more likely than private hospitals to have "financial stress" from trauma care. Any cuts in Medicaid, Medicare, or other programs that subsidize trauma centers would put the survival of many in jeopardy (Bazzoli, 1996). A survey of 66 trauma centers that closed found that uncompensated care, high operating costs, and inadequate reimbursement from medical assistance programs were primary factors in the closings (Dailey et al., 1992).

Attempts to control costs by "managed care" may be having an effect on prevention as well. Suicidal patients whose care was refused or attenuated by managed care personnel who did not see the patient have allegedly resulted in suicide completions (*60 Minutes,* 1997). Research is needed on the extent of the problem.

CLINICAL STUDIES OF TRAUMA AND SPECIFIC TREATMENT

Injury in America laid out a series of questions for research in the understanding and treatment of trauma (Committee on Trauma Research, 1985). Examples are: What happens to cells in shock and what can be done to prevent or reduce cellular dysfunction? How do metabolic systems respond to trauma and can interventions reduce harmful reactions or optimize reactions favorable to recovery? How does the immune system react and what can be done to control infection by augmenting the immune system or use of antimicrobials? What factors contribute to healing or failure to heal and can healing be enhanced therapeutically? What can be done to minimize nervous system damage and is nerve regeneration possible?

Answers to these and other questions depend on continued revision of models of anatomic systems at cellular, organ, and whole system levels based on animal as well as human studies. When a reasonable point of intervention is identified, a controlled clinical trial of a hypothesized effective intervention is warranted. Textbooks are available on experimental designs and statistical power issues in clinical trials and all of the issues cannot be repeated here (Fleiss, 1986; Stein, 1989).

In the simplest form of a controlled clinical trial, a change in procedure, medication, or whatever, is introduced in the treatment of a randomly selected experimental group while a randomly selected control group with the same medical condition receives the old accepted treatment, or a placebo in addition to the old treatment if the experimental treatment is new. If the effects for subsets of clinical conditions are in question, the experimental and control groups can be assigned within each group of patients with a given condition.

To avoid bias in measurement where possible, those treating the patient or obtaining measurements pre- and posttreatment should not know if the patient is in the experimental or control group. This is rather easily done in the case of drug therapy, but not in surgery or other hands-on treatment. At the least, the surgeons or others who administer obvious treatments should not be the persons to obtain measurements of outcome used in evaluation. Under certain circumstances, a crossover design can be used in which patients in an experimental group for a period are in the control group in a succeeding period and vice versa. For example, the effects of manual and mechanized ventilatory support on blood gasses were studied using such a design (Hurst et al., 1989).

Timing of treatment must also be considered in clinical trials. For example, based on animal studies, methylprednisolone was hypothesized to improve motor and sensory function of patients with acute spinal cord injury. In a controlled clinical trial, significant improvement was found among patients given the drug within 8 hours after injury, but not if delayed beyond 8 hours (Bracken et al., 1990). Although the treatment is not a cure, spinal cord patients treated within 8 hours were found better able to care for themselves and otherwise lead more independent lives. Further experiments using pharmacological approaches to improved functioning of spinal cord patients are under way (Smith et al., 1996).

Nonexperimental epidemiologic methods can be used to generate hypotheses regarding certain clinical issues. For example, the efficacy of surgical exploration of penetrating injuries of the spine has been questioned based on retrospective analysis of cases. The percentage whose nervous system function improved, remained the same, or deteriorated was similar with or without surgery. The proportion with complications such as infection and cerebrospinal fluid leakage, however, was significantly higher among those with surgery than without—22 percent versus 7 percent (Simpson et al., 1989). No randomized trials of surgical intervention for spinal cord injury have been done (Smith et al., 1996) and various contingencies make comparison of those treated and untreated by surgery problematic (Kiwerski, 1993).

Some clinical studies would benefit from appropriate use of multivariate analysis. For example, in a study of patients with vascular injuries in the abdomen, infection was related to low initial systolic blood pressure, number of blood transfusions, multiple injuries, and cross-clamped aorta during surgery (Wilson et al., 1989). A multivariate analysis, such as logistic regression, was not done, however, and might better isolate the potential contribution of each controlling for the others. A controlled clinical trial of the use of blood transfusions and surgical technique could be guided by the results.

Simple improvements in diagnostic tools may greatly improve clinical decisions. For example, assessment of the neurological status and possible effects of alcohol in unconscious patients is important. A device to measure concentration of alcohol in passive nasal exhalation of comatose patients was shown by epidemiologists and physicians working together to be almost perfectly correlated to blood alcohol concentration (Gerberich et al., 1989).

LONG-TERM CARE AND REHABILITATION

Many people who survive traumatic injury have lost abilities because of brain and spinal damage, lost digits or limbs, lost sensory function, and distortion of tissue from burn or other scars. These patients, and additional others, are affected psychologically, socially, and economically. There is substantial anecdotal evidence of fears of being injured again, of family breakup and disruption, of discrimination, and of economic deprivation (Kaufman, 1989). The quantification of these effects and factors that contribute to reduced dependency and productive and personally satisfying lives is a challenge to epidemiologists as well as other scientists. As noted in Chapter 2, one of the needs is more reliable and valid measures of various types of impairment of abilities and disability.

Injury in America identified numerous research issues in rehabilitation (Committee on Trauma Research, 1985) and these were expanded by a panel on disability (Pope & Tarlov, 1991). Examples are: What are the most effective methods of rehabilitation to restore activity and at the same time conserve the energies of the disabled? What are effective procedures and counseling in acute care that lead to reduction of scar contractures, muscular atrophy, and skeletal deformity as well as referral to rehabilitation and preparation of the patient for fit and use of prosthetic and cosmetic aids? What is the relative effectiveness of methods to control spasticity, optimize ventilation, improve cognitive function, and the like? What changes in the environments of persons with various handicaps would reduce their dependency or increase their productivity and satisfaction? How many persons are not receiving services that would benefit them, their families, or the community? What are the aspects of the medical care and rehabilitation systems, personal and family beliefs, or social situations of those in need of services that are barriers to use of services or benefit from them?

Studies of the posthospitalization outcomes of injury are limited by representativeness of samples, sample sizes, and methodological problems. Studies are usually confined to the patients discharged from one or more hospitals serving an urban area or region. To the extent that there is selectivity of hospitals by type of injury or severity, these studies may result in over- or underestimation of the extent of a given identified problem, limitations usually recognized by the researchers.

Although not representative of the injured population, follow-up studies of discharged patients are useful in development of criteria to identify while in hospital patients who will have problems and needs thereafter. In a study of discharged patients from two trauma centers, 80 percent had problems with posthospital self-care and an additional 12 percent, who could care for themselves, had problems with mobility or other physical activities. One year postdischarge, 23 percent continued to have problems with self-care and an additional 4 percent had continued mobility or other physical problems. Only 57 percent of those who had worked before the injury had returned to full-time employment one year postdischarge. Even among those with minor to moderately severe injuries of the extremities (AIS = 1–3), half to two-thirds who had been employed before their injuries had not returned to work after one year. Those with lower preinjury incomes were less likely to be working, controlling statistically for functional impairment (MacKenzie et al., 1988).

In another study, children up to age 18 in a children's hospital were followed for six months if they had one or more severe injuries (AIS = 4–5) or two or more moderate to severe injuries (AIS = 2–5). Of the 62 percent on whom follow-up data were obtained, about half had not returned to normal activities after six months. The authors stated that the results supported the need for more rehabilitative services, but they did not document the number and types of rehabilitation used for the children (Wesson et al., 1989). Without relating outcomes to type and degree of rehabilitation received, it is not possible to say that more such services would have made a difference.

Most of the longer term studies of patient outcomes are of small samples of patients during a few years postinjury. For example, in a follow-up study of 101 brain-injured patients 5–10.4 years postinjury, 63 were located (8 of these were deceased, including several undocumented mentions of suicide). Disability at follow-up was lower among those who had entered rehabilition earlier, but the study did not include persons with brain injuries who were not referred to, or did not use, rehabilitation facilities.

Among patients able to respond to the survey themselves, "significant others" (spouse, other relative, friend, etc.) rated the patients as more impaired than the patients rated themselves. Among major problems identified at follow-up were lack of social relationships (45 percent); unemployment (17 percent); and physical problems, dependency, and lack of motivation (21 percent). Needs for education, support groups, and supervision were stated but not quantified (Rappaport et al., 1989).

An interesting difference in findings from retrospective and cross-sectional studies when compared to a prospective study occurred in the attempt to find risk factors for postinjury use of acute-care facilities by patients with spinal injuries. Although such factors as level of lesion, years disabled, and cigarette use were significantly correlated to hospitalization when studied retrospectively and cross-sectionally, a prospective study found no such correlations. Hospitalization proved unpredictable prospectively, but outpatient facility use was correlated to age, years of disability, formal education, and dissatisfaction with medical care. Those in managed care programs for independent living were less likely to use outpatient care, suggesting that the programs may reduce the cost of medical care (Meyers et al., 1989).

When the psychosocial factors are assessed prior to hip fractures in the elderly, they are less predictive of institutionalization than in ex post facto assessments (Marottoli et al., 1994). Apparently, postinjury assessments are influenced by the injury experience.

In a study of 756 people with traumatic brain injury, the most important predictor of involvement in rehabilitation was not physical or demographic factors but the specialization of the treating physicians (Wrigley et al., 1994). If a physical medicine and rehabilitation specialist was involved in referral decisions, the patient was more likely to receive rehabilitation, controlling for injury severity and demographic factors. Research is needed on the extent to which medical teams without this specialty are aware of the opportunities and benefits of rehabilitation.

IMPROVING OUTCOMES

Models of rehabilitation have been developed which include not only the effects of drugs and physical therapy but also social support and transitional living centers. Research on effectiveness is needed at each stage of rehabilitation (Wood & Eames, 1989). To determine the effects of treatment and rehabilitation on outcomes, there must be some consensus on expected outcomes from particular interventions. For some types of injury, for example, traumatic brain injury, a consensus on priority of outcomes has not been attained. Clients, therapists, and third-party payers have different expectations (Garner & Finlayson, 1996). The effects on families are somewhat dependent on the preinjury status of family roles (e.g., Rivara et al., 1996).

There may be substantial selection bias in choice of therapies. Results of studies of use of catheters for bladder emptying of spinal cord patients are in substantial conflict as to extent of complications (Smith et al., 1996). Clearly, individual economic situations that affect availability of skilled caretakers and living conditions would have a substantial effect on use and maintenance of catheters and infection opportunities. Such factors would also affect affordability, and likely systematic use, of prophylactic antibiotics for urinary tract infections.

One promising approach to mobility of spinal-injured patients is the use of electrical stimulation. Most studies find improvements in patient physiology and mobility but the attrition rate is high. The complexity of the current technology and the effort required from the patient relative to the noticeable improvement often discourage the patients (Smith et al., 1996). Research is needed on the degree of improvement that would motivate patients to continue with the effort as well as the psychological effects of possible shattered hopes when the therapy fails to meet expectations.

The practice of physical therapy has evolved as the mix of problems presented to rehabilitation facilities has changed and the models of the functioning of the central nervous system (CNS) and musculoskeletal system have been improved by theory and research. Increased survival of persons with CNS damage presents a major challenge to physical therapists (Gordon, 1987; Pinkston, 1989). Technology for potentially improving aspects of impairment must be studied relative to traditional methods of hands-on movement and exercise. The relative effectiveness of available and new methods can be discerned in controlled clinical trials.

For example, one study compared the consequences of three types of therapy among patients with incomplete cervical spinal cord injuries—physical exercises supervised by a therapist (PET), electrical neuromuscular stimulation (NMS), and biofeedback using an electromyogram (EMG). The patients were randomly assigned to four groups and the sequence of the different therapies was varied among three groups—EMG-PET, EMG-NMS, NMS-PET—while the fourth group received only PET. Baseline and subsequent measurement of outcomes was done by persons unaware of the group assignment. Although improvements in function were found among all four groups, there were no differences among the groups (Klose et al., 1990).

The evaluation of therapy and rehabilitation for impairment from trauma is substantially dependent on the reliability, validity, and prognostic predictability of measures of impairment. Epidemiologists can contribute to the development of quantified scales of such outcomes as sensation, motor ability, and balance. One such study, for example, indicated the importance of early identification of discrepancies in sensation and motor ability as diagnostic tools for patients with spinal injury (Bracken et al., 1977–78).

The Glasgow Coma Scale is useful in acute care decisions but is not strongly correlated to long-term functioning (Zafonte et al., 1996). A battery of quantitative tests of sway among brain injured patients has been shown to be sensitive enough to distinguish even minimal balance problems (Lehmann, 1990). Accelerometers that can be worn by the patient to monitor physical activity have been studied for reliability and validity (Kochersberger et al., 1996). Performance in an obstacle course is not adequately correlated to other balance and functional measures (maximum $R = 0.54$) to be used as a screening measurement (Means et al., 1996).

In addition to their use in diagnosis and rehabilitation, reliable and valid measurements could be important in prevention of repeated trauma. For example, falls are a problem among hospitalized and institutionalized patients. In a rehabilitation hospital, 12.5 percent of patients fell in a year, mainly from wheelchairs (Vlahov, 1990). The fracture rates of men in Veterans Administration nursing homes were 5 to 11 times those in the age-matched general population (Rudman & Rudman, 1989). Among the potentially worthwhile questions for research are: Do those with more adverse scores on sensory, motor, or activity scales fall more often, or are those with particular combinations of scores on the scales more likely to fall? How do scores on tests of sway predict falls, if at all?

Potentially even more serious injuries can occur to people whose impairments are not severe enough to prevent driving but are severe enough to increase probability of a crash. One study followed 22 brain-injured patients for five years after a physician, a neuropsychologist, and a driving specialist judged them fit to drive. Measurement of driving records and fitness was based on telephone interviews with the patients and "matched" control group of close friends and spouses of the patients. A neuropsychological test battery was administered to those who claimed to have driving problems. The authors concluded that the screening was adequate to identify those "fit to drive" (Katz et al., 1990).

Unfortunately, the study is wholly inadequate to reach that conclusion. The sample size is too small to obtain any statistical power in comparison of driving records. There were significantly more women than men in the control group. Self-report of crashes, violations, and other problems in driving is not an acceptable methodology without independent validation from driving records.

LENGTH OF STAY AND COSTS

The pressure from the managed care systems to reduce hospital stays may result in earlier or more frequent referral to rehabilitation facilities, which may in turn be pressured to release the patient to home or nursing home care. In a study that included patients whose impairment originated from both trauma and other conditions, length of stay was moderately correlated to an index of impairment of specific abilities (eating, toileting, bathing, mobility, etc.), referral source, and year of admission. Type of medical insurance, sex, race, other medical conditions, and "psychologic capacity" were not predictive of length of stay. Age was said to have a complex interaction with the other predictive factors and was not included in the prediction model (Stineman & Williams, 1990). The authors were appropriately cautious about generalizing the results to other facilities without similar research in those facilities. Matched for sex and injury severity, older patients require longer, more costly periods of rehabilitation to achieve the same degree of functioning (Cifu et al., 1996).

Despite the wide variation in patient needs and resultant length of stays, the DRG system has only one category for rehabilitation based on overall average cost, but exemption is allowed, which minimized the effects for hospitals that obtained exemptions. The system was used in the Veterans Administration (VA) to place its hospitals in competition for a set budget. A study from one VA hospital looked at the length of stay, readmissions, and referrals to nursing homes or home health care before and after the system was adopted. While length of stay decreased an average three days, the discharges to nursing homes increased and those to home health care decreased significantly. The net effect may be increased costs, but costs were not assessed (Evans et al., 1990).

A study of the effect of prospective payment on treatment of hip fractures among the elderly (Palmer et al., 1989) resulted in lively debate regarding the relative efficacy and costs of rehabilitation in hospitals and skilled nursing care facilities (Lipson & Minassian, 1990). Comparison among facilities and the extent of referral to facilities may be influenced by home situations as well as medical conditions and costs (Palmer et al., 1990).

The effect of DRGs on who is treated where and who pays has been described as "squeezing the balloon." "Prospective payment systems hold the line on inpatient use and revenues, but outpatient services and spending rise dramatically" (Brown, 1988). Apparently, the relative effects of all the major potential factors on referral, outcomes in patient functioning, and costs have not been studied.

Certain programs have traditionally claimed to be cost-beneficial, that is, they return more in economic benefits to society than their costs. Vocational rehabilitation, for example, has a specific economic goal—to return the patient to gainful employment. If that employment returns more in taxes to the government than the cost of rehabilitating the person, then the investment clearly paid off, at least from the government's viewpoint, irrespective of the issues of intangible costs and benefits (more on this in Chapter 9). However, vocational rehabilitation has apparently not been studied in a randomized, controlled trial. Comparisons have been done of earnings before and after rehabilitation, but with insufficient follow-up to confirm that immediate postrehabilitation earnings were sustained. Also, types of rehabilitants were not compared, although change in types might change the cost–benefit ratios (Berkowitz, 1988). The decline in returns to investment as increased numbers of severely disabled persons are included in the program could sway the balance of costs and benefits to the negative. Costs exceed benefits among those with certain sensory disabilities in certain age groups, for example (Gibbs, 1988). Those who live by cost–benefit could also die by cost–benefit.

SUMMARY

Well-placed and organized emergency medical systems with staff experienced in treatment of trauma increases the probability of survival of the injured who survive the initial energy insult. Questions remain regarding the efficacy of certain treatments at the scene of injury. The existence of trauma centers, where probability of survival is increased, is threatened by evolving trends in organization and financing of medical care systems. Resolution of these issues, as well as clinical trials of acute care and rehabilitation regimes, would benefit from examination by epidemiologic methods.

REFERENCES

Baker SP, Gertner HR, Rutherford RB, and Spitz WU (1971) Traffic deaths due to blunt abdominal injuries. *Proceedings of the Fourteenth Annual Conference of the American Association for Automotive Medicine.* Ann Arbor: University of Michigan.

Basmajian JV, and Banerjee SN (eds) (1996) *Clinical Decision Making in Rehabilitation.* New York: Churchill-Livingstone.

Bazzoli GJ (1996) Factors that enhance continued trauma center participation in trauma systems. *J. Trauma* 41:876–885.

Berkowitz E (1988) The cost-benefit tradition in vocational rehabilitation. In Berkowitz E (ed), *Measuring the Efficiency of Public Programs: Costs and Benefits in Vocational Rehabilitation.* Philadelphia: Temple University Press.

Boyd DR (1983) Foreword. In Jacobs LM Jr, and Bennett BR, *Emergency Patient Care: Prehospital Ground and Air Procedures.* New York: Macmillan.

Bracken MB, Webb SB, and Wagner FC (1977–78) Classification of the severity of acute spinal cord injury. *Paraplegia* 15:319–326.

Bracken MB, Shepard MJ, Collins WF, Holford TR, Young W, Baskin DS, Eisenberg HM, Flamm E, Leo-Summers L, Maroon J, Marshall LF, Perot PL Jr, Piepmeier J, Sonntag VKH, Wagner FC, Wilberger JE, and Winn HR (1990) A randomized controlled trial of methylprednisolone or naxolone in the treatment of acute spinal-cord injury. *N Engl J Med* 322:1405–1411.

Brodsky H, and Hakkert S (1983) Highway fatal accidents and accessibility of emergency medical services. *Soc Sci Med* 17:731–740.

Brown LD (1988) *Health Policy in the United States: Issues and Options.* New York: Ford Foundation.

Cadigan A (1985) An evaluation of trauma center utilization in Chicago. Unpublished MPH thesis, Yale University.

Chakerian MU, Demarest GB, and Paiz A (1990) Burn DRGs: effects of recent changes and implications for the future. *J Trauma* 30:964–973.

Cifu DX, Kreutzer JS, Marwitz JH, Rosenthal M, Englander J, and High W (1996) Functional outcomes of older adults with traumatic brain injury: a prospective, multicenter analysis. *Arch Phys Med Rehabil* 77:883–888.

Committee on Trauma Research (1985) *Injury in America: A Continuing Public Health Problem.* Washington, DC: National Academy Press.

Dailey JT, Teter H, and Cowley RA (1992) Trauma center closures: a national assessment. *J Trauma* 33:539–546.

Evans RL, Hendricks RD, Bishop DS, Lawrence-Umlauf KV, Kirk C, and Halar EM (1990) Prospective payment for rehabilitation: effects on hospital readmission, home care, and placement. *Arch Phys Med Rehabil* 71:291–294.

Findley TW (1989) Research in physical medicine and rehabilitation. I. How to ask the question. *Am J Phys Med Rehabil* 68:26–30.

Fleiss JL (1986) *The Design and Analysis of Clinical Experiments.* New York: John Wiley and Sons.

Gann DS (1989) Presidential address—American Association for the Surgery of Trauma, 1988 Annual Session. *J Trauma* 29:1459–1461.

Garner SH, and Finlayson MAJ (1996) Traumatic brain injury. In Basmajian JV, and Banerjee SN (eds), *Clinical Decision Making in Rehabilitation.* New York: Churchill-Livingstone.

Gerberich SG, Gerberich BK, Fife D, Cicero JJ, Lilja GP, and Van Berkom LC (1989) Analyses of the relationship between blood alcohol and nasal breath alcohol concentrations: implications for assessment of trauma cases. *J Trauma* 29:338–343.

Gibbs E (1988) The vocational rehabilitation data base and the estimation of benefit cost ratios. In Berkowitz E (ed), *Measuring the Efficiency of Public Programs: Costs and Benefits in Vocational Rehabilitation.* Philadelphia: Temple University Press.

Gordon J (1987) Assumptions underlying physical therapy intervention: theoretical and historical perspectives. In Carr JH, et al. (eds), *Movement Science: Foundations for Physical Therapy in Rehabilitation.* Rockville, MD: Aspen Publishers.

Hurst JM, Davis K Jr, Branson RD, and Johannigman JA (1989) Comparison of blood gasses during transport using two methods of ventilatory support. *J Trauma* 29:1637–1639.

Jacobs BB, and Jacobs LM (1992) The effect of the new trauma DRGs on reimbursement. *J Trauma* 33:495–502.

Jacobs LM Jr, and Bennett BR (1983) *Emergency Patient Care: Prehospital Ground and Air Procedures.* New York: Macmillan.

Katz RT, Golden RS, Butter J, Tepper D, Rothke S, Holmes J, and Sahgal V (1990) Driving safety after brain damage: followup of twenty-two patients with matched controls. *Arch Phys Med Rehabil* 71:133–136.

Kaufman S (1989) Long-term impact of injury on individuals, families and society: personal narratives and policy implications. In Rice DP, and MacKenzie EJ (eds), *Cost of Injury in the United States: A Report to Congress, 1989.* San Francisco: University of California Institute for Health and Aging, and Baltimore: Johns Hopkins University Injury Prevention Center.

Kaweski SM, Sise MJ, and Virgilio RW (1990) The effect of prehospital fluids on survival in trauma patients. *J Trauma*30:1215–1219.

Kiwerski JE (1993) Neurological outcome from conservative or surgical treatment of cervical spinal cord injured patients. *J Paraplegia* 31:192.

Klose KJ, Schmidt DL, Needham BM, Brucker BS, Green BA, and Ayyar DR (1990) Rehabilitation therapy for patients with long-term spinal cord injuries. *Arch Phys Med Rehabil* 71:659–662.

Kochersberger G, McConnell E, Kuchibhatla MN, and Pieper C (1996) The reliability, validity, and stability of a measure of physical activity in the elderly. *Arch Phys Med Rehabil* 77:793–795.

Lehmann JF (1990) Quantitative evaluation of sway as an indicator of functional balance in post-traumatic brain injury. *Arch Phys Med Rehabil* 71:955–961.

Lewis FR (1983) Prehospital care: the role of the EMT-paramedic. In West, JG, Gazzaniga AB, and Cales RH (eds), *Trauma Care Systems.* New York: Praeger.

Lipson MJ, and Minassian P (1990) Differences in outcome: hospital rehabilitation vs skilled nursing facility rehabilitation. *Arch Intern Med* 150:1550–1551.

MacKenzie EJ, Siegel JH, Shapiro S, Moody M, and Smith RT (1988) Functional recovery and medical costs of trauma: an analysis by type and severity of injury. *J Trauma* 28:281–297.

MacKenzie EJ, Steinwachs DM, Bone LR, Floccare DJ, Ramzy AI, and The Preventable Death Study Group (1992) Inter-rater reliability of preventable death judgments. *J Trauma* 33:292–302.

Marottoli RA, Berkman LF, Leo-Summers L, and Cooney LM (1994) Predictors of mortality and institutionalization after hip fracture: the New Haven EPESE Cohort. *Am J Public Health* 84:1807–1812.

Martin GD, Cogbill TH, Landercasper J, and Strutt PJ (1990) Prospective analysis of rural interhospital transfer of injured patients to a referral trauma center. *J Trauma* 30:1014–1020.

Mattox KL, Bickell W, Pepe PE, Burch J, and Feliciano D (1989) Prospective MAST study in 911 patients. *J Trauma* 29:1104–1112.

Means KM, Rodell DE, and Sullivan PS (1996) Use of an obstacle course to assess balance and mobility in the elderly. *Arch Phys Med Rehabil* 75:88–95.

Messick WJ, Rutledge R, and Meyer AA (1992) The association of advanced life support and decreased per capita trauma death rates: an analysis of 12,417 trauma deaths. *J Trauma* 33:850– 855.

Meyers AR, Branch LG, Cupples A, Lederman RI, Feltin M, and Master RJ (1989) Predictors of medical care utilization by independently living adults with spinal cord injuries. *Arch Phys Med Rehabil* 70:471–475.

National Highway Traffic Safety Administration (1996) *Traffic Safety Facts 1995.* Washington, DC: U.S. Department of Transportation.

Oakes DD, Wilmot CB, Hall KM, and Sherck JP (1990) Benefits of early admission to a comprehensive trauma center for patients with spinal cord injury. *Arch Phys Med Rehabil* 71:637–643.

Palmer RM, Saywell RM Jr, Zollinger PW (1989) The impact of prospective payment systems on the treatment of hip fractures in the elderly. *Arch Intern Med* 149:2237–2241.

Palmer RM, Saywell RM Jr, and Zollinger TW (1990) In reply. *Arch Intern Med* 150:1551.

Pasquale MD, Rhodes M, Cipolle MD, Hauley T, Wasser T (1996) Defining "Dead on Arrival": Impact on a level I trauma center, *J Trauma* 41:726–730.

Petrie D, Lane P, Stewart TC (1996) An evaluation of patient outcomes comparing trauma team activated versus trauma team not activated using TRISS analysis. *J Trauma* 41:870–873.

Pinkston D (1989) Evolution of the practice of physical therapy in the United States. In Scully RM, and Barnes MR (eds), *Physical Therapy.* Philadelphia: J.B. Lippincott.

Pope AM, and Tarlov AR (1991) *Disability in America: Toward a National Agenda for Prevention.* Washington, DC: National Academy Press.

Rappaport M, Herrero-Backe C, Rappaport ML, and Winterfield KM (1989) Head injury outcome up to 10 years later. *Arch Phys Med Rehabil* 70:885–892.

Reines HD, Bartlett RL, Chudy NE, Kiragu KR, and McKnew MA (1988) Is advanced life support appropriate for victims of motor vehicle accidents: the South Carolina highway trauma project. *J Trauma* 28:563–570.

Rivara JB, Jaffe KM, Polissar NL, Fay GC, Liao S, and Martin KM (1996) Predictors of family functioning and changes 3 years after traumatic brain injury in children. *Arch Phys Med Rehabil* 77:754–764.

Rudman TW, and Rudman D (1989) High rate of fractures for men in nursing homes. *Am J Phys Med Rehabil* 68:2–5.

Schiller WR, Knox R, Zinnecker H, Jeevanandam M, Sayre M, Burke J, and Young DH (1988) Effect of helicopter transport of trauma victims on survival in an urban trauma center. *J Trauma* 28:1127–1134.

Schwab CW, Young G, Civil I, Ross SE, Talucci R, Rosenberg L, Shaikh K, O'Malley K, and Camishion RC (1988) DRG reimbursement for trauma: the demise of the trauma center (the use of ISS grouping as an early predictor of total hospital cost. *J Trauma* 28:939–946.

Schwartz RJ, Jacobs LM, and Yaezel D (1989) Impact of pre-trauma center care on length of stay and hospital charges. *J Trauma* 29:1611–1615.

Shackford SR, MacKersie RC, Davis JW, Wolf PL, and Hoyt DB (1989) Epidemiology and pathology of traumatic deaths occurring at a Level I trauma center in a regionalized system: the importance of secondary brain injury. *J Trauma* 29:1392–1397.

Simpson RK, Venger BH, and Narayan RK (1989) Treatment of acute penetrating injuries of the spine: a retrospective analysis. *J Trauma* 29:42–46.

60 Minutes (1997) HMO: managed or mangled. New York: CBS News, January 5.

Smith K, Marino RJ, and Graziani V (1996) Spinal cord injury. In Basmajian JV, and Banerjee SN (eds), *Clinical Decision Making in Rehabilitation*. New York: Churchill-Livingstone.

Smith RF, Frateschi L, Sloan EP, Campbell L, Krieg R, Edwards LC, and Barrett JA (1990) The impact of volume on outcome in seriously injured trauma patients: two years' experience of the Chicago trauma system. *J Trauma* 30:1066–1076.

Stein F (1989) *Anatomy of Clinical Research*. Thorofare, NJ: Slack, Inc.

Stineman MG and Williams SV (1990) Predicting inpatient rehabilitation length of stay. *Arch Phys Med Rehabil* 71:881– 887.

Trunkey DD (1983) Trauma. *Sci Am* 249(2):28–35.

Vlahov D (1990) Epidemiology of falls among patients in a rehabilitation hospital. *Arch Phys Med Rehabil* 71:8–12.

Waller JA, Payne SR, and McClallen JM (1989) Trauma centers and DRGs—inherent conflict? *J Trauma* 29:617–622.

Wesson DE, Williams JI, Spence LJ, Filler RM, Armstrong PF, and Pearl RH (1989) Functional outcome in pediatric trauma. *J Trauma* 29:589–592.

West JG, and Cales RH (1983) Methods of evaluation of trauma care. In West JG, Gazzaniga AB, and Cales RH (eds), *Trauma Care Systems*. New York: Praeger.

West JG, Gazzaniga AB, and Cales RH (1983) Do trauma systems save lives? In West JG, Gazzaniga AB, and Cales RH (eds), *Trauma Care Systems*. New York: Praeger.

Wilson DS, McElligott J, and Fielding LP (1992) Identification of preventable trauma deaths: confounded inquiries? *J Trauma* 32:45–51.

Wilson RF, Wiencek RG, and Balog M (1989) Predicting and preventing infection after abdominal vascular injuries. *J Trauma* 29:1371–1375.

Wood RLL, and Eames P (eds) (1989) *Models of Brain Injury Rehabilitation*. Baltimore: Johns Hopkins University Press.

Wrigley JM, Yoels WC, Webb CR, and Fine PR (1994) Social and physical factors in referral of people with traumatic brain injuries to rehabilitation. *Arch Phys Med Rehabil* 75:140–155.

Young JC, Macioce DP, and Young WW (1990) Identifying injuries and trauma severity in large databases. *J Trauma* 30:1220–1230.

Zafonte RD, Hammond FM, Mann NR, Wood DL, Black KL, and Millis SR (1996) Relationship between Glasgow Coma Scale and functional outcome. *Arch Phys Med Rehabil* 75:364–369.

9

INJURY EPIDEMIOLOGY AND ECONOMICS

In addition to the humane reasons for injury control, there are huge cost savings to be realized. The costs of medical care, rehabilitation, funerals, and lost productivity were $158 billion in the United States during 1985 according to a detailed accounting for that year, discounted to present value by 6 percent (Rice & MacKenzie, 1989). This so-called human capital cost does not include the intangible toll in pain, grief, social disruption, and disorganization. It also does not include substitution of economic productivity with caregiving to the injured by family members.

One of the most controversial uses of epidemiologic data is the assignment of economic costs to distributions of injury and disease, and the balancing of such costs against the costs of reducing risk. The controversy arises both from repugnance on the part of some people at the notion that all aspects of injury and death can be monetized and from widespread disagreement over the methods when monetization is attempted.

Epidemiologists who describe sets of injuries or assess risks usually do not concern themselves with economic issues directly (other than the cost of the study and efficient study designs), but those who study the effects of programs, laws, regulations, medical care, or rehabilitation often encounter economic arguments and research. The purpose of this chapter is to alert injury epidemiologists and users of the data to some of the terminology and issues in economic analysis of injury data related to decisions regarding injury control.

THE ECONOMIC CONTEXT

Neoclassic economists adhere to the philosophy that people choose the risks that they take and that almost any organized attempt to reduce the risk will result in failure. As mentioned previously, according to this theory, if people have an acceptable level of risk that they will tolerate, and their behavior offsets attempts to reduce risk, any attempt to reduce risk is a waste of money. As noted in Chapters 6 and 7, the studies that have observed individual behavior in situations where risk was reduced do not support the assumption that people offset risk reduction by more risky behavior, and many attempts at injury control have had a beneficial effect.

Most economists argue that the costs of any program, including attempts at injury reduction, should not exceed the benefits. Expenditures for injury control that exceed the cost of injuries reduced are inefficient, they argue, because there is a net reduction in the goods and services available to society (e.g., Anderson & Settle, 1977). To balance costs against benefits, it is necessary to place a monetary value not only on the direct costs (medical care, rehabilitation, funerals) and indirect costs (lost productivity), but also on pain and suffering.

The following data are necessary to estimate costs and benefits:

$a(i)$ = number of injuries of given severity i to which an intervention applies

$b(i)$ = cost of injuries by severity i (including monetized pain and suffering)

$c(i)$ = proportion of each severity level i or its consequences reduced by the intervention

d = reduced costs = sum of $a(i) \times b(i) \times c(i)$ where i = each severity level

e = cost of applying or incrementing the intervention (including intangibles such as inconvenience)

$f = d - e$ (that is, benefit less cost)

Some economists use d/e, the benefit to cost ratio, but benefit less cost is more useful for comparing interventions because the amount of savings is evident.

Many health professionals and others have adopted this economic viewpoint without carefully examining its philosophical underpinnings. An extensive bibliography of uses of cost–benefit analysis in health and medical decisions is accessible by computer modem through the WONDER system at the Centers for Disease Control and Prevention (Friede et al., 1993).

The welfare of society is the sum of the gross domestic product, according to the economic viewpoint. All dollars are equal, no matter what the consequences of their use. Money spent for addictive substances adverse to health such as cigarettes and alcohol is viewed as positively as money spent for injury reduction. It does not seem to matter to many economists that some of the gross demestic product is contributing to the destruction of life-sustaining elements of the planet, nor do they consider that many of the most valued aspects of life are not reflected in the gross domestic product (Self, 1977). Perhaps the best that can be said for neoclassic economics is that it is short-sighted.

In the extreme neoclassic economic view, every good, service, intellectual or emotional satisfaction, and health risk is purchased in a market with money or some behavior the value of which can be reduced to money. The "invisible hand" of the market governs supply and demand to produce the optimal social welfare, and government is necessary only to enforce contracts and protect the public from domestic criminals and extranational threats.

Others recognize that society is much more complex. Organized interests at least partly control some markets and others are generated by one-sided advertising. For example, in the 1930s and 1940s General Motors conspired with a tire company and an oil company to purchase and dismantle 46 mass transit companies that operated electric street cars in 16 states. Although the companies were convicted of antitrust violations, that did not restore the mass transit systems (Adams & Brock, 1987).

In product advertising, benefits are often overstated and risks are often not mentioned at all. Virtually no product advertising or user instruction gives a precise indication of risks of using a product—those that provide warnings state them in vague terms.

To do cost–benefit analysis, the monetary value of reduced risk that includes "pain and suffering" is usually assessed by research on "revealed preference," that is, implied value from behavior relative to risks, or by directly asking people what they would be willing to pay to reduce risks. To say the least, the research is problematic.

WILLINGNESS TO PAY

In the introduction of a study of product labels, the following statements were found: "Consumers take precautions whose benefits exceed their costs, and they forgo the other precautions. . . . To estimate the benefits of precautions the consumer must assess both the effect of taking the precaution on the probability of each possible injury that it protects against and the value of the resulting reduction in the risk of injury." Two pages later, introducing the labels for two products to be studied as to consumer intent to take precautions, the report says, "Because most readers may not be familiar with the four injuries and how they arise, we briefly describe them here" (Viscusi & Magat, 1987, pp. 43, 45).

How can one assume that the average consumer does a cost–benefit analysis on every product purchased based on the probability of injury if one assumes that readers of a book on risk, who are likely to have a better than average knowledge of risks, do not know the risks of injury from commonly used household products?

After attempting to assess the effects on intended precautions of particular labels that did not include quantitative estimates of risk, the researchers attempted to assess how much consumers would be willing to pay, per injury, to reduce them. A quantitative estimate of risk was included in information given to respondents during the willingness-to-pay phase of the study. The amounts that consumers were willing to have added to the overall costs of the products—an implied value of "$300,000 for gassings from bleach, $420,000 for child poisonings from bleach, $120,000 for hand burns from drain opener, and $360,000 for child poisonings"—were said to "appear to be excessive." The authors found it "implausible" that a relatively minor handburn would be valued at $120,000, "four times the respondents' average household income" (Viscusi & Magat, 1987, p. 93).

The point missed, of course, is that the individual does not have to spend four times the family income to reduce the risk. The cost of the product modifications is spread among all consumers and, in the aggregate, people may be willing to pay far more per product to reduce risk than economists' judgment of the worth of the risk. For the individual, the expenditure may be a few cents extra per product for household cleaners that will last weeks or months, a few dollars extra for a child's crib that may last for generations, or a few hundred dollars extra for a motor vehicle that will last for several years.

Also, contrary to popular belief, reduction of risk does not necessarily increase the cost of the product. In some cases the risk can even be reduced by reducing the cost of the product. It takes more material and thus costs more to make the front end of a vehicle sharp rather than smooth; protruding radio knobs, air conditioning controls, and gear-shift controls that penetrate the tissues of occupants in crashes cost more than smooth buttons (Robertson, 1990). Designers of a research safety vehicle in the mid-1970s estimated that, despite numerous features to enhance crash avoidance and crashworthiness, the retail cost of the vehicle if mass produced would have been no more than concurrently priced compact cars (DiNapoli et al., 1977).

Although it is claimed that the initial motor vehicle safety standards added several hundred dollars to the cost of new cars, the increases in producer prices of cars during the period of adoption of the standards was not as large as that for other durable goods. From 1964 to 1973, the producer price index for all durable goods rose 35 percent while the increase for cars was about half that, 17 percent (Robertson, 1983).

If purchasers have no quantitative information on risks of a product, and some manufacturers do not know the risks or do not attempt to reduce even those risks that would reduce or have no effect on the cost of the product, how can an economist argue that the consumers' use of the product is a "revealed preference" of the balance of costs and benefits? The issue is confounded further by the fact that the persons injured are often not the original purchasers of the product. Certainly the pedestrian who is struck by the sharp front of a vehicle had no say in its purchase. Based on the age of occupants injured, ownership of vehicles, and relationship of the injured person to the owner, about 75–80 percent of persons injured by motor vehicles were not party to the purchase (Baker, 1979).

Nevertheless, numerous economic studies attempt to assess valuation of life and limb by calculation of premiums in wages in risky occupations, demand for products that reduce risk relative to price, behavior implied to trade off risks and benefits, and surveys about people's willingness to pay for reduced risk. One summary of 29 such studies, about half of which were based on wage premiums relative to job risks, suggested a "willingness to pay" value of $2 million per life, about the average among the studies selected, although the results of individual studies ranged from $1 million to $3 million (Miller, 1989).

Another troubling aspect of cost–benefit analysis is the international implications. If the value of life and limb is based on the prevailing wages in a given country, there will be huge differences in the value placed on lives in different countries (Morrow & Bryant, 1995).

RISK–BENEFIT ANALYSIS

A variation of cost–benefit is so-called risk–benefit analysis in which historical death rates are used to argue that risks not exceeding them are acceptable. This point is most often made by physicists and engineers who believe public opposition to certain technologies such as nuclear power generation or types of disposal of military nuclear waste is irrational. One of the early advocates of this view said, "Automobile and airplane safety have been continuously weighed by society against economic costs and operating performance" (Starr, 1969). This anthropomorphic view of society makes no sense in the light of the history of either technology and the social processes that led to regulation or lack of regulation (Priest, 1988).

The translation of what has been tacitly accepted into what is acceptable is a prescription for disaster. Risk after risk could be added, each at or below the "acceptable" level, until a substantial number of the population is dead or disabled. As noted in Chapter 2, surveys of the public indicate that risks to the public that the government has accepted are not acceptable to the public.

Risk–benefit analysts can't have it both ways. On the one hand they say that risks with a history indicate what is acceptable, but on the other hand they are fond of lists of dollars spent "per life saved," calculated for a variety of employed or proposed countermeasures to risks, to illustrate governmental irrationality in risk management. One such array showed variation from $100 per life saved for expanded immunization in Indonesia to $200,000,000 per life saved for the control of radiation in "defense high level waste." Most of the injury-related countermeasures were in a range of $20,000 to $400,000 per life saved, but coal mine safety and other mine safety was said to cost $22,000,000 and $34,000,000 per life saved (Cohen, 1980). The accuracy of all of those estimates is unknown, but some were grossly misstated. For example, high school driver education was said to save lives, but it actually increases deaths (Chapter 5).

The implication of a list of costs per life saved is that efficient allocation of resources should be such that the costs would be similar if rational decisions were made. Sometimes appeals are made to ethical issues such as equity, that is, if the costs per life saved are different, some people benefit more than others from resource allocations. Others argue that the differences represent values placed on lives that have different values. For example, much more is allocated to protect the president of the United States than ordinary citizens (Shrader-Frechette, 1985).

Even if the estimates were accurate, the ages of the persons whose lives are preserved are very different among the technologies and programs. Cost per years of life preserved would result in a very different array for many hazards. The typical discounting to present value in cost analyses results in less value being placed on the lives of children. The previously noted list of costs per lives saved (Cohen, 1980) also calculated costs per 20 years of life preserved, but some of the technologies and programs affect mainly children and youth with more than 20 years expected life while others "save" lives of people who have a life expectancy less than 20 years.

In the 1990s, a widely publicized compendium of "500 life-saving interventions" more appropriately indicated cost *per year of life saved* (Tengs et al., 1995). The bibliography accompanying the list may be somewhat useful to persons in a position to recommend or initiate programs, but the list is of dubious quality and should not be the basis for decisions. Some of the research on which estimates are based is of doubtful validity. Many of the estimates are based on regulatory analyses by antiregulation economists or by government agencies. In at least one such agency, the National Highway Traffic Safety Administration, two regulatory analyses have been prepared on a given issue, one favorable and one unfavorable to the adoption of a given regulation. When the administrator decides which way the decision is to be made, the analysis supporting the decision is the one published. (See Chapter 10 for a critique of one such analysis—potential lives saved by a stability standard for motor vehicles.)

In addition, the noted list of 500 is not exhaustive. For example, only a small proportion of effective highway modifications are included and one of the most cost-effective—lighting roads at night at high-risk sites (Chapter 3)—is not mentioned. The cost-effectiveness of many of the technologies and programs mentioned on the list can be increased enormously by targeting them at high-risk populations or environments based on surveillance (Chapter 3). Depending on the extent that certain injuries are more or less likely to cluster, the cost-effectiveness would vary enormously from that listed.

For example, based on the cluster of motor vehicle crashes identified by surveillance in Browning, Montana (Chapter 3), the lighting and curb modifications that were installed in a two mile stretch of road cost about $6000 and the electricity to light the streets at night costs about $500 per year. The modifications undoubtedly paid for themselves in benefits to society in a few months.

Also, cost per year of life saved does not take into account the nonfatal injuries that would be prevented or severity reduced, which varies per life saved among technologies and programs. Somehow weighting the costs as well as pain, suffering, and other consequences of nonfatal health impairment and including them with the estimates of fatality reductions is very problematic. One book on risk–benefit analysis states that the weighting is "somewhat arbitrary" (Crouch & Wilson, 1982). The authors of that book advocated a thorough risk analysis before decisions are made, but they included Cohen's (1980) list of costs per life saved without the column for cost per 20 years of life.

Usually the attempt to account for nonfatal injuries is made by monetizing both fatal and nonfatal outcomes, which turns risk–benefit back into cost–benefit analysis. Some estimates of the cost of nonfatal injuries are based solely on the cost of medical care and lost work time. This discriminates against children and the elderly and does not include pain and suffering. It is also difficult to evaluate lost work time because some work is uncompensated. Moreover, 50 restricted-activity days for a given individual is likely to have a more severe economic impact than that of 5 restricted work days each for 10 people (Priest, 1988).

Another approach is to somehow adjust for quality years of life, which raises all sorts of issues (Baldwin et al., 1990). For example, do commodities consumed represent quality of life? If so, how does one deal with the quality of the commodities, which is not necessarily reflected in their price? Some analysts have pointed out that characteristics of people rather than what they consume are more indicative of quality of life (Culyer, 1990), but those qualities are not indicated in any pricing system.

Estimates of the quality of life can be obtained by questioning people, but all of the methodological issues of reliability and validity of self-reports are involved (Petitti, 1994). Risks with equal outcomes result in different responses by respondents if presented as gains rather than as losses (Kahneman & Tversky, 1979) or in other contexts (Loomes & McKenzie, 1990). People who have not experienced given disabilities themselves cannot give informed answers about the quality of life of persons with such disabilities and their families.

UNCERTAINTY IN COSTS OF INTERVENTIONS

Costs of product modifications and other injury control programs can be estimated more easily than benefits in some cases, but such estimates are often not done. Government budgets for highway modifications, regulatory agencies, and the like, are known. The total cost of regulations, however, is difficult to estimate—particularly when the regulations are performance regulations. For example, the government standard for energy absorption by steering assemblies during frontal car crashes did not necessarily increase costs. It could have reduced costs if it resulted in attention to designs that used cheaper materials.

Many programs that have been suggested or implemented to some degree have not included cost studies. Researchers who evaluate the effects of interventions seldom include cost estimates of the interventions. Also, the extant costs of products or their modifications, where known, should not always be accepted as though the least costly technology is used. For example, in Sri Lanka, burnt-out light bulbs are filled with kerosene and used as lamps, which increases fire risk compared to more sturdy, and costly, glass lamps (Berger & Mohan, 1996). In such situations, all the alternatives for lighting, including invention of a product as cheap as or cheaper than recycled bulbs, should be considered before assuming that the situation is determined by the economics.

It is often difficult to find data on the extent of implementation of many interventions. For example, a controlled experiment in which parents in an experimental group were counseled regarding infants' falls from tables, beds, and other heights, suggests that these falls can be reduced about 41 percent by physicians' warnings and counseling (Kravitz, 1973). To estimate the benefit minus costs that could be realized from expanding such counseling, however, we need data on the extent of counseling by physicians now. Apparently, no survey of physicians to determine the extent of such counseling and its cost has been done, nor is the willingness to counsel and the compensation expected for doing so known.

Also, certain costs that are not translatable into dollars are not known. Consider, for example, a proposal to reduce the high rate of involvement of teenaged drivers in severe crashes by raising the minimum licensing age to 18. What changes would occur in the daily routine of families with 16–17-year-old children who do not obtain licenses to drive as a result, and how does one assign dollar values to the changes?

Since no state has an 18-year-old licensing age, the exact effect of such a policy cannot be estimated. Research comparing fatal crash involvement of 16-year-old drivers in New Jersey, with a 17-year-old licensing age (except for an agricultural license at 16), and Connecticut, with a 16-year-old licensing age, indicates that about a 65–85 percent reduction in fatalities where 16-year-old drivers are involved would ensue from a 17-year-old minimum licensing age (Williams et al., 1983). The study found that the fatal crash rates of drivers 17–29 years old were comparable between the states, indicating no evidence that the reduction among 16 year olds was offset by increased driving by 17–29 year olds to transport 16 year olds not allowed to drive. Also, there were no offsetting rates of 16 year olds killed as pedestrians or bicyclists.

In 1995, there were 1833 people killed in the United States in or by motor vehicles where a driver was 16 years old. Since the fatal crash rate of persons in the age range of parents of 16 year olds is about 9 percent of that of 16 year olds, parent substitution of 16-year-old driving would prevent about 1251 deaths $[1833 \times (1 - 0.09) \times 0.75]$. To estimate nonfatal injuries by severity, the distribution of maximum abbreviated injury score was examined in the National Accident Sampling System–Crashworthiness Data System for 1993. Using the ratio of nonfatal to fatal injury distribution, the reduction in injuries expected from a 75 percent decrease in crashes by drivers less than 17 years old would be approximately AIS 1, 20,806; AIS 2, 4823; AIS 3, 2453; AIS 4, 658; AIS 5, 280; fatal, 1251. Since it is unlikely that every trip of a 16-year-old driver would be substituted by a parent or other adult, this is a minimum estimate.

The U.S. Department of Transportation has adopted the willingness-to-pay method of estimating injury costs (Table 9.1). Multiplying the numbers of injuries reduced times their estimated costs in Table 9.1, a reduction of about $4.8

TABLE 9.1. Costs by Abbreviated
Injury Scale (1994 U.S. dollars)

SEVERITY	COST PER INJURY
AIS 1	$ 5,000
AIS 2	40,000
AIS 3	150,000
AIS 4	490,000
AIS 5	1,980,000
AIS 6	2,600,000

Source: Federal Highway Administration, 1994.

billion in injury costs would have occurred from a 17-year-old minimum licensing age. The question remaining is whether the inconvenience of having 16 year olds unlicensed is worth amounts of money in that range. A survey of teenagers in Michigan, New Jersey, and New York, with very different rates of licensure, found very little effect of licensure on various activities. The increase in percentage of teenagers with jobs, comparing employment at age 15 and 16, was highest in New Jersey, where licensure at 16 was prohibited except in agriculture (Preusser et al., 1985).

The costs of law enforcement would probably not have to be incremented much, if any, to achieve the reduction. Most of the law's enforcement would be achieved by parents, who are unlikely to allow unlicensed drivers to use family vehicles.

The savings from increased age of licensure were first calculated, along with that for several other countermeasures, and submitted to the U.S. Congress in 1989 (Robertson, 1989). There has been no rush to enact legislation to realize the cost savings. There is serious doubt that many legislatures or other branches of government are interested in cost savings despite lip service to the contrary.

OVERLAP IN EFFECTS OF INTERVENTIONS

Often the same injuries would be prevented by more than one intervention. To the extent that there is such overlap in the effects of two or more approaches, the cost-effectiveness of each will not reflect the cost effectiveness of applying both at the same time. For example, as noted in Chapter 5, driving by 16–17 year olds is actually increased by high school driver education. Based on the numbers of students enrolled in 1985, a report to Congress noted that up to $2.2 billion in 1985 dollars would have been saved in that year if there were no driver education in high schools, including the $163 million cost of the program (Robertson, 1989). Since surveys of schools to determine the numbers of students enrolled have been discontinued, it is not possible to update those estimates.

Nevertheless, if the minimum licensing age were increased to 18, virtually all of the adverse effect of driver education would be eliminated. Raising the minimum licensing age to 18 and eliminating high school driver education simultaneously would not save the sum of the injury and program costs of driver education and the cost of injuries of drivers less than 18 because each of these policies would reduce the same injuries and deaths as the other. Only the cost of the driver education program could be added to the injury costs saved by raising the minimum licensing age to prevent double-counting of cost savings because of the overlap in injuries reduced.

This is a very obvious example of overlap in effects of countermeasures, but there are instances in which the effects of particular interventions and the overlaps of effects are less well known, even by those in a position to find out. In 1996, the administrator of the National Highway Traffic Safety Administration circulated a study of seat belt effectiveness based on linked police reports and hospital records from seven states. He claimed that the study showed seat belts would have prevented three of every five deaths of "unbuckled motorists," that is, seat belts are supposedly 60 percent effective, when used, in reducing occupant fatalities (Martinez, 1996).

The NHTSA also frequently issues reports on the involvement of alcohol in motor vehicle fatalities. In 1994, an estimated 32 percent of such fatalities involved a driver or other road user with a blood alcohol concentration of 0.10 percent by weight or more (National Highway Traffic Safety Administration, 1995). This information is often assumed to mean that reductions in alcohol use would result in a proportionate reduction in fatalities. Indeed, NHTSA has virtually ceased to issue standards for vehicle crashworthiness, rollover resistance, crash avoidance, and other factors, claiming that the majority of motor vehicle fatalities are related to nonuse of seat belts and use of alcohol (National Highway Traffic Safety Administration, 1994).

Since belt use is known to be lower among vehicle occupants with high blood alcohol concentrations (e.g., Foss et al., 1994), the effect of increasing belt use and reducing alcohol use cannot be additive because of the overlap. Indeed, correlation of alcohol use to Injury Severity Scores and hospital length of stay disappear when belt use is controlled (Anderson et al., 1990), indicative of confounding.

Also, if alcohol use is lower in drivers of later model cars—those that are more crashworthy (Chapter 7)—and belt use is higher in such cars, some of the fatalities attributed to alcohol and nonuse of belts may result from lack of crashworthiness of older vehicles. Alcohol involvement and belt use are known to be correlated to vehicle age. Also, alcohol use and aggressive or impulsive behavior may be attributable to some extent to a common precursor, which suggests the possibility that at least some of the aggressive or impulsive behavior would occur in the absence of alcohol (Chapter 4).

To illustrate the overlap of alcohol and belt use and the confounding of effects of other factors on assessment of the effects of belt use and alcohol, the regression model used to estimate the effects of vehicle modifications, belt use, alcohol, and other factors (Chapter 7), was examined in stages. First, regression coefficients of the effects of belt use and alcohol, separately and without control for other factors, were examined. They were then examined in combination without the other factors and in combination with the other factors. If the effects of belt and alcohol use are not confounded, the single estimates should not differ significantly from the effects in combination with other factors.

The regression coefficients and 95 percent confidence intervals are presented in Table 9.2. The estimates of belt use effects and alcohol effects, each alone, are greatly reduced when they are considered simultaneously. They are again reduced to much lower levels when the effects of safety standards, unrequired improvements in crashworthiness (NCAP), vehicle age, and vehicle size are all included. Note that the variance explained (R^2) is modest for seat belts and alcohol alone or in combination, but it is excellent for the full model.

Belt use was approximately 53 percent in 1991 (Datta & Guzek, 1990). If the remaining 47 percent of car occupants had been restrained, the occupant fatality rate of 1.6 per 100 million miles would have been reduced by about 21 percent. This is obtained by multiplying the coefficient in Table 9.2 by the percentage of unused belts ($0.007 \times 47 = 0.329$) and dividing the result by the death rate ($0.329/1.6 = 0.21$. The implied effectiveness of belts when used is 21/47, or 45 percent.

Alcohol at 0.1 percent by weight or more was found in about 23.4 percent of passenger car drivers in 1991 (Klein & Burgess, 1995). Multiplying the coefficient for alcohol (at or greater than 0.1 percent by weight) by the percentage of involvement ($-0.007 \times 23.4 = 0.164$) indicates that reducing such alco-

TABLE 9.2. Regression Estimates of the Effects on Car Occupant Death Rate per 100 Million Miles of Alcohol and Seat Belt Use Without and With Controls for Other Factors

	BELTS ONLY	ALCOHOL ONLY	BELTS AND ALCOHOL	ALL FACTORS COMBINED
Belt use, %	−0.034 −0.028, −0.039		−0.019 −0.026, −0.013	−0.007 −0.001, −0.013
Alcohol >0.1, %		0.070 0.059, 0.080	0.047 0.035, 0.060	0.007 0.001, 0.013
Standards				−0.260 −0.237, −0.283
NCAP publicity				−0.077 −0.044, −0.110
Calendar year				−0.017 −0.052, 0.019
Industrial production				0.029 0.015, 0.043
Expected from vehicle age				0.444 0.656, 0.232
Expected from wheelbase				1.066 0.612, 1.520
Intercept	3.47	−0.32	1.11	−0.793
R^2	0.35	0.39	0.46	0.92

95 percent confidence intervals are indicated beneath each coefficient.

hol involvement to zero would reduce the car occupant death rate by 0.164, which is 10 percent of the overall rate of 1.6.

Uncontrolled estimates of belt effectiveness and alcohol effects on fatal crashes are confounded by their covariation and the lower belt use and higher alcohol involvement in less crashworthy cars. The estimate of death reduction from seat belts, when used, in this study (45 percent) is similar to the 41 percent effectiveness found in research that compares who died relative to who was belted within vehicles with more than one occupant in similar seating positions—a methodology that obviously controls for vehicle crashworthiness as well (Chapter 7).

If alcohol were eliminated and belt use were 100 percent, almost two-thirds of car occupant fatalities would nevertheless occur. As a practical matter, both goals, however admirable, will not be attained. The hyperbolic claims by the government official responsible for objective consideration of the full range of options available for death and injury reduction are not justified by the empirical evidence.

Many of the fatalities that would be prevented by increased belt use or reduction of alcohol use are the same fatalities. Any cost–benefit analysis or estimate of cost per year of life preserved, such as comparing belt use laws and alcohol crackdowns as though they were additive, would be distorted.

COST-EFFECTIVENESS AND DECISION MAKING

There are many technologies, policies, and programs to reduce injury that produce a net benefit, even by the narrow criteria of human capital costs (Robertson, 1989). The failure to adopt them is not an issue of costs but of who pays versus who benefits and who decides whether or not the intervention is used. Analysis of ratios of cost to effectiveness, cost to benefits or cost to savings (where some costs and benefits are intangible) ignores feasibility of implementation because of ideological factors and concentrated interests that may oppose certain interventions.

In the United States, the gun lobby claims that unlimited "right to bear arms" is guaranteed by the Constitution, and few citizens are informed of the falsity of the argument (Christoffel & Teret, 1993). Since those injured by guns cannot be denied treatment, the false ideology is costly to everyone. In one major trauma center, for example, 79 percent of the costs for treatment of gunshot wounds was paid from taxes and an additional 19 percent was paid by insurers. Taxpayers and the insured paid for 98 percent of the treatment (Wintemute & Wright, 1992).

Policies such as government subsidization of bicycle helmet purchases, while accepted in Australia (Wood & Milne, 1988), may be difficult to implement in the United States. Although the majority of motorcyclists are in favor of helmet use laws, a vocal minority have been successful in gaining repeal in many states (Baker, 1980)—despite the data indicating huge economic losses (Hartunian et al., 1983; Robertson, 1989) and the evidence that the costs are paid with public monies. A detailed analysis of the costs of treatment and rehabilitative care of motorcyclists in a major trauma center found that 63 percent were reimbursed by tax-supported programs, mainly Medicaid (Rivara et al., 1988).

The failure of the Occupational Safety and Health Administration to extend relevant regulations to reduce farm injuries is partly due to the myth that farm owners bear the risk and can take precautions they deem appropriate (Kelsey, 1994). This ignores the effects of farm injury and its costs on farmers who qualify for Medicare or Medicaid, the latter when the farm goes belly up because the farmer can no longer work. Also, there are many injured farm workers who are not owners, are poorly paid, and cannot afford health insurance.

While, in the preceding instances, seemingly overwhelming ideological opposition or lobbying power drove the decisions, such power is not always as solid as it seems. No one familiar with Tennessee politics would have expected that state to be the first to enact a child-restraint use law, but it did, and other states followed. The gun lobby spent $6 million in an attempt to defeat gun control legislation in Maryland, but it was overwhelmingly defeated in a referendum in the 1988 election. The Brady Bill, providing for background checks on gun purchasers, survived the 1994–96 U.S. Congress, many of whose members were heavily beholden to the gun lobby.

Although there is some uncertainty in each of the estimates of potential for injury reduction discussed in this book because of variation in sampling error and the lack of good experimental design in some cases, there is no doubt that a substantial proportion of severe injuries could be reduced by a greater application of current knowledge. The potential cost savings, net of the cost of injury control programs, is in the billions of dollars for many interventions for which data are available. Usually the estimates of cost savings are far more sensitive to the difference in the estimates using the human capital and willingness-to-pay methods than they are to variation in estimates of effectiveness of a given intervention.

Even if all the benefits of a given risk-reduction technology or program could be estimated accurately, it is obvious that a great deal of resource allocation will not be made based on such an analysis. If the money in the federal budget allocated to programs for dealing with "defense high level waste" were reduced, it would not be allocated to private expenditures for safety of consumer products, much less immunization programs in Indonesia.

In those instances where a set of resources is available to a given decision maker or decision-making body, it certainly makes sense to attempt to allocate those resources to minimize human damage. One interesting issue for research is the extent to which cost–benefit or cost–effectiveness analysis actually affects decisions. In one study of future decision makers (graduate students in law and business), six experimental groups were given sets of information regarding policies to reduce motor vehicle injury, and their expressed preferences were compared to a control group given no information. The information given to the experimental groups was varied by attributable benefit, attributable risk, and relative risk. Generally, groups given data were much more likely than control groups to favor a regulatory policy (60 percent vs. 22 percent). Those given information on attributable risks and benefits in terms of injury reductions were somewhat more likely to favor regulation than those given relative risk information (64 percent vs. 52 percent). No data on costs were included, but responses varied significantly depending on attitudes regarding personal freedom and governmental regulation (Runyan and Earp, 1985).

Suppose that a set of local governments was randomly divided into experimental and control groups and each government in the experimental group was presented data on the benefits less costs of adopting a set of injury control measures while each one in the control group was presented the same injury control options without the cost–benefit analysis. Would the experimental communities be more or less likely to take action? If both groups took action, would the experimental group's actions be more efficient, that is, would the exerimental governments achieve more reduction of injury costs per dollar spent? Similar studies of injury control for workers in private corporations would be of interest, but the likelihood of gaining access to detailed data in enough companies would be problematic.

SUMMARY

The huge cost of injuries reveals the enormous potential for cost savings by injury control. Neoclassic economic theories of behavior are a barrier to application of approaches known to be effective. While many injury control programs pass the cost–benefit challenge, the methodological perils of placing economic value on life and limb can result in misleading conclusions. Costs of regulations, product modifications, and other programs, are often overstated. Some programs reduce the same injuries that other programs reduce, so that specification of the overlap is important to avoid duplication of effort.

REFERENCES

Adams W, and Brock JW (1987) Bigness and social efficiency: a case study of the U.S. auto industry. In Samuels WJ, and Miller AS (eds), *Corporations and Society: Power and Responsibility.* New York: Greenwood Press.

Agran PF, Dunkle DE, and Winn DG (1987) Effects of legislation on motor vehicle injuries to children. *Am J Dis Child* 141:959–964.

Anderson JA, McLellan BA, Pagliarello G, and Nelson WR (1990) The relative influence of alcohol and seatbelt usage on severity of injury from motor vehicle crashes. *J Trauma* 30:415–421.

Anderson LG, and Settle RF (1977) *Benefit-Cost Analysis: A Practical Guide.* Lexington, MA: D.C. Heath.

Baker SP (1979). Who bought the cars in which people were injured? An exploratory study. *Am J Public Health* 69:76.

Baker SP (1980) On lobbies, liberty, and the public good. *Am J Public Health* 70:573–574.

Baker SP, O'Neill B, and Karpf RS (1984) *The Injury Fact Book.* Lexington, MA: D.C. Heath.

Baldwin S, Godfrey C, and Propper C (eds) (1990) *Quality of Life: Perspectives and Policies.* London: Routledge.

Berger LR, and Mohan D (1996) *Injury Control: A Global View.* Delhi: Oxford University Press.

Christoffel T, and Teret S (1993) *Protecting the Public: Legal Issues in Injury Prevention.* New York: Oxford University Press.

Cohen BL (1980) Society's evaluation of life saving in radiation protection and other contexts. *Health Phys* 38:33.

Crouch EAC, and Wilson R (1982) *Risk/Benefit Analysis.* Cambridge, MA: Ballinger.

Culyer AJ (1990) Commodities, characteristics of commodities, characteristics of people, utilities, and the quality of life. In Baldwin S, Godfrey C, and Popper C (eds), *Quality of Life: Perspectives and Policies.* London: Routledge.

Datta TK, and Guzek P (1990) *Restraint System Use in 19 U.S. Cities: 1989 Annual Report.* Washington, DC: National Highway Traffic Safety Administration.

DiNapoli N, Fitzpatrick M, Strother C, Struble D, and Tanner R (1977) *Research Safety Vehicle Phase II, Volume II, Comprehensive Technical Results.* Springfield, VA: National Technical Information Service.

Federal Highway Administration (1994) Technical Advisory: Motor Vehicle Accident Costs. Washington, DC: U.S. Department of Transportation.

Foss RD, Beirness DJ, and Sprattler K (1994) Seat belt use among drinking drivers in Minnesota. *Am J Public Health* 84:1732–1737.

Friede A, Taylor WR, and Nadelman L (1993) On-line access to a cost-benefit/cost-effectiveness analysis bibliography via CDC WONDER. *Med Care* 31:JS12–JS17 (supplement).

Hartunian NS, Smart CN, Willeman TR, and Zador PL (1983) The economics of safety regulation: lives and dollars lost due to repeal of motorcycle helmet laws. *J Health Polit Policy Law* 8:76–98.

Kahneman D, and Tversky A (1979) Prospect theory: an analysis of decision under risk. *Econometrica* 47:263–291.

Kelsey TW (1994) The agrarian myth and policy responses to farm safety. *Am J Public Health* 84:1171–1177.

Klein TM, and Burgess M (1995) *Alcohol Involvement in Fatal Traffic Crashes, 1993.* Washington, DC: National Highway Traffic Safety Administration.

Kravitz H (1973) Prevention of falls in infancy by counseling mothers. *Illinois Med J* 144:570–573.

Loomes G, and McKenzie L (1990) The scope and limitations of QALY measures. In

Baldwin S, Godfrey C, and Popper C (eds), *Quality of Life: Perspectives and Policies.* London: Routledge.

Martinez R (1996) Letter to Highway Safety Data Users. Washington, DC: National Highway Traffic Safety Administration, April 12.

Miller TR (1989) Willingness to pay. In Rice DP, and MacKenzie EJ (eds), *Cost of Injury in the United States: A Report to Congress, 1989.* San Francisco: University of California Institute for Health and Aging, and Baltimore: Johns Hopkins University Injury Prevention Center.

Morrow RH, and Bryant JH (1995) Health policy approaches to measuring and valuing human life: conceptual and ethical issues. *Am J Public Health* 85:1356–1360.

National Highway Traffic Safety Administration (1983) *The Economic Cost to Society of Motor Vehicle Accidents.* Washington, DC: U.S. Department of Transportation.

National Highway Traffic Safety Administration (1994) Consumer Information Regulations; Federal Motor Vehicle Safety Standards; Rollover Prevention. *Fed Reg* 59:33254–33272.

National Highway Traffic Safety Administration (1995) *Traffic Safety Facts 1994.* Washington, DC: U.S. Department of Transportation.

Petitti DB (1994) *Meta-Analysis, Decision Analysis, and Cost-Effectiveness Analysis.* New York: Oxford University Press.

Preusser DF, Williams AF, and Lund AK (1985) Driver licensing age and lifestyles of 16 year olds. *Am J Public Health* 75:358.

Priest WC (1988) *Risks, Consensus, and Social Legislation: Forces That Led to Laws on Health, Safety and the Environment.* Boulder, CO: Westview Press.

Rice DP, and MacKenzie, EJ (eds) (1989) *Cost of Injury in the United States: A Report to Congress, 1989.* San Francisco: University of California Institute for Health and Aging, and Baltimore: Johns Hopkins University Injury Prevention Center.

Rivara FP, Dicker BG, Bergman AB, Dacey R, and Herman C (1988) The public cost of motorcycle trauma. *JAMA* 260:221–223.

Robertson LS (1983) *Injuries: Causes, Control Strategies, and Public Policy,* Lexington, MA: D.C. Heath.

Robertson LS (1987) Childhood injuries: knowledge and strategies for prevention. Springfield, VA: National Technical Information Service (PB88–172507/WHP).

Robertson LS (1989) Potential savings from injury prevention. In Rice DP, and MacKenzie EJ (eds), *Cost of Injury in the United States: A Report to Congress, 1989.* San Francisco: University of California Institute for Health and Aging, and Baltimore: Johns Hopkins University Injury Prevention Center.

Robertson LS (1990) Car design and risk of pedestrian deaths. *Am J Public Health* 80:609–610.

Runyan CW, and Earp JAL (1985) Epidemiologic evidence and motor vehicle policy making. *Am J Public Health* 75:354–360.

Self P (1977) *Econocrats and the Policy Process: The Politics and Philosophy of Cost-Benefit Analysis.* Boulder, CO: Westview Press.

Shrader-Frechette KS (1985) *Risk Analysis and Scientific Method.* Boston: D. Reidel.

Starr C (1969) Social benefit versus technological risk. *Science* 165:1232–1238.

Tengs TO, Adams ME, Pliskin JS, Safran DG, Siegal JE, Weinstein MC, and Graham JD (1995) Five-hundred life-saving interventions and their cost-effectiveness. *Risk Anal* 15:369–390.

Viscusi WK, and Magat WA (1987) *Learning about Risk: Consumer and Worker Responses to Hazard Information.* Cambridge, MA: Harvard University Press.

Williams AF, Karpf RS, and Zador PL (1983) Variations in minimum licensing age and fatal motor vehicle crashes. *Am J Public Health* 73:1401.

Wintemute GJ, and Wright MA (1992) Initial and subsequent hospital costs of firearm injuries. *J Trauma* 33:556–560.

Wood T, and Milne P (1988) Head injuries to pedal cyclists and the promotion of helmet use in Victoria, Australia. *Accident Anal Prev* 20:177.

10

INJURY POLICY ANALYSIS

In almost every sport that involves a ball, the good players learn to keep their eyes on the ball. The ball in injury epidemiology and injury control is energy, the necessary and specific cause of injury. The researcher who focuses on hypotheses specifying how concentrations of particular types of energy occur in contact with human beings is likely to produce the most useful results. If a hypothesized causal factor is substantially removed from the energy exhange in space or time, it usually has a weak or nonexistent correlation to injury rates.

An upsurge in interest in injuries began in the 1960s with the focus on energy and energy control as a primary path to injury control (Haddon et al., 1964). Members of Congress became aware of the new concepts and research, which led to the federal regulation of motor vehicles and other products (McCarry, 1972). As noted in Chapter 7, the initial regulations had a substantial effect on reducing certain injuries. This is not to say that regulation of products is always the most effective means of achieving injury control. Regulations specifying minimum standards often become an excuse for doing no more than the minimum. Regulations for other purposes, such as fuel economy, can have an adverse effect on injury rates if joint effects are not considered. Beyond the issuance of initial standards, agencies often bog down in minutiae, court battles, and defense from attacks by the regulated industries or antiregulation demagogues. A long list of practical and feasible regulations that have been neglected, such as propeller guards on boat motors to prevent slicing the bodies of swimmers (Vernick et al., n.d.), could be compiled.

Epidemiologic data on injuries can be used to estimate the potential consequences of alternative policies for injury control. By way of illustration in this chapter, estimated potential effects of three policies—a minimum standard for vehicle stability, product liability versus regulation, and alternative regulations to improve fuel economy and reduce injuries—are presented in "what if" analyses of policy.

UNSTABLE VEHICLES

In 1972, the National Highway Traffic Safety Administration successfully opposed the army's proposed sale of surplus Jeeps to the public because of evidence of instability of the vehicle. Nevertheless, the Jeep Corporation's civilian version, known as the CJ, continued to be sold—its commercials showing the vehicle going over hills with all wheels off the ground. Ford Motor Company, also a manufacturer of military Jeeps, in 1973 introduced for civilian use a jeeplike Bronco that was discontinued in 1978 (Snyder et al., 1980). In 1980, research and demonstration of the rollover propensity of the Jeep CJ-5 was featured on CBS's popular television program *60 Minutes.* The stability of other so-called utility vehicles was also of concern because of their high center of gravity relative to track width and resultant rollover rates, but attention focused on the Jeep CJ-5, which was the least stable. After hundreds of lawsuits, the CJ-5 was discontinued in 1984 and the CJ-7 in 1986.

Despite the demise of the pre-78 Bronco and the Jeep CJs, sales of utility vehicles increased from 132,000 in 1982 to 856,000 in 1988 (*Ward's Automotive Yearbook,* 1983–89). Researchers continued to document their high rollover rates (Reinfurt et al., 1981, 1984; Smith, 1982), but the government took no action other than to require a vague warning that the vehicles handle differently from other vehicles.

In 1986, Timothy Wirth, a Congressman, petitioned NHTSA to set a stability standard for all utility vehicles based on the strong correlation of the stability ratio (track width divided by twice the height of center of gravity) and the rollover rates among vehicles (Robertson & Kelley, 1989). In 1988, Consumers Union publicized tests of the Suzuki Samurai and petitioned the agency to prohibit its further sale based on its rollover propensity. These and other petitions were rejected by NHTSA.

In response to the Wirth petition, NHTSA argued that choice of a specific stability ratio would be arbitrary and that the agency was prohibited by law from prohibiting a class of vehicles (National Highway Traffic Safety Administration, 1987). Neither argument is valid. The death rate increases substantially as stability declines toward a static stability ratio of 1.2 g of lateral force, which is typical of utility vehicles but below the ratio of all but a few cars. The rollover death rate of the Jeep CJ-5 (stability 1 g) is 19 times that of cars; the CJ-7, pre-78 Bronco, and the Bronco II (stability 1.07–1.08 g) have rollover death rates 10 to 12 times that of cars, and the Samurai's (stability 1.12 g) rollover death rate is 6 times that of cars. In a regression analysis, stability explained 61 percent of the variation in rollover death rates among these and other utility vehicles (Chapter 4).

Setting the stability standard at a minimum ratio of 1.2 g of lateral force would be no more arbitrary than setting the blood alcohol concentration for drivers at 0.10 percent by weight. Since the standard could be met by lowering the center of gravity, widening the distance between the center of the tires, or both, the standard would not prohibit a class of vehicles. For example, the Jeep CJ-5 could have had a stability ratio above 1.2 by lengthening its axle by only 11 inches, and the other utility vehicles would have to be widened much less than that.

The Consumers Union petition to recall the Samurai was rejected on the grounds that the Samurai was not as bad as the Bronco II (National Highway Traffic Safety Administration, 1988). Subsequently, NHTSA announced that it would reconsider the rollover issue and specifically singled out the Bronco II because it is worse than the Samurai. In 1990, NHTSA rejected petitions that the CJ vehicles be recalled, saying that its rollover rate was only "slightly" higher than that of its peers. It subsequently also exonerated the Bronco II on similar grounds, stating that they were little different from peer vehicles. The leadership of the agency did not seem embarrassed by the logic of saying that a vehicle was not defective because it had an injury rate similar to vehicles with the same defect. Actually, those vehicles would have had no peers in rollover rates had the agency done something about vehicle stability when the issue was raised a decade earlier.

In June 1996, for the third time in a decade, the NHTSA administrator refused to adopt a standard for motor vehicle stability. He argued that the costs would exceed the benefits (National Highway Traffic Safety Administration, 1996).

The NHTSA prefers to measure stability by tipping a table with the vehicle on it and observing the angle at which the upper wheels lose contact (called the tilt table angle, or TTA) to $T/2H$, because measuring center of gravity can damage a vehicle and does not account for possible effects of suspension. It said a minimum TTA standard of 46.4 degrees would result in 61 fewer deaths and 63 fewer severe injuries, an estimate that doesn't pass the "smell test." The agency's own studies indicate that stability accounts for most of the variance in rollover percentage of single-vehicle crashes, controlling for behavioral and environmental factors (Harwin & Brewer, 1990; Mengert et al., 1989), and the death rate per vehicle of lower stability utility vehicles is 3–20 times that of passenger cars. Half of spinal injuries occur in motor vehicle crashes (Thurman et al., 1994) and 65 percent of the nonfatal motor vehicle occupant cases occur in rollovers (Thurman et al., 1995). The latter two referenced studies did not consider vehicle stability as a factor.

The agency measured $T/2H$ for numerous vehicles but TTA measurement was only done on a sample (Garrott, 1993). Although assembly of such measurements was discontinued by the agency in 1992, most of the vehicles on which the regulatory decision was based were not redesigned substantially before the 1995 model year.

To assess the effect of lack of adoption of the Wirth petition, a study was conducted of fatal crash rates per vehicle year of use for 1989–93 model vehicles in use during 1990–94. The 23 vehicles with known TTA up to 47.7 degrees were included to compare the results using TTA and $T/2H$.

The fatality data were extracted from the Fatal Accident Reporting System (Chapter 3). Vehicles in use, 1989–93 models during 1990–94, were obtained from published data (Insurance Institute for Highway Safety, 1995), and projected years of use were estimated from published vehicle sales (*Ward's Automotive Yearbook,* 1995), adjusted for known scrappage rates (Oak Ridge National Laboratory, 1984).

The effect of stability on fatal rollover rates per vehicles in use was estimated by logistic regression of the rollover per registered vehicles with nonrollover rates, wheelbase (distance from front to rear axle), and stability measures included as predictor variables. Nonrollover rates serve as a control for driver, vehicle, and environmental factors that affect fatality rates generally, and wheelbase has been correlated to rollover controlling for stability (Jones & Penny, 1990).

Table 10.1 presents the nonrollover and rollover death rates per 100,000 in use per year of the vehicles in the study, ranked from highest to lowest rollover rate. There is large variation in both death rates. The Amigo has a rollover death rate 16 times that of the Caravan/Voyager, although their nonrollover rates are similar.

The logistic regression estimates are presented in Table 10.2 separately for $T/2H$ (Model 1) and TTA (Model 2). $T/2H$ is significantly and strongly predictive of rollover when wheelbase and nonrollover rates are controlled; TTA is not. Rollover rates are significantly higher in vehicles with shorter wheelbases and in vehicles with higher nonrollover rates.

To project the deaths attributable to vehicle instability over the expected survival of vehicles, the number of vehicles remaining after scrappage in a given year of the 20 year period after manufacture was multiplied by the difference between the rate predicted from the regression analysis for a vehicle of that stability and a vehicle with the same nonrollover rate and wheel base but

TABLE 10.1. Vehicle Parameters and Death Rates per 100,000 Vehicles in Use, 1990–94

MAKE/MODEL	NONROLL	ROLLOVER	TOTAL	T/2H	WHEELBASE
89–93 Isuzu Amigo	7.9	35.8	43.7	1.11	92
90–93 Toyota 4Runner	5.0	20.3	25.3	1.08	103
91–93 Isuzu Rodeo	6.0	18.1	24.1	1.12	109
89–93 GEO Tracker	14.5	17.8	32.3	1.14	87
89–93 Jeep Wrangler	10.3	13.0	23.3	1.16	93
93 Ford Ranger	14.5	12.1	26.6	1.13	125
89–93 GM S/T Blazer	11.1	11.4	22.5	1.10	104
89–93 Nissan Pickup	15.1	11.2	26.3	1.16	116
91–93 Ford Escort	21.5	10.5	32.0	1.38	98
90–93 Nissan Pathfinder	3.5	10.0	13.5	1.07	104
89–93 GM S/T Pickup	16.5	9.8	26.3	1.16	123
89–93 GM 1500 Pickup	10.2	8.9	19.1	1.14	142
90–93 Ford Festiva	28.6	7.9	36.5	1.34	90
89–93 Ford F250 Pickup	5.6	6.9	12.5	1.11	155
89–93 GM Astro	8.1	5.7	13.8	1.11	111
89–93 Ford Bronco	4.8	5.6	10.4	1.06	105
92–93 Ford Aerostar	5.6	5.4	11.0	1.11	119
91–93 Ford Explorer	4.2	5.4	9.6	1.08	107
89–93 Ford F150 Pickup	7.4	5.3	12.7	1.15	139
89–93 Mazda MPV	6.2	4.8	11.0	1.16	110
90–93 GM Lumina Van	6.0	3.9	9.9	1.12	110
89–93 Chrysler D150 Pickup	10.9	3.2	14.1	1.28	115
91–93 Chrysler Caravan/ Voyager	6.0	2.2	8.2	1.18	119

a $T/2H$ of 1.2. Table 10.3 illustrates the calculation of preventable deaths by changing $T/2H$ using the 1991 Blazer/Jimmy ($T/2H = 1.10$) as an example. Based on the logistic coefficients in Table 10.2, the expected total rollover death rate of that vehicle is

$$\text{Expected} = \frac{1}{1 + \exp[-(-3.664 + (-5.236 \times 1.096) + (-.00435 \times 104) + (.0740 \times 11.1)]}$$
$$= 0.00011933$$

Substituting 1.2 for the $T/2H$ of 1.10 in the equation gives the expected rate at $T/2H = 1.2$ (0.00006923). The difference between the two rates (0.0000501) times the vehicles in use in a given year gives the estimate of preventable deaths in that year. Although the fractional numbers during a given year are expected values, the total is a realistic estimate. The 1991 Blazer/Jimmys would be expected to have approximately 107 fewer rollover deaths in the 20 year period after their initial sales if the $T/2H$ were 1.2.

TABLE 10.2. Logistic Regression Estimates of
Rollover Rates by Stability

	WHEELBASE AND NONROLLOVER RATES	
	COEFFICIENT	p
Model 1		
Intercept	−3.66	<0.01
T/2H	−5.24	<0.01
Wheelbase	−0.00*	<0.01
Nonroll rate	0.08	<0.01
Model 2		
Intercept	−9.43	<0.01
TTA	0.01	0.61
Wheelbase	−0.01	<0.01
Nonroll rate	0.03	<0.01

*>−0.05 but <0.

Had the minimum standard of $T/2H = 1.2$, proposed in 1986, been adopted beginning in 1990 and used in subsequent models, the estimated deaths that would have been prevented in the 1990–94 models with $T/2H < 1.2$ are summarized in the first column of Table 10.4. There are other vehicles with $T/2H$ less than 1.2 that were not included because of missing TTA. Nevertheless, approximately 5028 preventable rollover deaths are expected in the noted vehicles for lack of a rollover standard in that five year period. The Escort, Festiva, and Dodge D150 pickup are excluded from Table 10.4 because the $T/2H$ of each is above 1.2. The rank of vehicles by numbers of preventable rollover deaths is different from the rank of fatal rollover rates mainly because of differences in sales volumes. The rate represents the risk to the occupants, whereas the number of preventable deaths represents the loss to society because of the combination of rates and sales.

There is no sample of nonfatal injuries both adequate in clinical detail and large enough to estimate such injuries in specific makes and models of vehicles. By using ratios to deaths of hospitalized spinal cord and brain injuries, hospital days, and lost workdays in a sample of rollovers, an estimate of the extent of these outcomes was obtained. All rollovers ($n = 1893$) in the National Accident Sampling System–Crashworthiness Data System (Chapter 3) were examined for the years 1989–91 and the sampling ratio was used to estimate the national occurrence of these outcomes. The ratios of the specific outcomes to all rollover deaths were multiplied by the projected deaths attributable to $T/2H$ less than 1.2 to obtain estimates of reductions in those outcomes obtainable by a standard.

During 1989–91, a death count from the FARS data indicates a total of 28,347 people died in rollovers of passenger cars, vans, utility vehicles, and light trucks. The analysis of the national sample of all rollovers in such vehicles during 1989–91, with ratio to deaths in parentheses, indicated 13,949 hospitalized spinal cord injuries (0.492), 234,619 hospitalized brain injuries (8.3), 5.3 million hospital days (187), and 9.9 million lost workdays (349) among those employed. By using the ratios times the deaths preventable by increased stability (columns 2–4 in Table 10.4), it is expected that failure to adopt a standard applicable in 1990 models will result in approximately 2471 hospitalized spinal cord injuries, 41,726 hospitalized brain injuries, 940,129 hospital days, and 1.8 million lost workdays in the vehicles in Table 10.4 manufactured through 1994.

The effect on rollover fatalities of actually improved stability in a vehicle that did not change drastically in appearance is illustrated by the evolution in designs of the Jeep CJs and Wrangler. Figure 10.1 shows that first-event rollover and rollover that occurred after contact with another vehicle or object declined as the T/2H was gradually increased from 1.01 in the CJ-5 to 1.16 in the Wrangler. The nonrollover rate is similar among the Jeeps and is somewhat less than that of passenger cars.

The cost of changing vehicle parameters is known only to the manufactur-

TABLE 10.3. Projected Deaths Preventable During 1992–2011 in the 1991 Blazer/Jimmy Assuming $T/2H = 1.2$

YEAR	PROJECTED VEHICLES IN USE	PREVENTABLE DEATHS
1992	152,235	7.63
1993	151,623	7.60
1994	149,787	7.51
1995	147,339	7.38
1996	144,279	7.23
1997	140,454	7.04
1998	135,864	6.81
1999	130,356	6.53
2000	123,930	6.21
2001	116,739	5.85
2002	108,936	5.46
2003	100,674	5.04
2004	92,259	4.62
2005	83,844	4.20
2006	75,735	3.79
2007	67,932	3.40
2008	60,741	3.04
2009	54,009	2.71
2010	47,889	2.39
2011	42,381	2.12
Total		107

TABLE 10.4. Projected Rollover Outcomes Preventable by a $T/2H$ of 1.2 in 20 Years' Use, 1990–94 Models

MAKE/MODEL	DEATHS	SPINAL CORD INJURIES	BRAIN INJURIES	HOSPITAL DAYS	LOST WORKDAYS
Amigo	23	11	190	4,288	8,003
4Runner	135	66	1,120	25,240	47,106
Rodeo/Passport	66	32	545	12,282	22,921
Tracker	49	24	404	9,111	17,003
Wrangler	64	31	528	11,898	22,205
Ranger Pickup	736	362	6,113	137,724	257,035
Blazer/Jimmy (S/T)	696	342	5,776	130,127	242,857
Nissan Pickup	144	71	1,199	27,018	50,424
Pathfinder	131	64	1,087	24,488	45,703
S10/S15 Pickup	340	167	2,825	63,654	118,798
GM Light Pickups	592	291	4,910	110,625	206,461
F250 Pickup	178	88	1,479	33,324	62,194
Astro/Safari Van	327	161	2,713	61,129	114,085
Bronco	108	53	899	20,262	37,814
Aerostar Van	312	154	2,590	58,350	108,900
Explorer/Navajo	590	290	4,895	110,293	205,840
F150 Pickup	315	155	2,611	58,832	109,799
Mazda MPV	26	13	215	4,835	9,023
Lumina Van	78	38	644	14,506	27,072
Caravan/Voyager	118	58	983	22,143	41,326
Total	5,028	2,471	41,726	940,129	1,754,572

ers, but it is possible to relate the relevant parameters to base price of the vehicles. Ordinary least squares regression was used to estimate the effect of center of gravity height, track width, and wheelbase on the 1993 base price of vehicles in the study (*Ward's Automotive Yearbook*, 1993).

The base price of the 23 vehicles studied in relation to vehicle parameters is presented in Table 10.5. Track width and wheelbase are not related to vehicle price when the effect of center of gravity height is considered. For each 1 inch (2.54 centimeters) marginal increase in center of gravity height, there is an average $1446 increase in base price of the vehicle.

Based on the the projected 5028 preventable deaths in 5 years, each year's delay in adoption of a minimum stability standard of $T/2H = 1.2$ for light-duty vehicles in the United States resulted in the continued production of vehicles that will experience more than 1000 preventable deaths and huge costs from nonfatal injuries in rollovers. Although these results are based on vehicle models through 1994, there is no indication that the situation will change in future years. The government agency responsible for vehicle standards has failed in its duty to analyze the problem with due diligence (Frame, 1996) and the manufacturers have failed to act on what their own historic statements and experience would indicate (e.g., Stonex, 1961).

NHTSA's estimate of deaths prevented is based on a measure of stability (TTA) that is inferior in predicting rollover rates as well as several false assumptions. The agency falsely assumed that increased stability reduces only single-vehicle rollovers. It claimed that most crashes would occur whether the vehicle rolled or not despite clear evidence to the contrary (e.g., Fig. 10.1). It used only one model year when these vehicles are essentially unchanged in design for many years. And it failed to account for the total years of use prior to scrappage.

Stability can be increased by lowering center of gravity height, increasing track width, or both. If desired ground clearance means a high center of gravity, then appropriately increased track width can offset it. NHTSA argued that the 6 inch (3.24 cm) increase in track width necessary to stabilize some of the vehicles must be accompanied by a 10 inch (25.4 cm) increase in wheelbase to retain braking stability, but that is not true of lowered center of gravity. Further-

Fatal Accident Reporting System, 1988-94

FIGURE 10.1. Fatal crashes per 100,000 vehicles per year.

TABLE 10.5. Base Price of Vehicles in 1993 in Relation to Center of Gravity Height, Track Width, and Wheelbase in Inches

	COEFFICIENT	T	p
Intercept	−10,648	−1.32	0.203
Center of gravity height	1,446	4.59	<0.001
Track width	−114	−0.53	0.599
Wheelbase	−53	−1.63	0.119
$R^2 = 0.66$			

more, most of the vehicles would require less than a 6 inch (3.24 cm) extension of track to achieve $T/2H = 1.2$ given the same center of gravity. It is curious that the agency accepts a minimum ratio of wheelbase to track width to achieve braking stability but not a minimum track width to center of gravity height to achieve turning stability.

The NHTSA claims that required changes in track width and wheelbase would eliminate the "compact sport utility vehicle" class of vehicles, which the agency claims it is prohibited from doing by law. Aside from the fact that such vehicle classifications are arbitrary, the assumption is demonstrably untrue. The noted changes in the Jeep from the CJ-5 to the Wrangler did not eliminate the vehicle from the compact sport utility class and did not change the appearance appreciably. Extending the Wrangler's track width an additional 2 inches (5.08 cm) or lowering its center of gravity height 1 inch (2.54 cm) to achieve a $T/2H$ of 1.2 would not do so.

The official who signed the three *Federal Register* entries rejecting a rollover standard commented in a newspaper article that the total death rates in some of the less stable vehicles are less than average (Stepp, 1996). Although this is obviously true because some have longer than average wheelbases and lower than average nonrollover rates, as can be seen in Table 10.1, it is not an excuse for failure to reduce rollover rates where feasible and practicable. If a physician argued that we should not treat cancer because heart disease is declining, the comment would not be treated seriously even in a newspaper. The official who made the comment subsequently retired from the government and is now employed by the American Motor Vehicle Manufacturers' Association, a typical "revolving door" problem between industry and government in the United States. The government official who signed the rejection of the petition to recall the Samurai now works for the Association of International Vehicle Manufacturers, also a Washington lobbying organization.

The NHTSA's claim that the standard would be costly also is not supported by the Jeep's history and the vehicle price data. The 1993 Wrangler's base price, $11,410, is among the lower priced vehicles for sale in the United States.

The correlation of price to vehicle parameters indicates that a substantial increase in price is associated with raising center of gravity height when wheelbase and track width are controlled statistically. There is increased cost both in vehicle price and death and injury to ride high. While redesign of vehicles undoubtedly bears costs, the vehicles are periodically redesigned anyway, and it is not clear that increased stability would result in net increase in costs given the apparent higher marginal price of higher center of gravity.

Since the government no longer assembles data on vehicle stability, obtaining information on specific vehicles is difficult. Consumers Union has declared two vehicles "unacceptable," the Samurai and Trooper, but others as bad or worse have escaped adverse publicity.

REGULATORY FAILURE

The stability case is only one example of failure to adopt reasonable regulations. Multiunit trucks were less than 1 percent of registered vehicles but were 8 percent of vehicles in fatal crashes in the 1990s. Major aspects of the truck problem are braking capability, stability, and visibility at night. Trucks require longer distance for braking than cars and those with one or more articulation points are particularly unstable when the brakes lock. Also, trucks are struck at night more frequently, in the rear when they move slowly up grades and in the side when the headlamps of the truck are straight on the road, giving the impression to an approaching driver of another vehicle that the truck is entirely in its lane, although the trailer is across the road (Ervin, 1988).

The NHTSA attempted to require antilock brakes for tractor-trailer trucks in the 1970s but rescinded the standard based on claims that the technology was faulty. Such a standard has been adopted in Europe with no such problems being reported.

Despite the fact that research has found that double-trailer trucks have a risk of serious crashes more than twice that of ordinary 18-wheelers on the same roads (Stein & Jones, 1988), the federal government overrode state laws prohibiting two trailers, and trucks with three trailers are now being allowed. These trains without tracks, given their inherent lower stability, will no doubt further deteriorate the safety of the interstate highways, where they are most frequently used.

The visibility problem has been shown to be reduced substantially by reflective stripes around the outline of the truck trailers, and the force of crashes can be reduced by energy-absorbing underride guards. The government finally issued a standard for improved underride guards after two decades of delay. Virtually no trucks observed on the road have reflective stripes.

This history suggests that alternatives to regulation should be considered.

Regulation has some effect when applied, but component-by-component regulation requires a large and expert government bureaucracy, uncorrupted by bribes or the prospect of jobs in industry after retirement from government, and commitment from political leadership. Years of delay and neglect of cost-effective regulations usually occur when the regulatory agency is influenced politically. The issue is not partisan. The noted negligence on the vehicle stability issue in the United States by the Democrat administration of the 1990s was no improvement on the Republican antiregulation ideologues of the 1980s.

Lawsuits against manufacturers (tort litigation) are supposed to deter the design and manufacture of hazardous products and compensate the injured or their families. Although tort litigation has demonstrable effect in a few cases, it is applied spottily. When the hazards of products such as the Jeep CJs gain publicity, those injured in or by these products know there are grounds for lawsuits. A sufficient number of lawsuits filed may eventually deter the manufacturer sued from continuing production of the hazard, but apparently those producing products with similar characteristics without notoriety will not be deterred. Failure to provide technology such as air bags is even less often perceived by the injured as grounds for a lawsuit, and some courts have ruled that the federal passive restraint standard preempts the right to sue, despite the government's illegal rescission of the standard and the accompanying delay in implementation.

Tort liability laws have been under attack by corporations and their political supporters based on false claims of trivial lawsuits and increasing awards. Cases that became grist for the joke mill, such as that of the woman burned by McDonald's coffee, are often not trivial. The burned woman was served 180 degree coffee. She had third degree burns on 6 percent of her body and the needed skin grafts resulted in scarring of 16 percent of her body. McDonald's executives knew of about 700 complaints of burns but did nothing to reduce the risk (Nader & Smith, 1996).

Also, tort liability, even when applied, does not always fulfill the goal of compensation, particularly on a timely basis. Defense attorneys have a strong incentive to lengthen the negotiations, depositions, and court proceedings to maximize their fees. Many families suffer severe economic hardship for years and rehabilitation is often delayed while the litigation drags on (Kaufman, 1989). Less than half of the total monies involved in tort liability lawsuits end up in the plaintiffs' bank accounts (Research and Policy Committee, 1989).

Many of the faults of the present system might be ameliorated by blanket liability of the manufacturer for serious injuries. If, when the product was designed, the manufacturer knew that his or her company would be liable for all severe injuries, the cost of that liability could be balanced against the cost of applying technologies to minimize injury severity. If a certain payment to the injured persons or their estates were required to be timely, the injured or their heirs would have little incentive to sue and take the risk of obtaining nothing. Costs of litigation would be reduced and the injured could receive timely rehabilitation.

Furthermore, manufacturers occasionally assert that injury-reducing technology is not used when manufacturers fear that the evidence that risk could have been been reduced earlier would be used in lawsuits involving products that preceded the technology. The extent of the problem is undocumented, with only two states, New York and California, allowing such evidence to be introduced in trial. Clever lawyers in other states, however, often are successful in implying negligence on the basis of product improvements. Under blanket liability, the manufacturer would have no disincentive to improve the product's safety for fear of increased lawsuits.

Aside from objections from law firms that stand to lose income from such a system, the major objection is that manufacturers would be paying for injuries which were unavoidable in some cases and clearly the result of misuse of the product in others. No doubt this could happen, but not nearly as much as commonly thought. While the incidence of injury is caused by a wide variety of behavioral, environmental, and product-related factors, the severity is a simple function of the energy exchange with the human organism (Chapter 4). The amount of the energy exchange is largely determined by characteristics of products. Injury control analysts have specified numerous product modifications that would reduce severity (Robertson, 1983). For example, a research safety vehicle that was developed in the 1970s had improved pedestrian protection, improved energy absorption, and radar that detected imminent collisions and automatically applied brakes. The developers noted that it could be produced in large volume at a cost per unit no more than concurrent compact cars (DiNapoli et al., 1977). Twenty years later, no production vehicles have radar brakes.

Since the efficacy of blanket liability of manufacturers for severe injuries cannot be assessed without trying it, an experimental trial applied to manufacturers of motorized vehicles could be undertaken. These vehicles account for slightly more than half of severe and fatal unintentional injuries. A federal law applicable to such vehicles sold in interstate commerce would be necessary for an adequate test. Enactment by only a few states might not provide the incentives necessary for product modifications by manufacturers.

To reduce administrative costs and the likelihood of fraudulent claims, non-severe AIS 1 injuries (relatively trivial hairline fractures, cuts and bruises that usually do not require hospitalization) could be excluded. In order to estimate the potential blanket liability per vehicle of AIS 2–5 and fatal injuries, an estimate of the cost of injuries per vehicle was generated using national estimates of AIS 2–5 and fatal injuries in recently sold passenger vehicles. Government estimates of costs of injury by each AIS were used to calculate costs (Federal Highway Administration, 1994).

To estimate the cost of injuries in particular vehicles, the dollar amount for a given severity of injury was multiplied by the estimated number of such injuries associated with the 1990–94 model years of vehicles of these manufacturers involved in crashes during 1991–95 (Insurance Institute for Highway Safety, 1996). The ratio of Maximum Abbreviated Injury Scores (MAIS) for nonfatal injuries to fatalities for different classes of vehicles, from the National Accident Sampling System, was used to estimate cost per vehicle in 20 years of use, accounting for known scrappage rates as noted in the rollover study. The results are presented in Table 10.6.

The 20 year projected costs of MAIS 2–6 injuries among these vehicles vary from a low of $2128 per car for the Acura Legend to a high of $20,517 per car for the Chevrolet Camaro. The risk associated with a given vehicle is often not reflected in the base price. For example, the Mazda 626 has a death rate similar to the Cadillac Seville but is priced at less than half the Seville. Indeed, the low correlation of fatality rates and base price ($r^2 = 0.19$) suggests that crash protection is a minor element in the differential costs of vehicles. If manufacturers were spending substantial amounts to improve crashworthiness, the death rates would be more consistently lower in more expensive vehicles.

The total cost to consumers, base price plus injury costs, of supposedly low-priced vehicles varies hugely. Among vehicles with base prices less than $10,000, the total cost per vehicle will be $13,849 for the four-door Saturn SL but $25,457 for the two-door Hyundai Scoupe. Of course, the consumer sees only the base price. Those who experience severe crashes will disproportionately bear the brunt of the differences in injury costs. Insurance rates by make and model of vehicle do not reflect the differences seen here. The data make it clear that some vehicles would remain affordable if the manufacturers added anticipated injury costs to the base price of the vehicles rather than reducing the injuries by increasing crashworthiness or crash avoidance, but the prices of the more injurious models would have to be increased substantially to offset injury costs if the vehicles were not modified, potentially reducing sales. It is also clear that there is much potential for making those vehicles high in injury costs more crashworthy so that major increases in prices would not be necessary.

If manufacturers had to pay for the injuries of their products, would the injury rates decline? During an experimental period, say ten years, the effect of blanket liability on injury rates and vehicle costs could be assessed. To save government funds, NHTSA's now worthless regulatory divisions could be disbanded and the agency could be relegated to data collection and the support of nonvehicle aspects of injury reduction programs. The Fatal Accident Reporting System and the National Accident Sampling System should be retained to assess the effectiveness of a blanket liability experiment and to act as a resource to manufacturers to assess the risk of continuing to place hazardous vehicles on the roads.

If, during the ten year experimental period, the manufacturers failed to apply injury-reducing principles, the regulatory arm of NHTSA could be regenerated, possibly regaining some of its initial forcefulness with new personnel. An earlier reimposition of standards by the Congress would, of course, be possible if the manufacturers abandoned the standards that produced the gains of the past and took no action to reduce injury severity. If the experiment were successful, it could be applied to other products.

FUEL ECONOMY AND INJURIES

Injury is not the only effect of use of motor vehicles. If the fuel supply is greatly reduced by attrition of available supplies, political events, or natural disasters, fuel may become unavailable or prohibitively expensive. Following the oil boycott in the 1970s, the government adopted a policy to increase fuel economy of cars. Each manufacturer was required to attain a specified average fuel economy in the vehicles it sold in a given year and the average was increased incrementally. That policy has generated an ongoing debate on the effect of the policy on injury rates. Fuel economy is mainly affected by vehicle weight and horsepower. Manufacturers partially increased fuel economy by reducing weight and size, so-called downsizing of vehicles, and by reducing horsepower in the 1980s.

Based on the correlation of vehicle weight and injury rates, economists argued that the regulation increased injuries (Crandall & Graham, 1989). That analysis did not consider vehicle size, weight, and horsepower, which have differential effects on fuel economy and injuries. Distance available to decelerate in a crash as well as speed and energy absorption in the vehicle are the determinants of injury. Weight of the vehicle gives minimal, if any, protection in a single-vehicle crash and is protective in a multiple-vehicle crash only if the weight of the other vehicle is less, in which case it delivers greater force to the occupants of the other vehicle (Wood, 1997). Using data on fatal crashes of 1975–77 cars and 1985–87 cars, the effects of size (indicated by wheelbase), weight, and horsepower were analyzed in a regression equation (Robertson, 1991). As predicted by physics, reduced size was correlated to increased occupant death rates and reduced horsepower was correlated to reduced death rates. When these factors were controlled statistically, weight had little or no effect.

Using human capital cost of injury data in 1985 dollars (Rice & MacKenzie, 1989), a regression of injury costs by wheelbase and horsepower indicated an increase of $126 in injury costs per vehicle for each reduced inch of wheelbase and a decrease of $23 per vehicle for each unit of decreased horsepower during the average ten years of a vehicle's use. Fuel economy was increased by 1.07

TABLE 10.6. Occupant Death Rates per 100,000 per Year, Base Prices and Injury Costs in 20 Years Adjusted for Scrappage, 1990–94 Model Sold in the United States

MAKE/MODEL	FATAL RATE	BASE PRICE	INJURY COST	TOTAL
Acura Legend 4 door	5.22	$29,900	$ 2,127.99	$32,027.99
Jaguar XJ 4 door	5.43	50,300	2,211.64	52,511.64
Lexus ES 300 4 door	5.60	27,900	2,280.18	30,180.18
Chevrolet Caprice Wagon	5.82	20,100	2,372.26	22,472.26
Chrysler Town and Country Van	5.90	26,100	3,069.25	29,169.26
Chrysler Concorde 4 door	6.17	19,000	2,511.83	21,511.83
Lexus LS 400 2 door	6.24	47,000	2,543.34	49,543.34
Chevrolet Suburban 1500	6.54	20,000	3,404.36	23,404.36
GMC 2500 Pickup 4×4	6.62	17,100	3,444.22	20,544.22
Toyota Previa Van	6.66	19,200	3,469.14	22,669.14
Chevrolet Astro Van	6.68	16,200	3,478.44	19,678.44
Mazda 626 4 door	6.89	14,200	2,806.43	17,006.43
Cadillac Seville 4 door	6.89	37,600	2,808.52	40,408.52
Mercury Sable Wagon	6.96	19,100	2,836.12	21,936.12
Volvo 940/960 4 door	7.19	25,400	2,927.41	28,327.41
Plymouth Voyager Van	7.44	14,600	3,873.27	18,473.27
Lincoln Continental 4 door	7.49	34,000	3,052.12	37,052.12
Infiniti Q45 4 door	7.56	45,900	3,081.14	48,981.14
Jeep Grand Cherokee 4 door 4×4	7.61	20,200	3,959.83	24,159.83
Mercedes E Class 4 door	7.69	44,200	3,134.62	47,334.62
Pontiac Bonneville 4 door	7.77	20,000	3,166.85	23,166.85
Mitsubishi Diamante 4 door	7.85	22,900	3,198.68	26,098.68
BMW 5-Series 4 door	8.06	37,500	3,282.29	40,782.29
Dodge Caravan Van	8.14	14,100	4,236.76	18,336.76
Ford Taurus Wagon	8.17	17,300	3,327.01	20,627.01
Ford Explorer 4×4 4 door	8.20	19,900	4,268.98	24,168.98
Volkswagen Passat 4 door	8.61	15,300	3,509.16	18,809.16
Toyota Camry 4 door	9.16	15,600	3,731.36	19,331.36
Honda Accord 4 door	9.23	14,400	3,761.69	18,161.69
Jeep Cherokee 4×4 4 door	9.23	15,100	4,806.59	19,906.59
Ford Thunderbird 2 door	9.35	16,300	3,810.98	20,110.98
Nissan Maxima 4 door	10.02	21,500	4,082.96	25,582.96
Mazda MX-6 2 door	10.13	16,300	4,127.42	20,427.42
Lincoln Town Car 4 door	10.33	35,000	4,209.85	39,209.85
Ford Taurus 4 door	10.34	16,100	4,211.48	20,311.48
Mercury Sable 4 door	10.35	18,000	4,216.45	22,216.45
Ford Aerostar Van 4×4	10.50	18,500	5,463.32	23,963.33
Subaru Legacy 4 door	10.52	16,700	4,285.35	20,985.35
Mazda Miata 2 door	10.67	15,200	4,348.59	19,548.59
Saturn SL 4 door	10.68	9,500	4,349.14	13,849.14
Ford Aerostar Van 3 door	10.75	15,000	5,593.49	20,593.49
Cadillac DeVille 4 door	10.76	34,500	4,384.63	38,884.63

(continued)

TABLE 10.6. Continued

MAKE/MODEL	FATAL RATE	BASE PRICE	INJURY COST	TOTAL
GMC 2500 Pickup	10.77	15,300	5,604.81	20,904.81
BMW 3-Series 4 door	10.88	24,100	4,433.74	28,533.74
Subaru Legacy Wagon 4×4	10.97	23,100	4,468.88	27,568.88
Chevrolet Suburban 1500 4×4	11.03	22,200	5,743.63	27,943.63
GMC T15 Jimmy 4×4 4 door	11.22	18,800	5,838.57	24,638.57
Ford Explorer 4 door	11.30	18,000	5,880.10	23,880.10
Nissan Altima 4 door	11.40	13,300	4,645.89	17,945.89
Chevrolet 3500 Pickup	11.55	16,900	6,012.05	22,912.05
Chevrolet 2500 Pickup 4×4	11.59	17,100	6,033.48	23,133.48
GMC T15 Jimmy 2 door 4×4	11.77	17,400	6,125.42	23,525.42
Honda Civic 2 door	11.85	8,700	4,828.36	13,528.36
Honda Civic 4 door	11.90	11,500	4,847.43	16,347.43
Buick LeSabre 4 door	11.94	20,500	4,863.35	25,363.35
Buick Park Avenue 4 door	11.95	26,600	4,870.22	31,470.22
Chrysler LeBaron convertible	12.07	18,000	4,918.80	22,918.80
Buick Roadmaster 4 door	12.08	23,100	4,919.37	28,019.38
Ford F-150 Pickup	12.11	11,700	6,304.07	18,004.07
Ford F-250 Pickup 4×4	12.30	18,900	6,403.77	25,303.77
Mercury Grand Marquis 4 door	12.34	22,700	5,025.42	27,725.42
Ford Explorer 2 door	12.51	17,200	6,510.55	23,710.55
Ford Crown Victoria 4 door	12.83	20,700	5,228.41	25,928.41
Chevrolet Lumina 4 door	12.84	13,900	5,229.64	19,129.64
Oldsmobile 98 4 door	13.05	25,600	5,314.88	30,914.88
Oldsmobile 88 4 door	13.07	20,100	5,324.28	25,424.28
Mercury Capri 2 door	13.13	13,600	5,350.90	18,950.90
Nissan Pathfinder 4 door 4×4	13.36	20,400	6,955.43	27,355.43
Cadillac Eldorado 2 door	13.40	34,600	5,459.80	40,059.81
Dodge Intrepid 4 door	13.42	16,600	5,467.35	22,067.35
Hyundai Sonata 4 door	13.66	12,800	5,565.55	18,365.55
Ford F-350 Pickup	13.78	17,900	7,172.85	25,072.85
Lexus SC 300/400 2 door	14.09	35,100	5,741.65	40,841.65
Chevrolet T10 Blazer 4 door 4×4	14.11	18,400	7,342.33	25,742.34
Pontiac Sunbird convertible	14.38	15,900	5,859.21	21,759.21
Honda Civic Coupe 2 door	14.66	10,400	5,973.55	16,373.55
Chevrolet T10 Blazer 2 door 4×4	14.67	17,100	7,636.51	24,736.51
Plymouth Sundance 4 door	14.74	9,300	6,005.10	15,305.10
Jeep Cherokee 4 door	14.78	13,600	7,691.15	21,291.15
Chevrolet Corsica 4 door	14.79	11,900	6,027.03	17,927.03
Plymouth Acclaim 4 door	15.03	12,400	6,121.97	18,521.97
Chevrolet Caprice 4 door	15.08	18,600	6,142.48	24,742.48
Saturn SC 2 door	15.14	11,300	6,166.07	17,466.07

(continued)

TABLE 10.6. Occupant Death Rates per 100,000 per Year, Base Prices and Injury Costs in 20 Years Adjusted for Scrappage, 1990–94 Model Sold in the United States—Cont.

MAKE/MODEL	FATAL RATE	BASE PRICE	INJURY COST	TOTAL
Isuzu Trooper 4×4 4 door	15.26	20,100	7,943.32	28,043.32
Chevrolet Cavalier Wagon	15.29	10,200	6,226.92	16,426.92
Chevrolet 2500 Pickup	15.32	15,300	7,975.09	23,275.09
Ford Explorer 2 door	15.47	17,200	8,051.93	25,251.93
Dodge Spirit 4 door	15.58	12,400	6,346.24	18,746.24
Toyota MR2 2 door	15.81	19,300	6,441.92	25,741.93
Pontiac Grand Am 4 door	16.21	13,100	6,603.81	19,703.82
GMC 1500 Pickup	16.21	14,800	8,439.40	23,239.40
GMC 1500 Pickup 4×4	16.27	17,100	8,468.97	25,568.97
Ford F-350 Pickup 4×4	16.79	19,100	8,737.45	27,837.45
Isuzu Rodeo 4×4 4 door	16.86	18,300	8,773.34	27,073.34
Oldsmobile Bravada 4×4 4 door	16.89	25,800	8,792.64	34,592.64
Ford F-150 Pickup 4×4	16.93	15,000	8,812.29	23,812.29
Toyota Corolla 4 door	17.16	11,500	6,990.14	18,490.15
Ford Tempo 2 door	17.33	10,800	7,060.61	17,860.61
Mercury Topaz 4 door	17.53	11,400	7,142.19	18,542.19
Chevrolet 1500 Pickup	17.63	14,800	9,177.02	23,977.02
Toyota Tercel 2 door	17.66	8,300	7,194.83	15,494.83
Chevrolet 1500 Pickup 4×4	17.69	15,100	9,206.26	24,306.26
Chrysler LeBaron 4 door	17.70	15,000	7,210.74	22,210.74
Ford Tempo 4 door	17.90	10,800	7,292.95	18,092.95
Ford Escort Wagon	17.96	10,700	7,317.76	18,017.76
Chevrolet Lumina 2 door	18.27	15,200	7,443.66	22,643.66
Oldsmobile Ciera 4 door	18.57	14,700	7,563.71	22,263.71
Toyota Pickup	18.65	9,700	9,706.58	19,406.58
Ford Ranger Pickup	18.93	9,200	9,852.33	19,052.33
Buick Century 4 door	19.13	14,700	7,793.02	22,493.02
Ford Probe 2 door	19.53	13,200	7,957.56	21,157.56
Mitsubishi Eclipse 2 door	19.54	12,100	7,960.95	20,060.95
Mazda 323 2 door	20.14	7,800	8,204.07	16,004.07
Dodge Shadow 4 door	20.44	9,300	8,327.41	17,627.41
Chevrolet Cavalier 4 door	20.46	9,100	8,335.35	17,435.35
Plymouth Sundance 2 door	20.89	8,900	8,509.40	17,409.40
Pontiac Sunbird 2 door	21.06	9,900	8,578.92	18,478.91
Geo Prizm 4 door	21.24	10,400	8,653.66	19,053.66
Ford Ranger 4×4 Pickup	21.26	13,100	11,066.50	24,166.50
Mazda 929 4 door	21.47	29,600	8,746.75	38,346.76
Dodge Shadow 2 door	21.79	8,900	8,875.36	17,775.36
Chevrolet Cavalier 2 door	22.02	9,000	8,969.52	17,969.52
Eagle Talon 2 door	22.06	12,200	8,987.19	21,187.19
Chevrolet Beretta 2 door	22.08	11,900	8,994.54	20,894.54
Isuzu Pickup	22.42	9,000	11,667.30	20,667.30
Jeep Wrangler	22.46	11,400	11,691.62	23,091.62

(continued)

TABLE 10.6. Continued

MAKE/MODEL	FATAL RATE	BASE PRICE	INJURY COST	TOTAL
Toyota Pickup 4×4	22.54	14,100	11,730.54	25,830.54
Nissan Pickup	23.04	9,500	11,994.41	21,494.41
Toyota 4Runner 4×4 4 door	23.17	19,700	12,059.73	31,759.73
Honda Prelude 2 door	23.19	17,500	9,447.39	26,947.39
Nissan Pickup 4×4 2 door	23.53	12,900	12,249.48	25,149.48
Eagle Talon 4×4 2 door	23.99	18,200	9,771.20	27,971.20
Chevrolet S10 Pickup	24.15	10,900	12,571.52	23,471.52
Hyundai Excel 4 door	24.64	8,100	10,037.45	18,137.45
Plymouth Laser 2 door	24.76	14,200	10,086.73	24,286.74
Mazda Protege 4 door	24.99	11,200	10,180.02	21,380.02
Pontiac Sunbird 4 door	26.17	9,900	10,662.68	20,562.68
Isuzu Rodeo 4 door	26.39	19,400	13,738.16	33,138.16
Mitsubishi Pickup 2 door	27.04	8,900	14,074.07	22,974.07
Chevrolet K1500 Blazer 2 door	27.13	20,600	14,123.54	34,723.54
Hyundai Excel 2 door	27.40	7,200	11,162.54	18,362.54
Chevrolet S10 Blazer 2 door	27.44	15,300	14,282.73	29,582.73
Mercury Topaz 2 door	27.84	11,400	11,342.93	22,742.93
Dodge Stealth 2 door	28.86	18,900	11,755.62	30,655.62
Geo Metro 4 door	29.74	7,500	12,115.86	19,615.86
Chevrolet S10 Blazer 4 door	30.44	16,300	15,842.55	32,142.55
Geo Tracker 4×4 2 door	30.98	10,900	16,123.34	27,023.34
Geo Metro 2 door	32.81	7,000	13,367.24	20,367.24
Chevrolet Corvette 2 door	36.59	35,100	14,907.88	50,007.89
Hyundai Scoupe 2 door	39.17	9,500	15,956.66	25,456.66
Geo Tracker 2 door	40.13	10,600	20,890.32	31,490.32
Chevrolet Camaro 2 door	50.36	13,300	20,517.41	33,817.41

gallons per pound of weight reduction and 4.09 gallons per unit of horsepower reduction (Robertson, 1991).

Injury costs are substantially a function of vehicles that are undersized, overpowered, or both. Fuel consumption is mainly a function of horsepower and weight. A standard for average fuel economy leaves manufacturers free to continue to produce high-powered vehicles and offset the loss in fuel economy in their fleet by producing tiny "econoboxes," both of which increase injuries.

By using the data in Table 10.6, augmented by data on wheelbase, weight, and horsepower, the effects of these factors in the 1990s can be assessed. The regression equation for death rate per 100,000 passenger cars per year as a function of wheelbase (WB), curb weight (CW), horsepower (HP), number of doors (D), and price (P) is

$$\text{Rate} = 80.4 - 0.64(\text{WB}) + 0.002(\text{CW}) + 0.09(\text{HP}) - 1.87(\text{D}) - 0.0005(\text{P})$$

| Upper CI | -0.28 | 0.007 | 0.15 | -0.60 | -0.0003 |
| Lower CI | -1.01 | -0.004 | 0.03 | -3.14 | -0.0008 |

$R^2 = 0.50$

where CI refers to the 95 percent confidence interval. A logistic regression produced similar results.

As found in the analysis of earlier models, weight is not correlated to death rates significantly (95 percent CI overlaps zero) when wheelbase and horsepower are controlled statistically (Robertson, 1991). The number of doors is correlated to crash involvement and is a probably a reflection of drivers without children, who are more often out at night.

Vehicles with the same weight, horsepower, number of doors, and price will have an average reduction in occupant fatality rate of 0.64 per 100,000 vehicles per year for each increase of an inch in wheelbase. And vehicles with the same wheelbase, weight, number of doors, and price will have an average increase in fatal injury rate of 0.09 for each unit increment in horsepower. Since fuel consumption and fatalities are increased by horsepower, other things being equal, and more powerful engines cost more, reduction of horsepower would achieve conservation of life, fuel, and personal savings.

Critics of this analysis may argue that overpowered vehicles are overinvolved because of the way they are driven, but a vehicle cannot be driven at a speed far above the maximum legal limit if the capability to be so driven is not designed into the vehicle. Speeds above speed limits are sometimes deliberate, but unintentional speeding due to overpowered cars also occurs.

The distributions of horsepower in the the late 1970s, the late 1980s, and the early 1990s are shown in Figure 10.2. Some of the reduction in death rates in the 1980s may have resulted from reductions in horsepower during that decade. In the early 1990s models, horsepower was increased compared to the 1980s and, without airbags, the death rates probably would have increased. The rates could be reduced further, and more fuel conserved, by reducing the horsepower.

OTHER RESEARCH AND INJURY CONTROL EFFORTS

In 1985, a committee of the National Research Council/Institute of Medicine reported its review of the status of injury research and recommended that a Center for Injury Control be established at the Centers for Disease Control (CDC). The committee found that, despite the fact that injuries are among the major causes of years of potential life lost, for every dollar spent on cancer research (a total of about $1 billion annually in the early 1980s), the federal government was spending about 11 cents for injury research (Committee on Trauma Research, 1985).

FIGURE 10.2. Horsepower distributions in cars, by model years.

The Congress responded by transferring $10 million per year to the CDC from the Department of Transportation's (DOT) budget. This was inadequate to establish a Center and did not increase the total injury budget by much because some of the funds would have been used for research at DOT. Given the lack of quality of DOT research noted in this book, there was probably a net gain in research quality if not quantity.

Subsequently, the CDC budget was increased to about $20 million per year from the Department of Health and Human Services budget. In the meantime, the National Cancer Institute's budget was increased by about $600 million, partly for AIDS research. Some small increases in allocations for injury research also occurred in other federal agencies (Committee on Injury Control, 1988). Injury control was later elevated to Center status at CDC but the Center was attacked by the National Rifle Association for having the temerity to allocate a modest amount of funds for research on gun injuries. The Center's budget grows at a snail's pace.

Despite the relative lack of research funds, injury research has increased. In addition to research support, part of the CDC budget was allocated to "capacity building" in the states, such as improved injury surveillance systems. Several universities established centers for injury research and control, some funded by CDC and others by the National Institute for Occupational Safety and Health. Occasionally, these centers provide training for state and local health department personnel for a time. Corporate personnel receive some training in the occupational injury centers.

Private foundations occasionally show interest in injuries, but the commitment of dollars has been slow and minimal. A few union and management contracts have provided funds for joint committees to support research and improved surveillance of worker injuries.

These modest but important surges in interest and research funds are threatened by a federal budget crisis that was exacerbated by the deregulation of financial institutions and deficit spending in the 1980s. The problem is not just money, however. The programs that are launched are sometimes devoid of any sense of priority or knowledge of what is effective or ineffective. For weeks in the United States during 1996, the media drummed away with stories of government and private efforts to prevent children from being placed too close to air bags because of claims that about 30 children had been killed by the force of the bags. NHTSA, insurers, and safety groups joined in an Air Bag Safety Campaign. The "Safe Kids Coalition" had people in rest stops on highways attempting to convince people to place their children in back seats.

While there is nothing inherently wrong with such efforts, they are late in responding to an anticipated problem, they ignore the most effective means of protecting children, and there has been no comparable effort regarding much greater hazards to children. The risk to children too close to air bags when they deploy was known in the 1970s. Sensors to detect belt use were in use then and could have been modified to detect weight and position in seats and adjust air bag inflation rates. Several European countries have laws that require children to be seated in rear seats. Far more children are killed and maimed because child restraints are not used properly than are injured by air bags, but there have been no rest-stop campaigns to explain use of child restraints. None of this was mentioned during the air bag hysteria.

State and local governments, as well as private organizations at the local level, can make a substantial contribution to injury control. To do so, they must make use of data and knowledge of effectiveness of programs. Among the New York City Health Department's proposals for injury control was increased enrollment in high school driver education (Centers for Disease Control, 1991b), which, if successful, would increase injuries (Chapter 5). The CDC has successfully convened panels of experts to define an agenda for injury control (Centers for Disease Control, 1991a), but implementation is slow.

To implement what is known, it is necessary to understand organizational responsibilities and how to move organizations to action. When an injury problem is defined as a priority and countermeasures of known effectiveness are identified, it is obvious from some of the criticisms of certain organizations in this book that the implementation remains problematic.

Answers to the following questions may lead to increased action by those in a position to implement injury control. Who is in a position to take action (government agencies, corporations, voluntary organizations, etc.)? What are they doing now? What could they do in addition (or in substitution of currently ineffective actions)? What has been successful in changing the organization's actions in the past (information, embarrassment, demonstration of pluralistic ignorance)?

Whatever the strategies or tactics employed, there must be follow-up to see that the recommended changes were adopted. When an organization does successfully implement injury control, find ways to award recognition.

The concepts and methods outlined in this book and the referenced sources provide powerful tools for the identification of factors that could be controlled to reduce injuries. Surveillance identifies clusters of injuries geographically in some cases and in identifiable segments of populations in others (Chapter 3). There is wide variation among local areas in particular types of injuries (Bacon et al., 1989; Baker et al., 1987, 1988).

In an era of particularly strong antigovernment sentiment, it may be difficult for state and local governments to allocate resources to injury surveillance and control. However, taxpayers have shown willingness to support taxes for specific programs. In California, part of a special tax on cigarettes is being used for fire prevention as well as burn treatment and rehabilitation. In New York, the Public Health Law was amended in 1986 to provide for increased Medicaid reimbursement of hospitals to support poison control centers (Fisher, 1986). Florida and Kentucky adopted an additional $2 fine for each mile over the speed limit for speeding convictions, the funds to be allocated for research on spine and head injuries (State Health Report, 1997). Massachusetts is using its consumer protection laws to regulate handguns—banning the sale of cheap "Saturday-night specials" and requiring locking safeties on guns (*Nation's Health,* 1996).

One important consideration for state and local health departments, as well as other agencies such as highway departments, is the effectiveness of current expenditures. What is the scientific evidence that current activities are an important factor in the improvement of the public's health? Would alteration of some effort, from restaurant inspections to injury surveillance, for example, result in an increased threat to the health of restaurant patrons? This is a researchable question, but to find out, those in a position to make the change must be convinced of the importance of injury to the health of the population.

To the extent that enough surveillance has been done to specify targets for injury control efforts, attention should also be given to use of extant resources in ameliorative efforts. If the health department, a hospital trauma registry, or the police department identifies a set of intersections as points of high risk of injury, someone has to approach and convince the highway department that, for example, a year's delay in repaving a section of road and use of the funds to place flashing lights at the hazardous intersections should be done. As noted in Chapter 3, some highway departments approached by the injury control specialists in the Indian Health Service have been responsive when shown the data.

In a community in Sweden, a team of persons familiar with injury risks conducted "safety rounds" and identified the location of various conditions of buildings, walkways, playgrounds, and equipment, that were thought to increase risk of injury. Organizations in a position to change the conditions were contacted by mail and follow-up contacts were made if there was no response. In more than half the cases, the condition was modified or action was promised despite the lack of injury data showing the condition to be involved in injuries (Bjaras et al., 1990). Such efforts based on data from injury surveillance and other epidemiologic studies would increase the efficiency of injury control at reduced cost.

Local county and city health departments could become the lead agencies to acquire surveillance data and identify countermeasures that could be applied by relevant groups (Micik & Miclette, 1985). For this to happen, however, the Centers for Disease Control and Prevention, injury control research centers in universities, and state health departments must train local health department personnel in injury surveillance, countermeasure selection, and implementation. Without scientifically informed guidance, community coalitions tend to perpetuate the folklore of "accident prevention." Informed groups can promote changes if made aware of specific problems and remedies, as was done in Harlem (Chapter 5).

Familiarity with public health law may suggest a variety of ways that laws and their enforcement, such as laws regarding public nuisances and building codes, could be used to reduce risks revealed by injury surveillance (Christoffel, 1982; Christoffel & Teret, 1993; Graf, 1976).

Like all careers in public health, a career in injury epidemiology and control can be frustrating. It can also be enormously rewarding. Unlike those who work in cancer or heart disease, one does not have to wait a long time to find whether or not one's efforts are having an effect. The results of site-specific surveillance and targeted control efforts can sometimes be seen in a year or two (Chapter 3).

SUMMARY

The results of epidemiologic studies specifying factors that can be changed to reduce injuries can be used to project the effects of policies regarding those changes. Many current injury control efforts are administered by government agencies and private organizations that seem to have no system for establishing priorities and no systematic knowledge of policies and programs that are effective. Those who learn how, when, where, and who is injured are in a position to influence the setting of priorities. Those who also learn the approaches to injury control that are effective or ineffective are in a position to help rationalize the policy making process.

REFERENCES

Automotive News Market Data Book. Detroit: Automotive News, 1989–95.

Bacon WE, Smith GS, and Baker SP (1989) Geographic variation in the occurrence of hip fractures among the elderly white U.S. population. *Am J Public Health* 79:1556–1558.

Baker SP, Whitfield MA, and O'Neill B (1987) Geographic variations in mortality from motor vehicle crashes. *New Engl J Med* 316:1384–1387.

Baker SP, Whitfield MA, and O'Neill B (1988) County mapping of injury mortality. *J Trauma* 28:741–745.

Bjaras G, Danielsson K, Schelp L, Sjoberg D, and Skjonberg G (1990) Safety rounds in public environments: experience of a new tool for prevention of accidental injuries. *Accident Anal Prev* 22:223–228.

Centers for Disease Control (1991a) *Position Papers from the Third National Injury Control Conference.* Atlanta: Department of Health and Human Services.

Centers for Disease Control (1991b) Summaries: state and community-based injury control projects, applied methods injury surveillance projects, incentive grants for injury control intervention projects. Atlanta: Department of Health and Human Services.

Christoffel T (1982) *Health and the Law: A Handbook for Health Professionals.* New York: Free Press.

Christoffel T, and Teret SP (1993) *Protecting the Public: Legal Issues in Injury Prevention.* New York: Oxford University Press.

Committee on Injury Control (1988) *Injury Control: A Review of the Status and Progress of the Injury Control Program at the Centers for Disease Control.* Washington, DC: National Academy Press.

Committee on Trauma Research (1985) *Injury in America: A Continuing Public Health Problem.* Washington, DC: National Academy Press.

Crandall RW, and Graham JD (1989) The effects of fuel economy standards on automobile safety. *J Law Econ* 32:97–118.

Deppa RW (1986) Report of the Engineering Evaluation of All Terrain Vehicles (mimeo). Washington, DC: U.S. Consumer Product Safety Commission.

DiNapoli N, Fitzpatrick M, Strother C, Struble D, and Tanner R (1977) *Research Safety Vehicle Phase II, Volume II, Comprehensive Technical Results.* Springfield, VA: National Technical Information Service.

Ervin RD (1988) Injury risks posed by incompatibilities between trucks and other highway users. *Bull New York Acad Med* 64:816.

Federal Highway Administration (1994) Motor vehicle accident costs. Technical Advisory T 7570.2.

Fisher L (1986) New York State regional poison control centers injury control network legislation. *Vet Human Toxicol* 28:545–546.

Frame P (1996) Has Martinez dropped the ball at NHTSA? *Automot News,* June 24, p. 1.

Garrott WR (1993) Measured vehicle inertial parameters—NHTSA's data through September 1992. *SAE Tech Paper Series* 930897. Warrendale, PA: Society of Automotive Engineers.

General Accounting Office (1978) *Unwarranted Delays by the Department of Transportation to Improve Light Truck Safety.* Washington, DC: Comptroller General of the U.S.

Graf FP (1976) *Public Health Law Manual.* Washington, DC: American Public Health Association.

Haddon W Jr, Suchman EA, and Klein D (eds) (1964) *Accident Research: Methods and Approaches.* New York: Harper and Row.

Harwin EA, and Brewer HK (1990) Analysis of the relationship between vehicle rollover stability and rollover risk using the NHTSA CARDfile accident database. *J Traffic Med* 18:109–122.

Insurance Institute for Highway Safety (1990) Washington area car dealers still ignore belt display rule. *IIHS Status Report* 25:3–6.

Insurance Institute for Highway Safety (1996) Vehicle by vehicle death rate comparisons. *IIHS Status Report* 30:4–6.

Jones IS, and Penny MB (1990) Engineering parameters related to rollover frequency. *SAE Tech Paper Series* 900104. Warrendale, PA: Society of Automotive Engineers.

Kaufman S (1989) Long-term impact of injury on individuals, families, and society. In Rice DP, and MacKenzie EJ (eds), *Cost of Injury in the United States: A Report to Congress, 1989.* San Francisco: University of California Institute for Health and Aging, Baltimore: Johns Hopkins University Injury Prevention Center.

Kraus JF, Zador PF, Arzemanian S, Anderson CL, and Harrington S (1988) Motorcycle design and crash injuries in California. *Bull New York Acad Med* 64:788.

Litan RE, and Winston C (1988) Policy options. In Litan RE, and Winston C (eds), *Liability: Perspectives and Policy.* Washington, DC: Brookings.

McCarry C (1972) *Citizen Nader.* New York: Saturday Review Press.

Mengert P, Salvatore S, DiSario R, and Walter R (1989) Statistical estimation of rollover risk. Cambridge, MA: Transportation Systems Center.

Micik S, and Miclette M (1985) Injury prevention in the community: a systems approach. *Ped Clinics North Am* 32:251–265.

Miller TR (1989) Willingness to pay. In Rice DP, and MacKenzie EJ (eds), *Cost of Injury in the United States: A Report to Congress, 1989.* San Francisco: University of California Institute for Health and Aging and Baltimore: Johns Hopkins University Injury Prevention Center.

Nader R, and Smith WJ (1996) *No Contest: Corporate Lawyers and the Perversion of Justice in America.* New York: Random House.

National Highway Traffic Safety Administration (1983) *The Economic Cost to Society of Motor Vehicle Accidents.* DOT HS 806-342. Washington, DC: U.S. Department of Transportation.

National Highway Traffic Safety Administration (1987) Federal Motor Vehicle Safety Standards; denial of petition for rulemaking; vehicle rollover resistance. *Fed Reg* 52:49033.

National Highway Traffic Safety Administration (1988) Denial of motor vehicle safety defect petitions. *Fed Reg* 53:34866.

National Highway Traffic Safety Administration (1989–91) *National Accident Sampling System (NASS), Crashworthiness Data Subsystem, Analytical User's Manual.* Washington, DC: U.S. Department of Transportation.

National Highway Traffic Safety Administration (1989–92) *Fatal Accident Reporting System.* Washington, DC: U.S. Department of Transportation.

National Highway Traffic Safety Administration (1991) Technical assessment paper: relationship between rollover and vehicle factors. Washington, DC: U.S. Department of Transportation.

National Highway Traffic Safety Administration (1992) Rollover prevention. *Fed Reg* 57:242–252.

National Highway Traffic Safety Administration (1996) Federal Motor Vehicle Safety Standards; rollover prevention. *Fed Reg* 61:28550–28561.

Nation's Health (1996) Massachusetts takes a new aim at gun safety. Washington DC: American Public Health Association, December.

Newman R (1986) *Analysis of All Terrain Vehicle Related Injuries and Deaths.* Washington, DC: U.S. Consumer Product Safety Commission.

Oak Ridge National Laboratory (1984) Scrappage and survival rates of passenger cars and trucks in 1970–82. *Ward's Automotive Yearbook.* Detroit: Ward's Communications.

Priest GL (1988) Products liability law and the accident rate. In Litan RE, and Winston C (eds), *Liability: Perspectives and Policy.* Washington, DC: Brookings.

Reinfurt DW, Li LK, Popkin C, O'Neill B, Burchman P, and Wells JAK (1981) *A Comparison of Crash Experience of Utility Vehicles, Pickup Trucks and Passenger Cars.* Chapel Hill: University of North Carolina Highway Safety Research Center.

Reinfurt DW, Stutts JC, and Hamilton EG (1984) *A Further Look at Utility Vehicle Rollovers.* Chapel Hill: University of North Carolina Highway Safety Research Center.

Research and Policy Committee (1989) *Who Should Be Liable? A Guide to Policy for Dealing with Risk.* New York: Committee for Economic Development.

Rice DP, and MacKenzie EJ (eds) (1989) *Cost of Injury in the United States: A Report to Congress, 1989.* San Francisco: University of California Institute for Health and Aging, and Baltimore: Johns Hopkins University Injury Prevention Center.

Rivara FP, Dicker BG, Bergman AB, Dacey R, and Herman C (1988) The public cost of motorcycle trauma. *JAMA* 260:221.

Robertson LS (1983) *Injuries: Causes, Control Strategies and Public Policy.* Lexington, MA: D.C. Heath.

Robertson LS (1984a) Automobile safety regulations: rebuttal and new data. *Am J Public Health* 74:1390.

Robertson LS (1984b) Insurance incentives and seat belt use. *Am J Public Health* 74:1157–1158.

Robertson LS (1989a) Potential savings from injury prevention. In Rice DP, and MacKenzie EJ (eds), *Cost of Injury in the United States: A Report to Congress, 1989.* San Francisco: University of California Institute for Health and Aging, and Baltimore: Johns Hopkins University Injury Prevention Center.

Robertson LS (1989b) Risk of fatal rollover in utility vehicles relative to static stability. *Am J Public Health* 79:300.

Robertson LS (1990) Car design and risk of pedestrian deaths. *Am J Public Health* 80:609–610.

Robertson LS (1991) How to save fuel and reduce injuries in automobiles. *J Trauma* 31:107–109.

Robertson LS, and Kelley AB (1989) Static stability as a predictor of overturn in fatal motor vehicle crashes. *J Trauma* 29:313.

Sakiya T (1982) *Honda Motor: The Men, the Management, the Machines.* New York: Kodansha International.

Schachter L (1987) Update of ATV deaths and injuries. Memo to the Consumer Product Safety Commissioners, November 10.

Selvin S (1991) *Statistical Analysis of Epidemiologic Data.* New York: Oxford University Press.

Smith SR (1982) Analysis of fatal rollover accidents in utility vehicles (mimeo). Washington: National Highway Traffic Safety Administration.

Snyder RG, McDole TL, Ladd WM, and Minahan DJ (1980) *On-road Crash Experience of Utility Vehicles.* Ann Arbor: University of Michigan Highway Safety Research Institute.

State Health Report (1997) Florida, Kentucky funnel speeding fines into research on spine and head injuries. *Nation's Health,* February, p. 7.

Stein HW, and Jones IS (1988) Crash involvement of large trucks by configuration. *Am J Public Health* 78:491.

Stepp LS (1996) Truckin' to tragedy. *Washington Post,* March 1, p. D5.

Stonex KA (1961) Road design for safety. *Traffic Safety Res Rev* 5:18–30.

Thurman DJ, Burnett CL, Jeppson L, Beaudoin DE, and Sniezek JE (1994) Surveillance of spinal cord injuries in Utah, USA. *Paraplegia* 32:665–669.

Thurman DJ, Burnett CL, Beaudoin DE, Jeppson J, and Sniezek JE (1995) Risk factors and mechanisms of occurrence in motor vehicle-related spinal cord injuries: Utah. *Accident Anal Prev.* 27:411–415.

Vernick JS, Baker SP, Edmunds L, Kelley B, Smith L, Teret SP, and Zierler A (n.d.) *Motorboat Propeller Injuries.* Baltimore: Johns Hopkins University Injury Prevention Center.

Ward's Automotive Yearbook (1983–95) Detroit: Ward's Communications.

Warner KE (1983) Bags, buckles, and belts: the debate over mandatory passive restraints in automobiles. *J Health Polit Policy Law* 8:44.

Whitfield RA, and Jones IA (1995) The effect of passenger load on unstable vehicles in fatal, untripped rollover crashes. *Am J Public Health* 85:1268–1271.

Wood DP (1997) Safety and the car size effect: a fundamental explanation. *Accident Anal Prevent* 29:139–151.

INDEX

Abbreviated injury scale 30, 32–34, 54 55, 206, 223, 245–246
Abilities 127
Acceleration 13
Accident Facts 25
Accidents 3–4
Adolescents 119–121, 129
Advanced life support 198–199
Adulthood 123–125
Age 9–10, 23, 39, 90–91, 173, 209, 220
Agent 6–7, 167
Aggression 121–122
Aggressive drivers 114
Air bags 11, 17, 180, 188, 254
Aircraft crashes 41
Alcohol 15, 18, 53, 58, 60–61, 85, 88–89, 91–96, 121–122, 124–125, 130, 133, 147–148, 153–154, 158–159, 160–161, 178–180, 204–205, 217, 225–227
All-terrain vehicles 43–44, 168–170
Alzheimer's disease 127
American Motor Vehicle Manufacturer's Association 242
Anatomic Profile 33
Assaults 56, 65, 79–80, 92, 119, 121, 134, 144, 149, 154

Association of International Vehicle Manufacturers 242
Aspirin package 168
Asphyxiation 16, 51

Behavior 60, 99, 113–116, 127, 143, 155–156, 171–172
Biofeedback 208
Boat propellers 17
Bumper height 171
Bureau of Labor Statistics 25, 57
Bureau of Transportation Statistics 53
Burns 26, 34, 50, 133, 202

Cancer 2, 16, 39–40
Capture–recapture analysis 58
Carbon monoxide 18
Cardiovascular disease 39–40
Case finding 26
Causal analysis 85–88
    models 90–93, 102
Causation 5, 20, 88–89, 168
Cellular phones 96
Center for Auto Safety 114
Centers for Disease Control (CDC) 50, 56–57, 60, 64, 216, 256
    Center for Injury Control 2, 252–253

Center of gravity height 16, 170, 234, 240–242
Changeable factors 20
Child abuse 122
Childhood 117–119, 127, 170
Child resistant caps 187
Child restraints 17, 118, 143, 157–158, 254
Cigarettes 8, 14, 217
Clinicians 19
Coast Guard 58
Cohort 93
Community changes 133–134
Confounding 86, 89, 100
Consumer Product Safety Commission 43–44, 58, 168, 170
Consumers Union 234–235
Coroners 27, 56
Correlation 5, 89, 103–104, 175
Cost-benefit 144, 210, 216–218, 221, 227, 229, 235
Cost-effectiveness 227–229
Costs 44, 199–200, 202, 209, 215, 218, 221–224, 242–243, 245–251
Council of State and Territorial Epidemiologists 52
Counseling 127–128
Crash Outcome Data Evaluation System (CODES) 59
Crash tests 177–180
Cribs 181
Criminal justice 144

Data analysis 104–107
Data needs 18–19, 23
Daylight saving time 161
Dead-on-arrival criteria 200
Death certificates 19, 51, 56–57
Deaths 1, 25
Defects 188–189
Defensive driving 130
DeHaven, Hugh 12
Denial 120, 123
Deterrence 144–145, 148
Developmental stages 91, 117–119
Diagnosis-related groups (DRGs) 202, 209–210
Disability 21, 29, 35–38, 222
Drinking age laws 148, 158–159
Driver education 129–130, 161, 223–224, 254
Driver error 171
Driver licensing age 222–224
Drowning 2, 16, 41, 50, 63, 75–76
Drugs 17, 99–100

E codes 18–19, 50, 52
Economics 215
Education 133
Elderly 125–126, 132
Emergency medical service 63, 195–197
Energy 7–11, 21, 24, 167
    absorption 12–13, 17
    chemical 14
    electrical 15
    exchange 90
    mechanical 7, 11–14
    thermal 14
    tolerance 88, 171
Environment 167, 171, 183, 187–188
Epidemiology v, 1, 4, 215
    methods 5
    model 6
EPPINFO 65
Exercise 132
Exposure 41

Falls 2, 11, 13–14, 20, 25, 62–63, 77–78, 125–126, 128, 134, 208–209, 222
Fatal Accident Reporting System 53–54, 101, 114, 173, 176, 197, 236
Federal Aviation Administration 41
Federal Bureau of Investigation 56
Federal Highway Administration 97
Federal Motor Vehicle Safety Standards 172–177
Feedback 92
Firearms 2, 11, 118–119; see also Guns
Fire/burns 2, 8, 14, 58, 73–74, 89, 113–115, 118
Fireworks 133–134
Ford Motor Company 114, 234
Freedom of Information Act 59
Fuel economy 247, 251–252
Fuel tanks 89, 113–115
Functional Capacity Index 38

General Estimates System 55
General Motors 113–115, 176, 217
General Services Administration 177
Glasgow Coma Scale 31, 208
Gravity 12
Group behavior 135–136
Guardrail 66
Guns 8, 14, 17–18, 51, 95, 119, 123, 149–151, 153, 169, 227–228, 255; see also Firearms

Haddon, William, Jr. 8, 16, 49
Harlem 134–135

Hazard 16–18
Health care costs 2
Heart disease 2
Helicopters 199
Helmets 12, 17, 134, 145, 186–187, 227–228
HIV infection 2
Homicide 3, 50, 56, 65, 92, 121, 123, 144, 149
Horsepower 247, 251–253
Horses 136
Hospital Discharge Survey 51–52
Hospital records 30, 51–52, 56, 59
Hospitals 27
Host 6, 97
Human factors 113, 127

Impairment scale 35–37
Incentives 132
Indian Health Service 52, 64–66
Infectious disease 4, 6–7, 88
Injury 3–4
  bicycle 186–187
  case studies 169
  classifications 25
  clusters 50–51, 122, 255
  control 4, 7, 16, 62, 86
  distributions 39, 88
  factors and phases 8–9
  farm 57
  flow of cases 27
  football 28–29
  pedestrian 65–66, 128–129, 173–175
  police codes 54–55
  policy analysis 233–234
  preventable 240–241
  prevention 85
  rates 19, 39–45
  self-inflicted 81–82
  severity 19–20, 23–24, 29–35, 99, 185
  surveillance 19, 49–67, 255
  workers 181–183
Injury in America 203, 205
Injury Severity Score 30, 32, 34, 202, 225
Insurance rates 246
Intentional injury 3
International Classification of Diseases 18–19,
    33, 50–51
Intravenous fluids 198
IQ 126

Jeep Corporation 234
Journal of Political Economy 176

Lap/shoulder belts 11
  see also "seat belts"

effectiveness 183–185
  law effects 155–156, 160, 177–179
Laws 143–161, 256
Length of stay 209–210, 225
Life-saving interventions 220
Lighting 65, 172
Livestock 136
Lobbying 145, 227–228, 242
Logistic regression 32, 204

Mandatory sentencing 151–152
Mass 11
Medical examiners 27–28, 56
MEDLINE 24
Mileage 41, 101, 103, 176–179
Mine Safety and Health Administration 181
Mini/trail bikes 43
Motorcycles 16
Motor vehicles 2, 8–9, 11, 17, 53–55, 71–72,
    85, 103, 120, 134
  crashworthiness 87, 176–180
  horsepower 90–91
  size 90–91
  stability and rollover 91, 100–101, 107–108

N codes 18–19, 50, 52
National Accident Sampling System 54, 186,
    223, 238, 246
National Center for Health Statistics 25, 28, 51
National Crime Surveys 56
National Fire Data Center 58
National Health Interview Survey 25, 28, 35,
    52
National Highway Traffic Safety Administra-
    tion (NHTSA) 53–54, 59–60, 89, 103,
    114, 146, 176–177, 189, 220, 225, 234–
    235, 246
National Medical Care Utilization and Expendi-
    ture Survey 52
National Rifle Association 8, 253
National Safety Council 25–26, 130
Native Americans 124–125
Navajo Nation 65
New Car Assessment Program (NCAP) 178–
    180
Newton, Sir Issac 7

Occupational Safety and Health Administration
    (OSHA) 10, 57, 181–183, 228
Office of Management and Budget 181
Overlap in effects 224–227

Pedestrian behavior 154–155
Pediatric Trauma Score 34

Physical therapy 208
Physics 13
Playground 13
Pluralistic ignorance 135
Pneumatic antishock garment 198
Poisoning 34, 123
Police crackdowns 147–148
Police reports 29, 122
Policy 5
Posttrauma behavior 126–127
Potential life lost 39–40
Product design 168–170
Product liability 43, 244–245
Protective equipment 183
Psychopathology 120
Public health 144
    model 86
    research 1
Public Roads 97–98

Quality control 188
Quality years of life 221

Race 123–125
Railway fatalities 26
Reading lists v, vii
Refrigerators 181
Regression to the mean 146, 188
Regulation 43, 172–183, 220, 222, 233, 244
Regulatory failure 243–247
Rehabilitation 195, 205–209
Reliability 35, 38
Replication 147
Research objectives 18–19, 23–25
Research safety vehicle 218, 245
Risk 42–45, 120, 218–222, 229
Risk benefit 219–220
Risk compensation (homeostasis) theory 159–
    160, 174, 179–183
Risk factor 86
    surveillance 60, 160
Road modifications 63
Rules 143

Screening 133
Seat belts 54–55, 60–61, 225–227
    see also "lap/shoulder belts"
Selection bias 59, 130, 186
Sex 9–10, 90–91, 123–125, 153
Signalized intersections 159, 172
Sikhs 145
Smoke detectors 18
Snow, John 4

Snowmobiles 43
Speed 11, 17, 53, 90–91, 114, 156–157,
    172
Sports 143
Spinal cord injury 35, 204, 207, 238–239
Stairs 20
Statistical power 89
Statistics 24–25, 105–107
Strain 12
Stresses 12
Study designs 93, 145
    before–after 146–147
    case-control 94–98, 134, 186–187
    controlled experiments 94, 127–132, 152,
        198, 203
    cross-sectional 100–102
    double-pair comparison 185–186
    econometric 174–176
    ecological 102–103, 148–149, 199
    interrupted time series 147
    prospective 93, 98, 206
    retrospective 93, 96, 98, 206
Suicides 56, 121–122, 150, 169, 203
Surveillance 19, 49–67, 255
Swimming pools 17, 118

Technical strategies 16–18, 62–63
Telephone interviews 128
Television 131–132
Threat 121
Toxicology 15
Track width 16, 234, 240–242
Tractor-trailer trucks 170, 243
Transportation Research Board 157
Transportation Research Institute 53
Trauma centers 200–203
Trauma registries, 41
Trauma score 30–32
Traumatic brain injury 207, 238–239
Treatment 195, 197–200
    evaluation 201–202
Trucks 97, 170, 180

Unemployment 121
Unintended consequences 129, 157–161
Unit of analysis 93, 149
Unstable vehicles 234–243
Utility poles 18
Utility vehicles 16, 91, 170, 180, 240–242

Validity 35
Vans 16, 170
Vector 6, 97

Vehicle 6, 11, 167, 178
    size and weight 247, 251–252
    occupant death rates 248–251
Velocity 11–13
Veterans Administration 209–210
Violence 126, 149
Visibility 243

Washington Heights 135
White Mountain Apache Tribal Council 136
White River Apache Reservation 65
Willingness to pay 217–219
Wirth, Timothy 234
Worker's Compensation 57, 182
Worker education 131